Prevail Over Yourself

Achieving a Balanced and Healthy Life

Gym Bag Books

Prevail Over Yourself

Achieving a Balanced and Healthy Life

Alexander Babinets

Copyright © 2011 by Alexander Babinets.

Library of Congress Control Number:		2010902037
ISBN:	Hardcover	978-1-4500-4302-1
	Softcover	978-1-4500-4301-4

Credits:

Alexander Babinets, MA, Phys. Ed - author
Luba Grup, CPTN Certified Personal Trainer - coauthor, model for exercises demonstrations, illustrations graphic design
Liliana Grup - cover design
Rita Grup - model on the cover image and exercises demonstrations
Evgenii Babinets - tables and figures designs

This book was printed in the United States of America.

To order additional copies of this book, contact:
Xlibris Corporation
1-888-795-4274
www.Xlibris.com
Orders@Xlibris.com
56389

To my parents who gave me life,
to my children who gave my life a purpose,
and to my dear love Luba who makes my life possible.

CONTENTS

PART 3
Soul

PREFACE

I wrote this book not just to give you illustrations of exercises and rules to follow. I've seen too many people quitting. Those were the people who belonged to the top-notch facilities, who were prescribed amazing fitness programs, who joined boot camps, and even those who had long-term one-on-one personal training packages. It breaks my heart to see how many of you looking so enthusiastic at the beginning and later completely losing interest in pursuing your fitness goals. Gyms keep charging you their membership fees, but you—being locked into a contract, stuck at home or at work—will hope that the next day, then the next day, then the next day, will come back, and then you will continue what you started. For many of you, that day, unfortunately, never comes.

Sure, gyms like your money, and some of them even thank you for not coming since you are not using their equipment, lockers, aerobic rooms, parking, etc. The number of fitness clubs all over the world is continuously growing, but the number of sick and overweight people is not reducing but growing. That's what hurts me.

Gyms teach people how to exercise, use their equipment; they also provide classes, swimming pools and other amenities. But gyms don't teach their members how to actually stay mentally strong to accomplish their fitness goals. Of course you can always hire a personal trainer, but what if you cannot afford one?

A personal trainer will show you how to exercise with your body, but not many trainers can actually teach how to exercise with your mind and how to structure your thoughts to last until the end on your own.

Meanwhile, our competitive world of instant gratification keeps telling us that everything in life is supposed to come to us easy, with little or no effort. We no longer need to walk—we have cars, elevators, escalators, etc. We no longer need to do our house duties—machines do it for us. And we don't even need to cook anymore. We have cheap fast food available on almost every corner. Now we even have so-called "magic" exercising machines advertised on TV or quick "magic" ten-minute workout programs, and we don't need to go to our gyms. Soon, these machines will be exercising for us, and we will be just watching them.

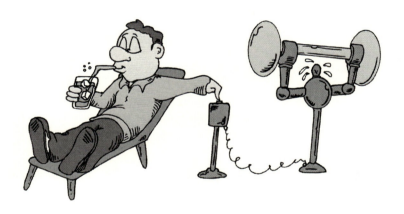

Since 1984, the number of fitness clubs in United States grew from 7,000 to 29,000, and the number of members joining these clubs grew from 15 million members to 41 million, but the sad part is that the number of overweight and obese people also grew from 30% in 1984 to 65% in 2006. Obviously, something is wrong with this picture, and we definitely need to look for better ways how to stop killing ourselves, because with the number of overweight people, the number of sick people and deaths grew too.

We have gyms everywhere now. We also have hundreds of weight loss clinics and programs advertized on TV, radio, or in the mail. But neither of these helps us to reduce the percentage of overweight people. It just keeps growing.

With drastic technology development, physical labor is almost eliminated from our lives.

Is this good for us? It feels good, but what comes later? Millions of people get sick, lack self-esteem and communication skills, develop fears and nervousness, and live with suffering and pain. After all, we end up with heart attacks, strokes, depression, and mental illnesses.

Our bodies have muscles, and we need to use them. If we don't, our muscles will get weak, and then we lose not only our appearance but also confidence in ourselves, and worst of all, we lose our health. Our muscles are our second heart, and they provide all the physiological processes in our body. All these processes deteriorate with time if we don't get physically active.

Just several decades ago we only had gyms for bodybuilders and athletes. Regular people did not need them because life was so much more physical—walking, bicycling, climbing stairs, doing house duties, gardening, and much more. Will we ever go back to those times? I highly doubt it. We cannot reverse the progress, and gym business would not be doing so well if there was a chance. We don't have much of a choice anymore how to get physically active except for dedicating a specific time for it. Our life is filled with duties that exclude physical effort except for only a few professions.

My intention in writing this book was to help you persevere. Many people when making their fitness resolutions set their goals too high, try to commit to more than they are ready for, lack support from family and friends, or just don't have the resources for accomplishing their goals. The quick-fix programs, such as diets, or any short-term commitments in many cases are setting us up to fail. Quick fixes have temporary power even though they sometimes work. Most of these quick fixes set us up for dependency on them, emotional and physical discomfort, since they are forcefully applied to us. Many of our life's bad habits eventually diminish or "melt away" all our achievements. Ninety percent of those who succeed in losing weight unfortunately gain it back within a year due to lack of their mental strength.

Habits that we develop through our life have a tremendous pull and effect on us. Many times it is very hard to learn new habits and see life in a completely different perspective.

Many people consider their fitness resolutions as terms, and every term, obviously, has an end. Instead, these resolutions should be viewed as lifestyle changes. It requires breaking some habits, restructuring thoughts, and sometimes even reconstructing life. It is one thing to achieve your goal, but a totally different thing to maintain it.

To find inner strength and the power within you not to give up requires much more than just a quick fix. We need to train our mind, just like we train our muscles. Before making any commitments in life, we need to feel strong enough to follow them. We need to learn how to develop independence from outer sources, resist temptations, stay positive, and believe in our own power. When we are on a quick-fix program, we submit to the power and the rules of that program. Even if we succeed, this success usually ends with the program itself and does not train our own power within. As soon as we stop being influenced by it, we may feel lost and confused again.

When we perform physical exercises, our muscles get strong, and when we need our muscles, we will use them in our daily life. Our mind can also be trained and can get strong. With a strong mind, any goal is achievable, but if our mind is weak, we will quit every time. Year after year, jumping from gym to gym, we will be making all sorts of excuses: "I don't like that gym," "It's too far for me," or "I am too busy this year." And the list goes on and on. These are just procrastinations. Our mind needs to be trained together with the muscles to be able to resist all that.

From generation to generation, history repeats itself, and people do the same mistakes as they did hundreds of years ago. But we should be able to learn from previous generations on how to make our lives better, not only by buying a larger TV or a more comfortable couch. We should be able to learn how to use our bodies to enjoy more things in life, stay physically active throughout all ages, and at fifty-five feel the same as we were at twenty-seven. (Not that some of us feel good at twenty-seven.) At any age, we can do something to improve our lives.

People who exercise regularly live longer. But it is not the longevity which I am going to talk about in this book. I am for the *quality* of all those years, months, and days that we live. Regular exercise produces happy hormones and heals a lot of not only physical but also mental problems, and this is what enhances the quality of our life. We can enjoy our day regardless of the weather or time of the day; we can resist the negativity and influences of other people and see the world as a beautiful place and be more confident that our life is going to be the way we want.

As we grow up and get older, our values and interests change. But few things stay the same—we always want to have nice bodies, to be healthy, and to feel good. We also want to be reassured that we will have enough strength to achieve what we want in life. Our daily tasks and emotions often provoke us to procrastinate and look for excuses.

By exercising your mind and acquiring personal inner strength, you can discover the endless possibilities within yourself. You will see how strong you can be. You will never quit anything you start. Your body will do anything what your mind tells it to.

People do not quit their fitness resolutions because they don't have enough equipment or they can't find the right program. They usually quit because of the lack of willpower, self-discipline, or patience. These three powerful components are the keys in achieving anything in life.

Once you acquire the inner strength, you will be able to perform any activity for as long as you need to and until you reach your goal.

The power to control our mind and ability to alter our thoughts separates us humans from any other living kind. Our possessed habits can be relearned, since most of them are acquired through influence. We have ability to choose which habits to keep and which to give up.

With the help of willpower, self-discipline, and patience, our bodies and our lives can be unrecognizably changed. We can rebuild our figures to perfect proportions, change the way we perceive things, and also redirect our life to where we really want.

This book is not just about exercise. I was always looking for a balance between exercise and other important things in life. I never wanted my exercise program to be just a time sucker. I wanted it to help me achieve everything else in life, fight my fears, overreactions, and unnecessary emotions.

Nobody wants to be just a gorgeous dummy. We also want to grow as humans, producers and achievers, so at the end of our life we could say, "I lived my life the way I dreamed it!"

INTRODUCTION

There is nothing in this world more valuable than our health. A healthy poor is much happier than a sick king.
—old folk saying

*   *   *

Work, school, family, kids, our own laziness—excuses, excuses.

It is nice to come home, slip your feet into your slippers, sink in a comfortable chair, turn on the TV, and watch your favorite show. Years go by. Muscles are slowly weakening, waist disappearing. And one day, when a broken elevator forces you to use the stairs, you suddenly realize that something has happened to your body. You used to fly through three floors in one breath, but now twenty steps got you out of order. And what is that pain under your ribs?

Moments like these make many people think and decide,

"Something must be done about it. It can't continue like this. Tomorrow I'll go to the park, join the gym, or put the treadmill in my basement."

*   *   *

"I have a good job, live in a comfortable apartment, and have everything I need. But every time I look in the mirror, I get so agitated—only five years ago, I was size 8, now it is 12, and my skirts keep getting tighter and tighter."

"I'm thirteen years old. I am the skinniest in my class. No matter how much I eat, my arms still look like sticks. Food does not make me any stronger or better looking. I can still do only few push-ups, and at school's track and field, I am always the last one."

How to lose weight? How to get strong? How to get rid of all aches and pains? How to build muscles? How to develop self-esteem? How to look and feel younger? From generation to generation, people keep asking these questions over and over again.

In the meantime, our life is becoming more and more comfortable and convenient. We drive cars and use elevators, escalators, dishwashers, laundry machines, remote controls, cell phones, you name it. Everything is available quickly, easily, and with little effort, and the idea that achieving some objectives might require commitment, strength of character, or physical labor seems to have been forgotten.

Nearly one-third of the adults in United States and Canada are obese (BMI over 30). A new study finds that nearly half of kids nationwide are now overweight (32 percent) and obese (16 percent). Researchers found that the hearts and livers of some children these days are in worse condition than of some forty-five-year-old adults.

Diabetes, stroke, hypertension, osteoporosis, coronary heart disease, cancer, and other diseases directly related to obesity health problems kill millions every year.

Are we people foolish or crazy, and why don't we care?

We actually do. According to a survey done by the IHRSA (International Health, Racquet and Sportsclub Association), nine out of ten Americans believe that regular exercise is essential to stay healthy and manage their weight. Obesity affects about one in four adult Americans, and during any one year, over half of Americans go on a weight-loss diet or are trying to maintain their weight.

Why is then the number of overweight people still growing?

The survey conducted by American Sports Data Inc. showed that people have become nonreactive and insensitive to the obesity epidemic. While they claim to understand that being overweight or obese is not healthy, 65 percent of respondents stated, "Not everyone can be thin, some people are just overweight." This response represents a frightening notion that many Americans are either becoming satisfied with their lack of physical health or they do not seem to understand the connection between lack of physical activity and poor health condition.

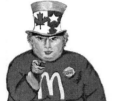

A growing belief in instant gratification has led people to believe that it's all right to be fat, happy, and sassy.

Junk food manufacturers and fast-food restaurants have lowered nation's standards by total invasion with advertising on TV, radio, and in the mail. Sedentary lifestyle—such as video games, television, and Internet—has made matters even worse.

Too many diets, too many different opinions on how to lose weight make Americans confused. Misleading information on TV, mail, and radio about so-called "magic" machines, "magic" pills, or "magic" diets have brought even more confusion since none of these approaches brought any stable results.

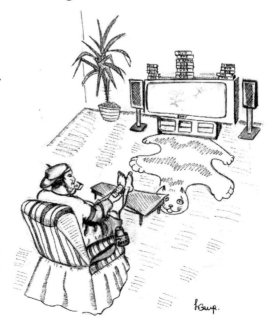

Life starts to move faster, and activities that require thought, time, focus, healthy eating, and exercise are left avoided or sacrificed. Americans need to be reeducated so that they'll make the time that's required to enjoy a healthy living.

Part 1

Mind

CHAPTER 1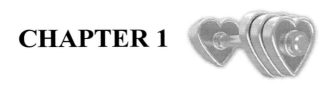

WHY PEOPLE QUIT

At the beginning of January when another New Year's resolution campaign kicked in, I decided—this time I'll do it! Enough is enough! Inspired by a new flyer from a local gym, I said to myself, "I am going to start exercising at home." I had my day off from work; my kids were with my wife at her friend's house, and I took a bus to the closest sports store to buy some clothes and fitness equipment.

A salesperson met me at the door, politely asked what I was looking for, and after I answered, invited me to show around. To buy some clothes was an easy part—I got a couple of baggy-looking T-shirts, and that was it. But the equipment part was "fun." The saleslady suggested that it would be a good idea to start with adjustable dumbbells so I can vary the weight for different exercises.

I lied to her that I was very strong, and she recommended buying sixty-pound dumbbells. I paid at the cash register and went to pick up my dumbbells. The saleslady asked if I needed any help. "No," I said and grabbed the dumbbells lying on the shelf. First time I thought they were attached. I pulled again. They moved but didn't come off. The saleslady wondered if I was OK. "Oh yeah," I squeezed through my teeth and started rolling the dumbbells off the shelf. When the weights went down, I thought I was going to die. The dumbbells were slowly nailing me to the floor. "Let go!" my whole body was screaming. "Let go right now!"

But I didn't. Through my tears I smiled to the saleslady and headed to the exit. While I was walking like a duck through the long aisle of the sports store, I felt my arms getting longer and longer.

I did accomplish my "first fitness goal"—successfully making it to the end of the aisle of the sports store with my dumbbells.

I brought my dumbbells home on the taxi because I was too embarrassed to go on the bus. After I came home, I put my dumbbells in the corner of my bedroom, and they are still there—shiny, beautiful ones . . . untouched.

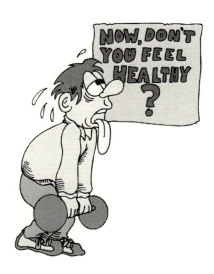

More than half of those who join fitness clubs and majority of those who try exercising at home give up on their commitments after six to eight weeks. Over 90 percent of those who have lost twenty-five pounds or more return to their previous weight within the next year.

Why do people quit?

I started asking people this question about twenty years ago, and this is what I heard:

"Because of my work schedule."
"Because of my family life."
"Because of my children."
"I am too busy."
"I am too young."
"I am too old."
"I don't have the time."
And there were many other similar reasons.

My intention was to help these people to persevere, but I could not fix their problems because they were too personal, and I had no authority over them.

Later, as I learned more and more about us, humans, I discovered that most of the answers that I've heard from people were not the real reasons for quitting. The actual problem lay much deeper, and those real reasons were hidden inside of people's minds. In order to discover them, we need to understand who we are and what our mind is. Reading more and more about human psychology made me realize that majority of people quit for the same reasons—the reasons have nothing to do with our everyday life:

1. *Reactiveness*

As human beings, we are responsible for our lives, and our behavior is a function of our decisions. We have the initiative and the responsibility to make things happen, but not all of us are the same. Some recognize this "response-ability," and some don't. Those who do recognize it do not blame the consequences of their behavior on the circumstances, conditions, or other people. However, some of us decide to be controlled by these circumstances, acquiring some very sticky habits. In making such choices, these people become hasty and *reactive*. They get easily influenced by instant gratification and comfortable laziness. Even the weather conditions affect them. If the weather is good, they feel good; but if the weather is bad, it affects their attitude and performance. *Reactive* people also get affected by other people. When other people treat them well, they feel well, but when other people don't treat them

23

well, they become defensive and protective. Reactive people are driven by their feelings, emotions, and conditions of their environment. Pursuing goals requires resisting to temptations and influence of the circumstances that is not characteristic of reactive people. They are usually self-centered and concentrate on immediate satisfactions, getting easily distracted when pursuing their goals.

2. *Fears*

Fears hold people back from making new decisions and accomplishing their goals. They may feel dependent on their fears and hold on to these negative thoughts.

Why are we afraid? In many cases, fear is survival. It is our natural response when we face danger. For example, you are crossing the street and see a car coming right at you; fear of death will make you run to save your life.

But many of the fears are consequences of our imagination and are not real. Roll back your thoughts into your past and try to remember how many things you were afraid for no reason. Some people, even in their adult years, still carry on the fears from their childhood. Consciously, they realize that these fears are not real, but when faced with the cause of their fear, they still react. A good example is the fear of mice. Mice are no danger to people; consciously, it is understood, but many people are still afraid of them even when they are an adult. Why is that? Because many times, these responses occur outside of our conscious mind. Trying to logically approach our fears does not always help. In many cases, reasoning with a fear does not change anything. For the subconscious mind, it does not make a difference what is real or what is not. Once faced with danger, it believes it again and again.

Fears create attitudes that produce procrastinations, poor time management skills, and avoidance. Subconscious fears originate deeply inside of our minds, and we often try to "hide" from them. Many fears pollute our minds, immobilize us, prevent us from transforming our ideas into actions, or cause various physical problems. Some of the fears make us avoid people or lead us to making mistakes.

Why do people continue to live with their fears? Because facing fears creates anxiety, and people rather pretend that their fears don't exist than acknowledge them. Many people avoid thinking about their fears because fears are often viewed as a form of weakness or inadequacy. They think that such avoidance will make their fears disappear.

Some fears bother us throughout our life and prevent us from following our dreams.

Can we change it, or are we forever slaves of these negative thoughts? While it can be difficult to completely get rid of some of our fears, dealing with many of our fears can be learned. We have the ability to keep most of our fears under control. But until we discover our fears and bring them into light, we will not relieve ourselves.

The most common fears preventing us from pursuing our goals are the following:

- Fear of failure
- Fear of success
- Fear of risks
- Fear of rejection
- Fear of unknown

Fear of Failure

Some of us carry out this fear from childhood. Fear of failure is the greatest obstacle preventing us from our successes. Some of those who have failed before may never regain their confidence because they often associate their failures with themselves or their inability to produce tasks. We all make mistakes and fail sometimes. This is just a part of being a human. And we should never associate our personality or self-esteem with our failures. Those failures have nothing to do with us. Nobody is born to be a loser or a winner, and nobody knows everything or can predict everything. Some people are stronger and some weaker. Some have more knowledge and experience and some less, but nobody is an actual failure. For example, if you failed your exam, it doesn't mean that you are not capable of learning this subject again. Or if you failed your job interview, this also doesn't mean that you are a loser. Each and every failure should be anticipated as a <u>stand-alone event</u> and not as a pattern of your actions or part of your personality.

From 1878 to 1880, Thomas Edison, the electric bulb inventor, worked on at least *three thousand* different theories to develop an efficient incandescent lamp. Most of these theories have failed, but Edison viewed each of his failures as the next step to success and never linked them with his own self-esteem.

Our schooling system and our society unfortunately consider failures as something to be ashamed of. As a consequence, we are subconsciously growing up habituated with a fear of trying anything new or taking risks. We would often rather stick to our old habits, even if they are bad, than take a step toward a better life. Trying new always involves risk of failure. But if we stop taking risks, our subconscious mind may close up and put our entire life's progress on hold forever.

Successful people are also going through their ups and downs, and they are also experiencing similar life problems like any of us. But what successful people don't do is allow these problems interfere with their goals, slow them down, or discredit their previous achievements.

Fear of Success

We may want to ask ourselves a question: "If success is about getting what you want, what could be frightening about it?" Despite of how paradoxical it may sound, but fear of success exists. While consciously we all want success, our subconscious mind does not always agree with this statement. It often tries to oppose and overpower our desires to attain the success:

"What if I don't deserve the success?"
"When I am successful, there is too much responsibility out there."
"When I am successful, people are going to judge and criticize me."
"When I am successful, I am going to lose my friends."
"Other people will suffer because of my success."

In order to overcome this fear, we need, first, to be fully aware of its existence. Otherwise we will feel powerless and will be working toward our successes with halfway strength.

Of course, just acknowledging the fear doesn't make it disappear. But if we properly evaluate each of our fears, we can better understand ourselves. Then we can gradually relay our subconscious feelings so they can work with us instead of taking our power away.

Fear of Risks

Risks are associated in our society with a danger or a threat. Risk of injury, risk of getting ill, risk of heart attack, risk of death, etc. From our childhood, we've been programmed to be cautious about almost everything, and we try avoiding risks. Then many of us grow up without even having an opportunity to try anything new, to be different, or at least to be sure to be able to change anything in life. Then being adults we keep sinking in every day's sameness and getting used to our repetitive routines. Life goes by, and we subconsciously accept that we are simply not designed for progress, and every day should be the same. Same mornings, same afternoons, and same evenings. Same, same, same.

We watch how other people progress in life and assume, "Ah, they're just lucky!" Consciously we wish to do what other people could, but our subconscious mind tells us, "Don't risk! It's better to be safe than sorry." And then we give up.

If we continue living without taking any risks, we may completely lose our confidence in ourselves and then start doubting our ability to function successfully at all. If our mind does not receive an important message, "I can do it," our self-confidence gets wasted because of insufficient use and will slowly get into the state of atrophy. When a situation arises when we need our self-confidence, it will be useless to serve us.

Begin to visualize risks as opportunities and not as dangers. Take smaller risks to build your self-confidence slowly. Practice your positive self-talk to immobilize your fears. Eventually your subconscious mind will learn new approaches to help you take bigger risks.

Fear of Rejection

We start learning about pain of rejection from childhood. This fear follows us through our adolescence and even adult years. Today's lifestyle has created boundaries and invisible fences between people. This leads to an emotional isolation that allows us very little connection with each other. We restrict ourselves with communications by Internet, text messaging, and at best, by phone. Social skills and verbal communications between people are left only for certain occasions. Lack of these skills has led to developing fear of rejection. We all like to be liked and look for approval from others so we can be more confident about ourselves. Fear of losing favor or being disliked can block us from pursuing our goals.

G.A. *I grew up in a family where education was valued the most, and until about thirty years old, I was working hard toward my career. Studying through university years, I haven't had many close relationships with females because of my constant lack of time. After I graduated and got my diploma on hand, I suddenly realized that it was the time for something new in my life—maybe that new relationship.*

There were some nice girls in my class, but my communication with them was limited to only discussions about homework and projects. The idea of actually approaching them personally and asking to go out never crossed my mind before.

We were preparing for the graduation party, and this was a good chance for me to explore my new desires. But I had absolutely no idea of how to do it. Asking for someone's help about that subject looked embarrassing to me, but I knew that I had to do something. Many of my friends were already either married or dating, and this was challenging me. I felt like this was my time.

I shared my secret with my best friend, and he pushed me into something that I will never forget. He said that he read this idea on the Internet: I had to give him a hundred dollar bill as collateral and agree for him to keep it if by the end of our graduation party I was not going to be out with one of our school girls. I really liked that idea, and after we laughed about it, I went to prepare for the party.

At the party, I lost all my communications skills and almost fainted when I tried to approach the first girl. Trying very hard to talk, I felt like I had a ball in my throat. "What if she says no? What if my friends see or hear when she says no?" was going through my mind. I tried to ignore these thoughts, but every time I was about to make a new attempt, my tongue was glued to my lips again.

Did I take a girl out? Of course I did, and my buddy had to give me my hundred bucks back. But this was one of the most infuriating experiences in my school life. This was more frightening than any of my exams.

Fear of rejection creates a feeling of inadequacy. We may feel like someone is always looking over our shoulder, judging and evaluating us. We often find ourselves hesitating in making choices or applying halfway efforts when pursuing our goals.

People who are afraid of being rejected don't always perceive it as fear. They sometimes identify this feeling as a desire to be a nice person, and they spend enormous amount of time and energy trying to please others. By doing so, these people are neglecting their own desires and never have enough time to accomplish their own goals.

Fear of rejection is engaged by subconscious thinking. Hearing no hurts, and we as humans always try to avoid the risk of being hurt.

But our subconscious mind still can sabotage us without even a need for a valuable reason.

Fear of Unknown

I remember the first time I took my kids to Disney World in Florida. When we went to the amusement park, my kids started dragging me to go with them on all sorts of rides. But I wasn't so great at handling motion simulators and roller coasters, so I refused to go. My kids got disappointed, but still kept bugging me to join them. They were so excited and thrilled that step by step I started to get excited too. I've never been on any of those rides and did not even have a clue what they are and how I would feel if I decided to go.

I promised my kids that I will try it the next day and started doing my own research. In the evening, I went on Internet on YouTube to see the videos of the rides that my kids went on, and my fear totally disappeared. There was nothing threatening in what I saw, and all rides looked like fun.

Next day my kids and I had so much fun together that I completely forgot about my motion sickness. I slowly "graduated" from easy rides to the most advanced ones, and my kids were very proud of my "accomplishments."

*   *   *

The origin of each of our fear is different, and as such, we should deal with each of them differently. However, we should remember that most of fears are invented in our minds, and nothing is more fearful than the fear itself. The best way to overcome our fears is trying to alter our thoughts. We need to recognize all our fears, so our self-defeating beliefs move from our subconscious into our conscious. Then we will be able to effectively deal with our fears.

Some fears disappear as we grow up and some when we get into new relationships. Many fears can be completely dissolved by love and support of our parents, spouses, family members, or friends. Some people are spiritually strong, and some are weak and look to others for support.

We may never completely eliminate some of our fears, but our ability to keep fears under control helps us to live a more joyful life.

We can also approach our fears by recognizing that our life always has two parts: the *good* and the *bad*. The bad part is where all our fears originate. Many people expect only good things from life, ignoring learning how to deal with the bad. Not accepting the bad as part of our life and unwillingness to face problems leads to many disappointments, frustrations, nervousness, and eventually develops some of our fears. Many parents indulge their children by allowing them to experience only good things in life and not teaching them how to deal with pain, failure, rejection, illnesses, or hardship. As a consequence, the child grows up not prepared for life and not knowing how to accept the bad.

We humans should be able to recognize that not acknowledging the bad does not make it disappear, but expecting and respecting it helps deal with stressful situations and destroys our fears at their origins.

What Helps Overcome Fears

- *Recognize your fear and accept that it exists.*
- *Analyze if your fear is real or imaginary.*
- *Dismiss imaginary fears.* It is not always easy, but if you practice, eventually you will learn how to approach most of your fears.
- *Roll back in time to understand the origin of your fear.* Sometimes, when you remind yourself what brought you fear, you may realize the insignificance of your worries.
- *Share your fears.* Your best friend, parents, your spouse, or even your children could help you to deal with your fears. Be cautious in sharing your fears with fearful people though because they can reinforce your fears even further.
- *Replace fearful thoughts with positive ones.*
- *Avoid negative people and negative events, movies, books.* Spend time with positive, courageous, and risk-taking people. You will absorb these qualities into your life. Negative people can be very fearful and insecure.

- *Do things you are afraid of.* Very often going "against" your fears helps to make them disappear. For example, if you are afraid of public speaking, doing it repeatedly may help overcome this fear. First, speak in front of a small group and gradually take bigger steps. Eventually, you may lose your fear.
- *Replace negative feelings* such as "I am scared" or "I can't do this" with positive and encouraging statements such as "I am brave" or "I want to do this." Repeat them every time you experience fear.
- *Have faith.* Fear and faith are inversely proportional. The more faith you have, the less you fear. Many heroic events happened in the name of faith. Faith can completely dissolve your fear.

From the very moment we start transforming our thinking from subconscious to conscious (trying to understand why it happens), all our fears begin losing their strength. Subconscious mind wants us to be afraid and believe in terror, but consciously, we can do many things to ease our fears. It is always less frightening when we know our fears. Then we can put them under the "spotlight" and start analyzing. Often we may find that many of our fears are just harmless ghosts of our imaginations.

3. *Negative feedbacks*

We all sometimes receive different feedbacks from other people, parents, teachers, friends, family members, etc. The impact of these feedbacks varies depending on how we are willing to accept them. Some of these feedbacks can reinforce our spiritual power, and some can destroy. Negative feedbacks can be caught up by our subconscious mind, and as a result, we may stop believing in ourselves or give up every time we meet challenges.

"You're an idiot!"
"You're a fat pig!"
"You're an ugly bastard!"
"You could never accomplish anything!"
"You're a loser!"

"You're weak!"
"You don't know how to do anything!"

Many of us heard these words in childhood, and sometimes even when we are adults. They are very powerful. Some people absorb them very personally and later on, in adulthood, still allow these words control their lives.

But the feedbacks are often based on our emotions and not on values and facts. Emotions change. The one who gives feedback often forgets what he said much sooner than the one who receives it.

Negative feedbacks are our fears, and the way to deal with them is the same way as we deal with our fears.

Willpower-training exercises reinforce our resistance to negativity. When one knows his/her self-worth and it is proven by values and not led by emotions, it builds strong statements in his/her subconscious mind to persevere.

4. Dependency on others

Dependency on others or too comfortable surroundings sometimes degrade self-worth and self-esteem. For example, housewives who depend on their husbands for everything may experience lack of self-esteem and willpower to pursue their own goals.

Many wealthy families grow their children secluded with only pleasures and do not let them acknowledge hardships and difficulties. Under these circumstances, the child—later adult—does not know how to experience the production of his own creation. He/she may feel useless and worthless trying to achieve something due to lack of these skills. Meeting with difficulties in attaining some results, these people are subconsciously programmed to rely on others and quit.

5. Resentment of discipline

In some families, discipline is harshly taught by the parents toward their children. As a result, children may grow up regarding the discipline of any kind as limitation of freedom. Throughout their lives, they perceive discipline as something unpleasant and frightening. Fear of change holds them back from making serious decisions or achieving some goals.

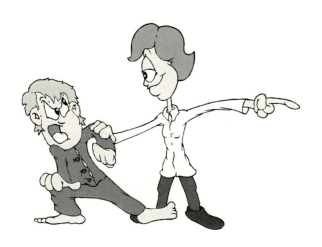

6. *Temptations*

Overpowering temptations seen on TV, shopping malls, restaurants, newspapers, fliers, etc. distracts the attention and weakens the will of many people. Being influenced by it, they usually blame the lack of time, circumstances, or other people for their failures.

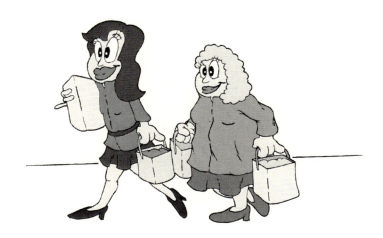

7. *Emotions*

When we go through our everyday life, we deal with different things. Often there are things that we don't expect and don't plan on doing that day that fall out of the blue: somebody called you with a bad news, you're stuck in traffic, your child got sick, your car broke down, etc.

How do we usually react? We often forget about what we planned for the day and start doing things that trigger our emotions first even if those things are sometimes not really important and can be done later. As we get more and more occupied with doing things that trigger our emotions each day, we may forget about our big goals and life plans.

Some days we may get so emotional that we don't even need a valid reason for quitting. We come home, sit on the couch, and say, "I just don't feel like doing anything."

8. *Ignorance*

You wake up one morning and finally decide: "I am going to change my life! I am going to exercise, eat right, learn how to deal with my stress, and be happy!" You go buy appropriate books, watch inspiring movies or TV shows about people like yourself.

Something happens down the road, and for no particular reason, all those exciting things slowly start fading out in your mind. You still realize that changing your life would be nice, but something inside of you tells you, "Ah, forget it! Not right now! Maybe someday later." When you turn on the TV show that used to drive you to do good things, you don't feel so excited about it anymore. You go to your favorite fast-food restaurant, sit down on the table, make your first bite of the bad-tasting good sandwich, and think, "Tastes good! Feels good too! Can't be that bad." And all you were thinking before about changing your life simply gets ignored. Deep inside, you still realize that you need to change your life, but something that lies even deeper tells you otherwise: "Maybe this is bad . . . but I just like it that way . . . Not now! Maybe later! At least not today!"

Days go by, life goes on, and nothing gets changed.

*　　*　　*

When people pursue their goals, very often they quit because they get influenced by various things. These things corrupt people's minds, allowing them to procrastinate or look for excuses. Once they failed, they start looking for easier and easier solutions or fall for quick-fix short-term programs. These programs are usually based on producing only results and not on developing people's own willpower or self-discipline. Consequently, at the end of every quick fix, people go back to their previous state of thinking and rely on success only with influence from the outer source and not from within themselves.

Only by developing personal willpower, self-discipline, and patience can we possess our own thoughts and gain the ability to make decisions. Only then we can no longer be influenced by our own weaknesses, weaknesses of others, or circumstances.

CHAPTER 2

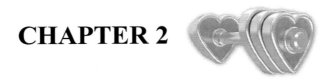

MIND WORKS

Our mind is very divertive. Literally speaking, there are always two different people "living" inside of us. We often contradict ourselves and our own decisions. One side of us is always fun loving and pleasure seeking, and the other side supports serious commitments in life and discipline. Many times we feel like being on the crossroads—one side of us advises us to go one direction while the other one turns us another way.

The side that is looking for pleasures has tremendous power over us. Most people live being ruled mostly by it. It's obvious. We live only once, and whatever comfortable, convenient, and enjoyable attracts us. We don't want to become slaves of difficult routines or not having time doing things that we love to do.

But the other side of us realizes that to be productive in life requires effort and commitment. So what should we do? Should we battle the pleasure side in order to achieve something? We probably could, but then it would be a quick fix, and as we know, all quick fixes have temporary power. Eventually, at the end of every quick fix, our mind will swing back, and all our achievements will be diminished. A good example of this is diets. Dieting is a restriction of our pleasures. If we didn't know that the diet will end, we would never start it. The success of produced results this way zeros down very rapidly.

Our pleasure side is not our enemy, and we should never blame it for not succeeding in life. If we did not have pleasures, we would not be humans. We hunt for pleasures throughout our lives whether we realize it or not. We make sacrifices or suffer sometimes for the purpose of future pleasures. So we should never be trying to take away our pleasures. Instead we should be looking for ways to add more of them and try acquiring the ability to enjoy more things in life. In order to do that, we need to understand how our mind works. Then we can make our pleasure side work toward our successes and not against them.

Let's look at our pleasure side as our child that needs parental guidance. That child lives inside of us and is part of us. Contradicting with him is like contradicting with ourselves. No matter how spoiled this child may look sometimes, we should never ignore his opinion or disvalue his wishes. Our role as parents is to direct his actions and educate him instead of creating more conflicts. We also need to know what he is about and understand his nature before we try to discipline him or change his behaviors. Here is what he (your pleasure side) will tell you sometimes when you try to be productive:

1.   This idea is not a good idea.

Your pleasure side is very conservative and pessimistic to any improvements. It sometimes may try to discourage you from them.

"It's too difficult."
"It's too complicated."
"It takes too long."
"It's not worth it."

2.   Success is boring.

In order to remain in control, pleasure side will always try to bring up the negativities in successful people:

"Successful people are dull."
"Rich people are miserable."
"Skinny people are anorexic."
"Eating healthy is not fun."
"Exercising is a waste of time."

3.   This is not for me.

Every time you look for ways to improve yourself or get successful, your pleasure side will try to overpower you and convince otherwise:

"I am too old for this."
"I will never lose weight because of my body type."
"I will not last."

These attempts are nothing but trying to prove to you that the problem why you cannot succeed in life lies within your personality and that you are lacking some kind of ability to turn your desires into reality. To make this statement even stronger, your pleasure side will try to draw your attention to all your failures and mistakes. This, in the end, may develop a sense of insecurity and disbelief in yourself. If you obey, you will lose your enthusiasm and eventually give up.

4.   Let's do something else.

Achieving something in life requires not only acquiring some information. To understand something, we need to study it, plan it, organize and practice, and this takes time and effort. Every time you try to concentrate and work on that, your pleasure side will try to convince you to do something else instead or skip difficult steps. For example, when you need to perform some practical exercises to develop certain skills, the pleasure side will tell you, "I understand how to do it. Let's just think about these exercises. Let's do something fun instead." It will try to do anything to redirect your thinking. Your pleasure side has enormous amount of options on how to take your attention away on any occasion. Always remember that.

"Let's watch TV."
"I am hungry."
"I am tired."
"I am not in a good mood for this."
"I need to do this . . ."
"I need to do that."
"I want to go there."
"I need to go shopping."
"I need to call my friend."

5.   Let's do it later.

Your pleasure side will always try to put your plans on hold and find a variety of reasons to logically approach this idea.

"Before I join the gym, I need to look better."
"I don't have proper clothes to start exercising."
"I need to do some more research."
"I'll start next Monday."
"I need to finish something else first."

Despite all these bad things that your pleasure side does to you, never try to crush it. Instead, look for cooperation and compromise. Most of the diets, boot camps, and other quick-fix programs are intended to defeat the pleasure side. They create an enormous conflict with it, thus with your own self. Unless we learn how to avoid these conflicts, these programs will never work for us. We will always be jumping from one quick solution to another without any permanent and visible results.

Self-Talk

Thousands of thoughts are going through our minds every day, and based on these thoughts, we make our daily decisions. Inside of our minds we not only think but also talk. This is called a *self-talk*, a powerful tool that we can use to succeed in life. This talk never stops inside of our minds. "I am hungry," we go and eat. "I am tired," we go and rest. "I want to do this . . ." and we start doing that. Inside of our minds we always receive messages and then act upon those messages.

Many of these messages are repetitive and programmed in our mind subconsciously. We are not always exactly hearing them, but they are still doing their jobs. Some of them help us to succeed and some distract us from those successes. But they are all "trained" by us and "doing what they are told." This is how we develop our habits.

If we want to change our habits, we need to "retrain" our subconscious mind by repetitively doing things that develop a new habit. This is done through our self-talk.

But before we start talking ourselves into something new, let's realize how our subconscious mind works and what we need to do to control it.

We have to always remember that our subconscious mind has a tremendous power over us. How often we get influenced by it without even being aware? How many times we impulsively buy things that we don't even need, and how much time we uselessly spend instead of catching up with things that are long-time overdue. This happens because we subconsciously obey to our pleasure side and listen to one of the commands described earlier. Often when we try to do something productive, our subconscious mind puts us back on the couch in front of our TV and gives us millions of reasons to do that.

Regardless of its power, our subconscious mind still belongs to us, and we have the power to control it. We just need to know the rules that our subconscious mind operates with. Then we can apply these rules to change our habits.

Rule number 1. Present tense

Our subconscious mind always works from *present tense*. If you want to overpower it, your self-talk commands need to be said in present tense. For example, if you say, "I have to go to the gym" and you are presently watching TV, your subconscious mind will immediately oppose you: "I am busy, I am watching TV." So instead of saying "I have to go to the gym" or "I need to go to the gym," say "I am going to the gym." This way you are forcing your subconscious mind to immediately switch from one activity to another. As you practice your self-talk more and more, your subconscious mind will obey you and will follow your actions. Try "I am having a soup" instead of "I am having a cookie," and you will feel the power of being in control.

As you say your command (and it is in present tense), don't delay your action or start doubting your decision because your subconscious mind will immediately flip you over and "knock you down" making you "having a cookie" instead of "having a soup." You have to show your subconscious mind that "I am having a soup" is your action and not just your words. If you don't act on time, your subconscious mind will act for you. It has to feel your power and know who is in control. That control cannot be just your words; it has to be your actions.

Start with small and easy things and slowly graduate to more difficult ones, but always act upon your words. If you don't, your subconscious mind will never "take you seriously" or believe you and will not obey you.

If you repeatedly say things in the present tense and act upon your words, your subconscious mind will remember these things, and eventually they will become your new habits. Eventually, you will reach the point where there will be no difference for your subconscious mind "having a cookie" or "having a soup."

Rule number 2. No negativity

Second important rule to remember is that negative approach never works with subconscious mind. As soon as you say no to any of your habits or behaviors, you will be creating a conflict with yourself for the simple reason that the subconscious mind is part of you. Contradicting with it is contradicting yourself. Say "I am not having a cookie" when you really want it, and you will position yourself directly against yourself. You will feel it. Then your subconscious mind will send messages to your emotional and physical receptacles, and you will eventually be overpowered by it and give up.

If we want to break our habits, going against them is totally useless because these habits are developed by pleasures, and they give us pleasures. They are very powerful. Much better way is to learn new habits that are just as pleasurable so we can replace old ones. Leaving "empty spaces" where our old habits "lived" will eventually lead to going back to them.

Rule number 3. Be specific

Third rule in dealing with your subconscious mind is to be specific when giving your commands. Subconscious mind can only respond to one message at a time. When you say "I am having a soup" or "I am having a cookie," it can only respond to one of these commands. You have to always address exactly what you want. If you repeat your statements over and over again, your subconscious mind will start working toward your new desires. You will be amazed how fast you can progress. But always be specific.

Anything we want in life can be available to us if we possess the ability to transform our subconscious thinking to our conscious. In simple words, it means to open up our mind to understand our subconscious and make intentional efforts to improve it.

Some habits can be very difficult to change, but millions of people do it every day. And anyone can do it. It really all depends on how you "slice" everything in your head and which things in your life you give more value. You might get different advices on what to do, but eventually, it will still come down to evaluating your own thoughts. No one can control what goes through your mind.

Only you.

Power of Words

When you have your self-talk, be careful in selecting your words for it. They are not just words but also your thoughts and later your actions. Some words can make your subconscious mind work for you and some against you. Remember, your subconscious mind does not like to obey and wants to always be in control.

Never use "I have to," "I must," or "I should" because by doing this you are letting your subconscious mind know that you are weak and have no control over your behaviors. Use "I am" or "I choose." Your subconscious mind has to hear your choices in a forceful and positive manner. Only then it senses your power and obeys you.

Never say "I will try." "Trying" is a weak thinking and doesn't put you in full control. Do things instead of just trying them. Only then you will move with full force and determination.

Never say "I think I can do this" because what you are actually saying by this is "I am not fully sure that I can do this." Say "I know I can do this" and feel it. "*Knowing* that you can do this" give you full power while "*thinking* that you can do this" takes some of that power away.

Where you go from where you are right now is only up to you.

CHAPTER 3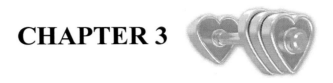

BRAIN POWER

Our brain has two sides. Both sides have different functions and deal with different kinds of problems. That's why we sometimes "hear" controversies inside of our minds.

Left side of our brain is more logical and deals with words, examination, investigation, breakdowns, and sequential thinking. It is very dominant and likes to keep things under control.

The right side is more creative, intuitive, and sometimes can get spontaneous. It likes dealing with pictures and imaginations. This is the one that allows us to have dreams, visualize them and go after them. The right side helps us to put things together and figures out the relationship between those things. It is holistic, free of boundaries and limitations, and is able to deal with simultaneous thinking.

The left side is very logical, but at the same time very conservative, which means it does not like the change. When we procrastinate or look for excuses in order to delay our actions, the left side always finds logical explanations for it. We know how sometimes we hide behind those explanations. "I am not ready to quit smoking because I am still under a lot of stress." Or "I am not ready to join the gym because I have a lot of projects at work." Or "I eat sweets in the middle of the night because I just can't sleep." All these sound pretty logical, but these are also procrastinations. By having explanations to our procrastinations, we are *consciously* giving values to them. Then we, ourselves, get influenced by these values and eventually give in to their power. Our mind senses that power and later accepts it subconsciously. Subconscious thinking becomes very hard to change.

Every time we want a change in our life, we need the help of the right part of our brain. Being inventive and proactive, the right side will always push us to achieve something.

Best if we could use both sides in balance, but unfortunately, most people live ruled by the left side. Change is often uncomfortable and requires strength of character and willpower. These qualities are developed by the right side of our brain.

How can we reinforce the right side of our brain?

Since it is creative, inventive, and imaginary, then we, obviously, should be trying to draw upon these capacities. We need to aim practicing and experiencing situations in our everyday life, which will emphasize and strengthen those capacities. Here are some exercises below. They are simple but very powerful and will put your right side immediately at work. Have a piece of paper and a pen. Expand your imagination to the maximum:

1. In your thoughts, step out of your present time and see yourself five years from now. If your life continues going this way, do you like what you see? Are you happy? What did you achieve? Are you healthy? Do you have everything you wanted?

   What would you change now, in your present, to make your life better in five years?

2. You hear on the radio that an enormous meteoroid is going to hit the Earth in sixty days, and we are all going to die. How would you restructure your priorities in life?

What would you do first, second, third, etc.?

3. Your doctor told you that you have cancer that has no cure, and you have only thirty days to live? When you die, how do you want to be remembered? What do you want to be said on your funeral by those whom you loved, your friends, or simply people whom you knew or worked with? What would you tell them before you die? How would you act toward those who are in a strained relationship with you? Would you try to fix those relationships? In your thoughts or on the paper, make a sample speech for each of these people and what you would like to hear from them.

4. You home is burning in fire. What would you take with you while getting out of that fire?

5. You know that you may have a very serious health problem two years from now, but you have the power to prevent it.

   What would you do?

These exercises will help you to learn how to imagine things and then put your thoughts into action. Of course, in these types of situations, we act different—more immediate, because we realize the need for our actions. But by using your imagination, you can purposely create any circumstances to reinforce any of your everyday actions. Our mind is a very powerful tool. It can either make us immobile and sluggish or successful and dynamic. These capabilities are in our hands, more specifically in our heads. The powerful steering wheel of life lies there—inside of our brain, and both sides, left and right are the hands holding that wheel. In order for our life to get directed where we want, we need to try using both sides in balance. Otherwise our life will be just like a car directed only left or only right going into *endless boring circles*.

* * *

Inside of our minds we visualize things, and we have the power to choose the way to see it. We have ability to control that, and the volume of that control directly depends on the volume of our imagination. What we can visualize in our minds later can become our everyday thoughts and then gradually transform into real actions toward our goals. Thought is real, halfway physical and alive. Everything in our life starts from a simple thought. Thoughts move our progress, thoughts make our dreams come true, and they are our initial actions. The most complicated mathematic formulas are created by simple thoughts and visualization of things. Airplanes with millions of parts in them started with visualization of the paper airplane that we all make in our schools.

How can we train ourselves to achieve what we want in life? How can we go on without doubt? Some of our goals look so big, unreal, and mysterious. And there are so many everyday obstacles that distract and weaken us.

Step-by-step, from small achievements to larger and more complicated ones is the way to go. When a child learns to walk, he makes his first step wobbling and unsure. But moments later something happens, and he decides to go ahead and risk walking. He may immediately fall, but does he give up? Inspired by his tiny success, he gets up and tries again and again until his walking gets right.

Our mind is very mysterious, and we still don't know how to realize the full capacity of it, but one thing we know for sure that if we want to achieve something in life, we need to imagine it first.

Placebo Effect

Here's the article from *Wikipedia*, a popular Internet source, about *placebo*. Note that some paragraphs are rephrased for your easy reading.

"A *placebo* is a trick used in medicine when a patient is given a fake pill, told that that it may improve his/her condition, but not told that that pill was fake. Such a medical intervention may cause the patient to believe the treatment will help him/her to recover, and this belief may produce an actual therapeutic effect, causing the patient to feel better. This phenomenon is known as the *placebo effect*.

The placebo effect points to the importance of the perception and the brain's role in physical health. This effect has been used not only with pills, but also with creams, inhalants, injections, and many other therapies. Medical devices such as ultrasound can act as placebos too.

The physicians (family doctors) have even been called placebos. A study found that patient recovery can be speeded up by words "You will be better in a few days," or "The treatment would certainly make you better" rather than negative words such as "I am not sure that the treatment I am going to give you will have an effect."

The placebo effect may be a component of pharmacological therapies: Pain-killing and anxiety-reducing drugs that are infused secretly without an individual's knowledge are less effective than when a patient knows they are receiving them. Likewise, the effects of stimulation from implanted electrodes in the brains of those with advanced Parkinson's disease are greater when they are aware they are receiving this stimulation. Sometimes administering or prescribing a placebo merges into fake medicine.

The word *placebo* came from Latin. It actually means "I shall please." In 1811, it was defined as "medicine adapted more to please rather than to benefit the patient." The placebo was first used in the eighteenth century. In 1785, it was defined as a "commonplace method or medicine." Placebos were widespread in medicine until the twentieth century, and they were sometimes endorsed as "necessary lies."

The effect of placebo treatments has been studied for the following medical conditions:

- ADHD
- Amalgam fillings
- Anxiety disorders
- Asthma
- Autism
- Benign prostatic enlargement
- Binge eating disorder
- Bipolar mania
- Cough
- Crohn's disease
- Depression
- Dyspepsia and gastric motility
- Epilepsy
- Erectile dysfunction
- Food allergy
- Gastric and duodenal ulcers
- Headache
- Heart failure, congestive
- Herpes simplex
- Hypertension: mild and moderate
- Irritable bowel syndrome
- Migraine prophylaxis
- Multiple sclerosis
- Nausea: gastric activity
- Nausea: chemotherapy
- Nausea and vomiting: postoperative (sham acupuncture)
- Pain
- Panic disorders
- Parkinson's disease
- Pathological gambling
- Premenstrual dysphoric disorder
- Psoriatic arthritis
- Reflux esophagitis
- Restless leg syndrome
- Rheumatic diseases
- Sexual dysfunction: women
- Social phobia
- Third molar extraction swelling (sham ultrasound)
- Ulcerative colitis
- Vulvar vestibulitis

Placebos are produced by *expectancy* effect, where fake pills or substances are believed to be a drug. The expectancy effect can be enhanced through factors such as the enthusiasm of the doctor, differences in size and color of placebo pills, or the use of other inventions such as injections. In one study, the response to a placebo increased from 44% to 62% when the doctor gave them with "warmth, attention, and confidence." Expectancy effects have been found to occur with a range of substances. Those who think a treatment will work display a stronger placebo effect than those who do not, as evidenced by a study of acupuncture.

Because the placebo effect is based upon expectations and conditioning, the effect *disappears* if the patient is told that their expectations are unrealistic or that the placebo intervention is ineffective. A conditioned pain reduction can be totally removed when its existence is explained. It has also been reported of subjects given placebos in a trial of antidepressants that "once the trial was over and the patients who had been given placebos were told as much, they quickly deteriorated."

A placebo described as a muscle relaxant will cause muscle relaxation, and if described as the opposite—muscle tension. A placebo presented as a stimulant will have this effect on heart rhythm and blood pressure, but when administered as a depressant—the opposite effect. The consumption of caffeine has been reported to cause similar effects even when decaffeinated coffee is consumed. Perceived muscle stimulants such as fake creatine can increase endurance, speed, and weight-lifting ability. Placebos can help smokers quit. Perceived allergens which are not truly allergenic can cause allergies. Inventions such as psychotherapy can have placebo effects. The effect has been even observed in the transplantation of human embryonic neurons into the brains of those with advanced Parkinson's disease.

Because placebos are dependent upon *perception* and *expectation*, various factors which change the perception can increase the magnitude of the placebo response. For example, studies have found that the color and size of the placebo pill makes a difference, with "hot colored" pills working better as stimulants while "cool colored" pills work better as depressants. Capsules rather than tablets seem to be more effective, and size can make a difference. One researcher has found that big pills increase the effect while another has argued that the effect is dependent upon cultural background. More pills, branding, past experience, and high price increase the effect of placebo pills. Injection and acupuncture have larger effect than pills. *Proper adherence to placebos has been found to decrease **mortality**.*

Motivation may contribute to the placebo effect. The active goals of an individual change their experience by altering expectation symptoms and by changing their behavior.

The placebo effect can work selectively. If an analgesic placebo cream is applied on one hand, it will reduce pain only in that hand and not elsewhere on the body. If a person is given a placebo under one name, and they respond, they will respond in the same way on a later occasion to that placebo under that name but not if under another."

Placebo Effect and the Brain

Functional imaging upon placebo shows us the link between our imagination and brain functionality. If we humans can realize our perception into reality to eliminate not just a simple pain but also many life-threatening diseases and even death, why then do we sometimes feel that we can't achieve our goals? Why do we only look at the things that we want instead of having them? The placebo effect clearly displays that if we put our thoughts together and strongly believe, we can practically achieve anything.

The placebo effect is proven not only in medicine but also in psychology in many books. "Fake it until you make it," or purposely changing the image of yourself described further is one of those tricks that people use.

A placebo effect phenomenon is a pure indication of the power of our brain, its capacity, and our ability to achieve what we imagine.

Nocebo effect

"In the opposite effect", describes Wikipedia, "a patient who does not believe in a treatment may experience a worsening of symptoms. This effect is called *nocebo*. This word also has a Latin origin and means "I shall harm." Nocebo effect can be measured in the same way as the placebo effect, e.g., when someone receives a fake pill, substance or sham treatment, results may report a worsening of symptoms. The recipients may nullify the treatment by simply having a negative attitude toward the effectiveness of the substance prescribed and the mentality toward the ability to get well".

This is the same effect we experience when we disbelieve in our capabilities and in what we can achieve in life. If we concentrate our attention on our mistakes and failures, we will always be applying nocebo, and our life will be limited.

CHAPTER 4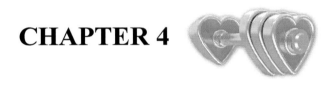

TURNING YOUR DREAM INTO REALITY

We all dream about something. If our dreams stay unrealized, we regret, consciously or unconsciously. While everyone has an ability to turn his dream into reality, not everyone understands how. Some dreams take longer time to realize and with more effort and some with less. But if we look carefully at the patterns of achieving almost anything in life, we can recognize little difference between small and big dreams. Yes, big dreams require more planning and preparation, more willpower, self-discipline, and patience, but this is all the difference. Sometimes we just think that it is too complicated, making it look complicated, and then everything else along the way gets complicated, and those dreams don't come true. But life is pretty straightforward and simple. In most cases, if one person could achieve something, so can another. Make it simple; see it simple. If you choose your direction and keep going there, one day you will be there no matter what. Sometimes you may feel that there is nothing there or you are headed to a dead end, but . . . just keep going, keep pushing. Complicated will eventually become simple, you will see; hard will become easy, and unknown will get familiar. There is no other way.

Every dream destination is just as simple as any road trip, and it depends only on how far your road trip is. Let's do this comparison together and look what we need to go on the road trip, and then try applying those rules to all our other dreams.

Here you go:

For our road trip, we need first *a map* of the most effective route. Without a good map, we would be lost and would not know where to go.

After we highlight our route on the map, we *prepare everything* we need for the trip: clothes, food, water, cutlery, toiletry, gas for the car, etc.

Once we start driving, we *visualize* our final destination in our thoughts. Although we don't see it yet, we assume that it's there.

We also know that if we keep driving at a *certain speed*, we'll get to our destinations on a certain day and at a certain time.

Focusing on the road ahead will help us avoid accidents, frequent stops, and it will also get us to our destination on time.

Now, let's look at the similarity of our road trip with any other dream.

1. *A map of your dream*

We as humans have many of these maps in our thoughts. When you choose your map, make sure that it is not the map of all the things around you. It has to be the map of the way *you want it to be*. If we were to choose the map for our road trip, we would not go by the small roads or confusing ways. We would surely choose the shortest ones and the fastest. But again, this is your dream, and you choose how to "drive." Do not include in the map of your dream the circumstances of your surroundings, somebody else's opinions, and other sorts of distractions that will diminish your focus. You have to have a clear vision (map) of your destination as if there was nothing else there to distract your view.

2. *Assume and believe*

Visualize your dream and always keep it in your thoughts. Assume and believe that your dream destination is real and that it is already there. Don't see it as "maybe" or "probably," but truly believe that it is there. Believing is always seeing something that *does not exist yet*. If that something already exists, then it becomes *a fact* and not a belief anymore. Most people are afraid to experiment or take chances because they don't believe enough. When distractions or difficulties come along the way, these people lose the sight of their dreams. Focusing on what you want and keeping a picture of your dream in your thoughts is the main key in achieving your goal.

Don't ever doubt yourself or question if you can do it. The only things you won't be able to do are the ones that *you think* you can't do. When you have a good feeling about something, trust your guts, and those things will always come out good. As soon as you start doubting yourself, you subconsciously start working with halfway efforts, and things won't work out. Put your mind together and start thinking better of yourself—give yourself more credit and believe that you can do anything, no matter how ridiculous or impossible your idea may look to others. By statistics, many outstanding ideas came out of ridiculous thinking. That includes most of our technological inventions. Be proactive, dare to try things, and most of all believe in yourself and trust your guts. Discard the opinions of those who don't believe in you, and go with a full feeling that you will accomplish your goal. That goal may not be accomplished the way you picture it, but it doesn't matter. The end result is what matters the most.

3. *Figure out the date*

Most people did not realize their dreams simply because they never planned them. What would happen with our road trip if we did not plan the dates for it? We would never know when to start driving or when to arrive.

Plan your dream precisely. Stick to the committed date but be realistic in timing and allow time for setbacks.

4. *Prepare yourself*

Carefully prepare yourself, and have everything you need to make the way to your dream less frustrating. If we did not prepare for our road trip and took everything we need, imagine how many unnecessary extra stops we would have to make.

5. *Break it down*

Break down your plan into months, weeks, and days. "A thousand-mile journey starts with one step." Treat every step as an important one. A child first learns how to turn over, then how to sit up, to crawl, and only then how to walk and run. This is true in all areas of our development. Each and every step is important, cannot be skipped, and takes time.

It is the same as in our road trip. When we plan it, we want to know how many days it would take us to get to our final destination. At the end of each day, we would sit down and analyze how much is left to drive.

6. *Focus*

Temptations, procrastinations, and all sorts of excuses can throw you off your schedule or can even make you fail. Just like on the road trip, if we would make many stops, we would probably get to our destinations much later (or never). Notice how focused you have to be when you drive, especially on the highway and how much can happen in less than a second if you lose your focus. When you go after your dreams, you have to stay just as focused, and sometimes very little time can decide a lot.

7. *Expect delays*

Anything can happen along the way. Anticipate it. We are only humans, and all make mistakes, get tired, or get sick. Other people and circumstances can also cause some delays. Do not get frustrated, and direct your energy constructively on the solution to problems and not on the problems themselves.

8.   *Finish what you start*

The last miles of the road trip often are the hardest to drive. But in order to get to any destination, we need to learn how go until the end. Anyone can start, but not everyone can last until the end. All our previous efforts will be a waste of time if we are not able to go to the finish line.

9.   *Get excited and enjoy the process*

When we are positive and happy about things that we do, we always perform better and more efficiently. Negative thinking slows down the process in achieving our goals or can even discourage us from pursuing them at all. Not everything along the way is enjoyable, but negativity only makes it worse.

When we are trying to achieve something, we may look for shortcuts in order to save some time and effort, expecting to be able to skip some of these steps, but with the same effectiveness and results. By doing so, we are, in the end, shortcutting the natural process. We are missing not only important ingredients to get to our dream destinations but also the experience in achieving our next goals. When a child learns how to walk, he does not skip some of his steps in order to learn walking faster. Each and every step needs to be taken, and shortcutting in achieving our goals only results in disappointments and frustrations.

I remember myself neglecting these principles many times—in my childhood and even when I was already an adult. Always believing in my possibilities and eager to succeed, I often found myself blinded by passion and excitement—I sometimes skipped some steps in my planning and went straight to accomplishing my goals. But I've learned that it is not always the faster you start, the faster you go. Many times, if your goal is big, you need to dedicate a lot of time to proper planning. Good planning helps making the process of achieving your goal less painful. Yes, planning can get boring and might drain a lot of your time and energy, but every minute spent on it pays off. It can result in saving you days, months, or sometimes even years.

CHAPTER 5

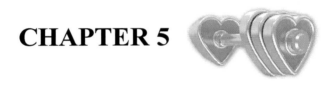

TIME MANAGEMENT

G.T. *I joined the gyms for the third time. At the beginning, everything was fine, but then I got so busy that I just couldn't find time for my workouts. I am running my own business, have three kids, need to cook, take care of my house, family, and other things . . . I don't think I can handle it . . .*

L.Z. *I want to retire in five years, and this is my main focus right now. I understand that I need to exercise, but I just don't have the time. When I retire, I am sure things will get better . . . Then I'll be able to spare some time for myself.*

F.H. *I have a full-time job, and I'm also going to evening school four times a week. Saturdays, I take my kids to piano lessons, and Sundays I go to church. How can I stick the workouts in my crazy schedule? It's not that I don't want to, it's just I can't find the time.*

These are typical problems, and finding time to exercise in our speedy life is never easy. We all realize that health is important to us, but when it comes to managing the time, we get lost in everyday tasks, and exercise routine often becomes our last priority. Partially it happens because of poor planning, but the main problem lies much deeper.

In our lives we are surrounded by our principles and values that make us happy. Those things are work, family, hobbies, pleasures, religion, friends, etc. The circle of these things forces us to play with our time and spread it among those things. If we want to add something new into our life and we don't know how to manage our time properly, things can get really out of order. We may sometimes wait for the miracle to happen or expect that new time will be found somehow later by itself. Already habituated with old habits, we may get frustrated and eventually give up on anything new.

How to find time to exercise when there is only twenty-four hours in a day and our schedule is already 100 percent filled with other important things?

Here are some ways:

1.   Something's gotta give

We obviously cannot stretch the time, and some of our daily activities might need to be sacrificed, some shortened, and some moved to other days.

Let's look at one example: let's say, you have four different activities in your evening schedule, and these activities already occupy 100 percent of your evening time. Take a close look on each of these activities and see where you can cut corners. Sometimes we spend too much time on watching useless TV programs, endless conversations on the phone, chatting on Messenger, Facebook, or Twitter. And then we complain that we don't have the time. It is not always the time that we don't have, but sometimes, we are not willing to sacrifice that time for something that is more important.

2.   Combining activities

I wrote most of this book using my BlackBerry during my cardio workouts. Yes, it was a little uncomfortable, and I would probably prefer doing it in a comfortable chair in front of my large screen monitor, but this was the only way that I could find time for it in my busy schedule.

Cardio workouts are pretty suitable for reading, watching movies, making phone calls, text messaging, e-mailing, and web browsing from phones.

Latest cardio machines (figure 1) in many gyms are now equipped with TV monitors built in them. Some stationary bikes have even capability of web browsing and e-mailing.

Personalised TV

iPod and iPhone allow audio/video selections and to watch videos, movies and shows on the LCD screen

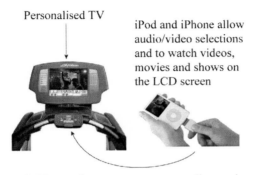

Figure 1. Entertainment on gym cardio equipment

If your gym does not have these machines or you prefer to do your cardio at home on your own treadmill or elliptical machine, there are few other options (figure 2). You can strap your laptop to your cardio machine. This system is relatively inexpensive, available on the Internet, and allows you to do some things on your computer while doing cardiovascular exercise.

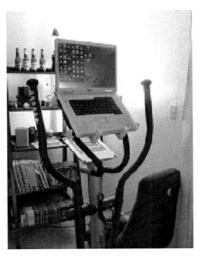

Figure 2. Attaching laptop to home cardio equipment

With today's technology and development of iPads, iPhones, and BlackBerries (figure 3), it makes it even easier to have fun while exercising. You not only can call or chat on the Internet, but also watch a movie or a TV show, or use Internet on your laptop or iPad providing that it is equipped with internet mobile stick.

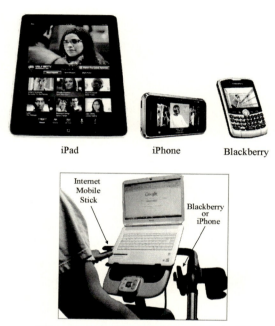

iPad   iPhone   Blackberry

Office away from office while doing cario in the gym

Figure 3. Using communication devices during cardio workouts

If you like music, you can definitely incorporate listening or watching it. Music is a great motivational tool. When I go for my run and plug my ears with my music, I am not really running there—in my thoughts I am either performing on stage or going crazy in front of that stage where my favorite band is playing. This makes my run feel shorter than it is and much more enjoyable.

3. *Prioritizing*

Have you ever looked in the viewfinder of the camera with manual focus? When you spin the lenses, you can change the focus depending what you want to see sharper. If you focus on the closer objects, they look sharp while the farther ones look hazy and unclear. By changing the focus again, you can make farther objects look sharper, while closer ones get hazier.

We humans have those lenses in our minds, and when we browse through the things that we need to do, we can actually sharpen the images of more important things and do them first. In the ideal world, by doing this, we would be able to completely keep our lives under control. But we have emotions, and our emotions sometimes can affect our ability to change our focus.

One time my wife and I were walking through the shopping mall. We were headed to our gym for a cardio workout. Browsing through store displays, I noticed a nice GPS for our truck. I asked my wife if we could stop for a minute to find out some details about it, and she agreed. Forty minutes later we kept asking for more and more questions about that GPS, and when we looked at the time, we realized that we don't have any of it left for our cardio. We gave up on buying the GPS and also on our workout and ran home to get ready for work.

We often create urgencies like that and then blame the circumstances for not having enough time. These urgencies rise up like monsters in front of us and change our focus. Very often they aren't critical and not even important at a particular moment.

Often we give up on the things that we have to do and do the things that we want to do. This is how we procrastinate. At these moments we are deeply searching in our minds trying to find any reason to win our procrastination. We look for excuses, blame somebody else, or simply feel sorry for ourselves. Slowly but surely we are giving in to the force of circumstances and decide, "I don't have the time!" As we repeat this statement, it gets stronger day by day supported by new excuses. Subconscious mind accepts this statement, and then we completely give up.

4. Fair time distribution

Some parents involve their kids in multiple extracurricular activities and then completely forget about themselves. Running from karate lessons, piano rehearsals, dancing classes to art schools or singing practices, these parents by the end of their day end up being completely emotionally and physically drained. This leads to a disproportional life—a busy and happy kid with a sick and tired parent. Loving your child does not necessarily mean getting him busy at the cost of your health. This could be balanced by equally spreading time between child's activities and parent's activities. Parents who take care of themselves are healthy and agile and can spend more quality time with their children, bonding their relationship instead of giving up these relationships to too many extracurricular-activity teachers. In addition, parents who lead a healthy lifestyle will also set an example for their children to follow lifelong healthy habits.

*　　*　　*

Everyone values different things in life. Time to exercise can be found, but only if we look it and try to prioritize things. If there is a will, there is a way. *Important things in our lives <u>are not always urgent</u>, but they are important, and we need to do them, so we don't go behind our schedules. <u>Urgent things are not always important</u>, and often we purposely make them look important by acting emotionally.* Ability to realize what to do first and see further in life is given to us humans through our self-awareness. We are not only driven by our emotions or habits, but we also have a capability to predict some consequences of our behavior. Refocusing "our lenses" on preventive matters instead of impulsive-urgent-emotional ones gives us the power to possess ourselves and control our values.

CHAPTER 6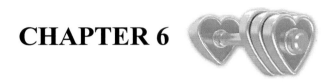

PATTERNS TOWARD SUCCESS

I started writing this book about five years ago. Some days I was writing one page a day, some two, and sometimes I went weeks or months without writing. Time went by, and on my computer, I've collected a pretty large file with a number of pages. One day I decided to start working on the publishing of this book. After I reviewed all my work, I was shocked with the inconsistency of the information. I could not put pages together and could not make any chapters. After long hours of thinking it over, I realized that I had only two choices: give it up or rewrite my book again.

I sat down and remembered all my previous achievements, and all that inspired me and gave me a new strength. I recognized that if I just repeat the patterns that led me to accomplishing my previous goals, then I can easily accomplish this one.

There are different patterns that people follow while achieving their goals. By learning from our past, we improve our patterns, and then these patterns become our footprints of life. We walk these footprints over and over again to make things happen, and every time it gets better and better. We become skilled and experienced.

Thought is the most significant step in our successes. It's like a match to a fire. It initializes everything and gets us up into action. Thoughts build foundations to our dreams, and just like a foundation of a house, thoughts keep our dreams steady, alive, and safe.

We still don't know how much potential our mind has. Studies have shown that our brain is working only on 5%-10% of its own capacity. Where is the other 90%? How much can we do? *New Worlds* and *Guinness World Records* prove again and again that we are way far from the exact answer. There are many cases when doctors prescribed a complete disability for someone, but he recovers and performs better than ever. Sometimes deadly diseases turn around and give up to the power of the mind. How fast can we run? How strong can we be? How much can we achieve? We don't know. But what we do know is that our mind has tremendous power and sometimes makes miracles—something that seemed unreal yesterday and impossible, today becomes a reality. If we put our thoughts together, we can go against all odds and predictions, against rules and even common sense.

1. Allow yourself to dream

Didn't we all wish to have superpowers when we were little? Sometimes we dreamed and pretended achieving anything we wanted!

We grew up. Life taught some of us to give up on superpowers, quit dreaming, and accept the reality. But some of us kept dreaming.

What is the reality? Is it a cruel world with fake friends, bad people, pollution, wars, and limitations? Or is it a beautiful place filled with love, honesty, trust, joy, happiness, and endless opportunities? It depends on what you believe. Many of us go through life successful, live with love and happiness. But some of us accept that life is tough and unfair. These are the consequences of our thinking. Without a thought we cannot move to one or another direction. Our actions are controlled by our thoughts. If we think that life is hard, it will be. If we think that certain things are possible and certain things are not, that is how it is going to be! Once we start thinking a certain way, we subconsciously build our attitude toward the way we think, and then start doing things that we think of. When we watch TV, read books, browse the Internet, or listen to the radio, we also concentrate our attention on the things that we think of. Then our attitude gets supported by new information and becomes stronger and stronger, leading us to do more and more things toward our present attitude.

By changing your beliefs, you can change your reality, and you can achieve practically anything you want. There are millions of facts showing us how many people went above and beyond their possibilities. Are they any different from the rest? Yes and no! The fact is, they always kept on dreaming! They believed in their "superpowers" and held on to their dreams.

Just a couple of decades ago we could not imagine that almost everyone of us will have a cell phone and wireless Internet. Fifty years ago this fact probably looked impossible. A hundred years ago nobody would believe that people will be walking on the moon or spend months in space. Now humans are developing the system so anyone can go to space just for a trip. Impossible? What is really impossible? We ourselves in our minds create those barriers and then live surrounded by them.

Allow yourself to dream, and dream to the fullest, not about something that is a bare minimum for you or something that you would settle for, but about something that you really want—your ultimate dream, your best wish, and your greatest desire which is also your purpose in life. Don't settle for anything less or inhibit someone else's dreams.

2. *Don't let failures and mistakes stop you from dreaming*

OK, let's say you've finally decided to allow yourself to dream and made your first few steps. But as soon as you started to get excited about it, suddenly everything turned around in a totally opposite direction, and all your effort not only zeroed down but got into a big minus. Is your dream gone? Is it going backward? No, it's still going forward. Look at the hockey or football players, how many times they have to go back and forth the field trying to win the game. And none of their games is still a guaranteed success. Is losing a disappointing experience for them? Of course it is! But do they give up? Day after day they train again and again to have another chance to experience that wonderful moment of victory, the experience that makes the effort of all years of training worthwhile.

3.   *Measure your success right*

> *Success is not measured by what you accomplish but by the opposition you have encountered, and the courage with which you have maintained the struggle against overwhelming odds.*
>
> —***Orison Swett Marden***

Success is often mixed up with the level of achievement. It is not how much you achieve, but the amount of difficulties that you are going through while making that success. Only then it feels that you achieved the success. In simple words, the more difficult it is for you to strive for your success, the bigger is your success.

Let's say you decided to become a *successful* runner. How would you measure your success? Most likely by winning a race? But whom are you racing with? With people who've never run before or those who are like yourself who want to be good at it too? You would probably be the first if you race with those who never ran before, but how big would the level of your success be? The level of achievement and the level of success are two different things. The level of achievement in this case will be higher, but the level of success is not that great. It may look like you are achieving a lot winning the race against those who never ran before, but will this race challenge you? Will you really feel that you achieved a lot?

If you decide to run against runners like yourself, you will have fewer chances to win, and your level of achievement in this case might be lower, but the success will be much higher.

I remember my college years when we went on basketball competitions. There were suppose to be fifteen teams participating in those competitions, and we were training very hard. Winning any of the medals would be as a great success then. But when we arrived, it appeared to be that only three teams including ours could participate in those competitions. We won the second place. Yes, level of our achievement was great—we came home with silver medals. But when we were driving home in our bus, nobody was even talking because we did not really feel that we achieved anything.

Next year we went on the same competition and won third place out of nineteen teams. This was the greatest success in our basketball history. Our bronze medals had much more value for us than the silver ones last year.

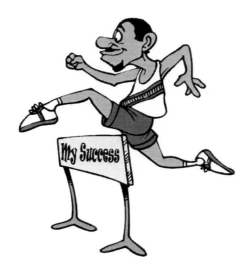

4. *Change your image*

Having an image of yourself is seeing or visualizing yourself in a certain way.

The way you see yourself inside of your thoughts is the way you will eventually become in the future. This happens for a reason described earlier—your thinking creates your attitude, and then your attitude leads to your actions. You do things based on your attitude and then become what you thought of yourself initially.

Everything starts from thinking, and if you want to change yourself and your situation, you must first start thinking of yourself the way you want to be. This idea is also known as **"fake it until you make it"** or as **"act as if."** It imitates confidence and produces success. The purpose of it is to avoid getting stuck on being not confident and also overcoming the fear of not being confident.

Wikipedia describes it like this: "It is a common device in rap music, where performers will often make records and music videos presenting themselves as successful, handling large amounts of cash, and showing off obvious signs of luxury like expensive clothing and excessive jewelry, even when this record or video is their first release and made when they have not yet achieved the success they display."

Those who consider themselves as losers usually support their image by thinking of their failures and mistakes done in the past. As time goes by and more mistakes or failures are made (often the consequence of such thinking), these people may never learn how to succeed in life. In order to be successful, we first need to change the image of ourselves and start seeing ourselves as winners. Then instead of mistakes and failures, our focus will be readdressed to our successes and achievements. Our attitude will change our actions and will lead us to more and more successes.

For example, when it comes to your body, don't concentrate on the parts that you don't like on yourself when you look in the mirror. There is no good use in doing it. It will only corrupt your confidence. Look at the parts that you do like and visualize all the other parts becoming just as good soon. This type of thinking will lead you to act toward your desires. Don't try to wonder how this is going to happen. Just keep thinking about it, and you will see how your thoughts will gradually explore you into your actions.

5.   *Attitude*

Looking at my past, I can recognize that everything good that happened to me was when I had a good attitude. If I kept my hopes up, everything went fine. Opportunities found me by themselves, and I did not even have to do much. I was like a magnet attracting all the good things to myself. Sometimes I could not believe how easy I could accomplish extremely difficult tasks. But as soon as I allowed myself to go down and get emotionally low, I immediately attracted all the negativity. I tried to reason with that condition by working harder, but instead of improving, everything was only getting worse. Slowly through the years I've learned that things rarely change for the better if you are not better yourself. The vibes of your attitude very deeply penetrate in everything you do. If you are positive, everything works out, but as soon as you get negative, everything starts going to waste. And the interesting thing is that pretending or faking your feelings doesn't work. I tried to force a smile on my face when I felt like crying just to hide my feelings, but things rarely turned out for the better. Trying to pretend what you feel is almost like trying to get a new body-paint job for your car when its engine is broken.

I am not trying to disagree with the fact that it is sometimes difficult to keep a positive attitude. We occasionally get stuck on our negative emotions, and in some way, these types of emotions even comforts us. There are times when we feel even inconvenienced to get positive. But there is nothing good or comfortable about negative attitude. It does not get us anywhere further than our new mistakes, broken relationships, failures, and health problems. Positive attitude helps us to prosper in life, live longer and happier.

Having a positive attitude does not necessarily mean being always uplifted, feeling energized and cheerful. Sometimes not having a bad attitude is good enough. Extracting the *good* from any situation in life and trying to always see "glass half full" and not "half empty" is a skill. This skill allows us to work our lives around ourselves and get what we want, instead of wasting time on endless and useless negative speculations.

Sometimes, being negative, we wait for something positive to happen. We try to convince ourselves that if those positive things happen to us, we would definitely change our attitude. But in life, it does not work that way. While we are hoping for something good to happen, we keep spreading negative vibes around ourselves, and those vibes attract more negativity. The positive things only start shaping up when we turn around our feelings first. It's almost like switching on a different radio frequency. The feeling of good has to come first from our inside—from within our own thoughts. Then our surroundings start "reading" those vibes and bring us all the good that we deserve. The amount of that good received depends on how strong we believe in "the happening" and how long we can hold on to it. If we emotionally switch back and forth from negative feeling to positive ones, we only get more confused. Staying on positive "frequency" is a skill that we develop with willpower training.

The most difficult task is to stay positive when negative things surround you. Anyone can be positive when everything is all right, but it is much harder when it is not. But our mind has tremendous reserve for development.

Here are some attitudes that may lead you to fail:

Perfectionism
Perfectionism is really a subconscious fear of being mediocre. Nothing in our life is perfect, and nobody is perfect. Perfectionist attitude creates unwillingness to accept that fact. "If I can't do it perfect, I might as well not do it at all" thinking leads to procrastinations and avoidances. Trying to escape from taking opportunities, risks, or sometimes just being lazy, we say, "Oh, no, this is not for me, it has to be perfect." Because perfectionism is viewed in our society as a positive trait, we often accept it and allow ourselves to hide behind this "screen" and procrastinate.

All or nothing
"All or nothing" attitude is very similar to perfectionism and also paralyzes our efforts to pursue our goals. "All" is often viewed as something big and received quickly, but to achieve "all" requires doing small and repetitive tasks. When we say, "It's all or nothing," we subconsciously reject doing those tasks and as a result often end up with "nothing." This extremist attitude prevents us from attempting to start anything and also develops many of our previously explored subconscious fears. These fears lead us to quit.

"All or nothing" attitude is multiplying our negative physiological powers. Many of our goals will stay unrealized, and having this attitude, we will be working against ourselves.

There is only one right way

When we search for ways to achieve our goals, we want them to be done in the most efficient way, and this is only normal. But what if those ways are not right at our hands or not within our capabilities? What if we simply can't afford those ways? "There is only one right way" attitude is another technique that our subconscious mind uses to make us procrastinate and hide from "the truth." There are usually various alternatives to achieve the same goal. But we often choose to ignore those alternatives so we can procrastinate and escape from pursuing our goals.

Poor me

This attitude makes us avoid doing things that are difficult or require concentration. Feeling sorry for ourselves locks us in the state of mind that gives us a feeling that we are just *not capable, not lucky*, or simply *don't have access* to ways of accomplishing our goals.

It could always be worse

It is interesting how our society is "trained" to love bad.

Why do many people like watching TV news? Are the people really being attracted to horrible events that TV news hosts display? Not exactly. In most cases those events make a person feel that he/she is not in the most terrible situation and "there could always be worse." But does this type of thinking helps us progress in life? Many times it does totally the opposite—it shuts you down by a comfy feeling that "my situation is not that bad."

It doesn't mean that we should never think like that. Realizing that "it could always be worse" many times can be helpful. But we also have to be aware that this feeling can also completely immobilize us and make us settle in life, preventing from further progresses and achieving what we want. It is one thing to appreciating what you have, and it is completely different to getting used to the idea that in life "it could always be worse."

The same thing can happen when we want to improve our body. We look at others who are in worse shape than us and conclude, "I am not that bad." But compared to who?

In order to succeed in life, we should be applying "it could always be better" more often.

6.   Create a sense of urgency

If you remember the sample exercises given in chapter 3, "Brain Power," and now you understand what to do to reinforce the right side of your brain, by using your imagination, you can come up with similar situations in life to help yourself achieve your goals faster. Naturally, when people make choices for the sequence of doing various things throughout their day, they often choose easy and pleasurable things first, leaving the difficult ones later. That "later" often never comes because of either so-called "constant lack of time" due to more pleasurable things, or purposely created procrastinations, leaving doing difficult things for "later . . . later . . . and more later."

If in your mind, you purposely make _important things look and feel urgent_, you will always do them first. Some time down the road while pursuing your goals, you will see how doing difficult things will feel enjoyable to do, and those difficult things may not be as difficult anymore because you will acquire a new skill—how to overcome difficulties, which is emotionally always rewarded by extraordinary feeling of accomplishment. The more difficult things you accomplish, the greater the feeling of that accomplishment. It just amazingly makes you feel worthwhile.

Create the need for you to act. Imagine things, and make your actions look like emergency so your right side of your brain will force you to do things. Pretend that you don't have a choice, have very limited time for it, or expect your dream to be taken away from you. Play with your mind, use _present tense_ and _be specific_ in your self-talk.

7.   Learn how to handle the pressure

We are all experiencing pressure every day. The level of that pressure varies depending on where we are and what we do. Some people have more pressure at work, some have more at home, and some—at work and at home.

Not all people know how to do handle the pressure well. When we focus on the problems, the pressure rises, but if we try to refocus and think of the solutions to those problems, then we can reduce it. For example, we are often pressed by time. We feel that we are always going behind our schedules, getting frustrated when we get stuck in traffic, or delayed with our meetings or plans. What are our natural reactions to that? Very often, blaming everything on circumstances, other people, something else, and in the end, getting caught by our emotions. This leads to wasting time instead of concentrating on solving problems.

The best thing that I've learned about dealing with pressure is to expect it. The pressure is unpleasant, and everything unpleasant becomes even more unpleasant when it comes unexpectedly. The amount of pressure is much greater when you are not ready. This is very easy to prove if you just imagine someone trying to scare you from behind. But if you know that that someone is there, behind you, you will not react the same way.

This does not mean that we have to be always feeling uptight and scared of something bad coming because it will only create a bad attitude, and by doing this, we will only increase the pressure instead of reducing it. We have to learn how to expect the pressure without being afraid of it and accept it more like a challenge and not as a distraction.

8. *Love the change*

In our life, we are very easily getting used to comfortable things and immediately become possessive of those things. We create our *comfort zones* and subconsciously adopt them. These zones become our world, principles, and our "lenses" through which we often view everything. When we want to achieve something in life, and it requires leaving our comfort zones, we procrastinate, look for excuses, or simply defend ourselves with a variety of reasons. Time goes by. We keep hoping that something will change by itself, or our circumstances will adjust to what we want. But nothing changes, and one day, we realize that we are already too old for a change. We genuinely regret about wasted time and wish that somebody would help us to go back to our past so we can revise our lives. We understand that if we would have made those changes we would attain so much more additional pleasures in our lives. We would be happier, more fulfilled, and satisfied with our accomplishments.

Going forward in time in my imaginations helps me to see my mistakes that I have the power to prevent right now. In the future, I can tell myself what to do and what not to do and what I need to change to get what I want. I love the change. Change makes me alive and allows me to make my choices. Without a change, our life would stop being interesting and exciting.

Yes, change sometimes is uncomfortable, but it is very rewarding in the end. When we want to change something in our life, we often have to go through difficulties. But difficulties make us valuable individuals. Only going through them can we recognize ourselves for who we really are.

9. Make it a priority

Have you ever noticed that some people read nice books, watch deep and meaningful movies, and never learn from them? Why people sometimes say one thing and do the total opposite? Because we all live ruled by our habits "surrounded" by different priorities. If our priorities contradict with priorities of the books we read or movies we watch, we'll never learn from them. Those books will occupy our minds for a while, movies will entertain, but nothing gets learned or changes *until we want that change*. It is not enough just to acquire information. We need to set a new priority and commit to it.

Committing does not only mean knowing it, understanding, and accepting, but, most importantly, living it, practicing, and continuously advancing. When we set our priorities, we decide what we want, then restructure our lives and act upon our decisions.

The way I look at the word *priority* is as *prior-it*, which means whatever your priority is, it must be done prior something *it*, and *it* is everything else you do. If other things interfere with your priority, those things are done later. We always do our main priorities first.

But what happens when we have too many priorities and they all look like main ones? Which ones do we do first, and what do we do to avoid confrontations between our priorities to help succeed in life? We need to learn how to manage and balance them.

Let's look at our priorities as bank accounts and imagine that if we put an effort to act upon any of our priority, this will be equal as making deposits into that account, and if we take advantage of any of our priority, it will be equal as withdrawing from that account. For example, if you spend most of your time at work and rarely see your family, you are making a lot of deposits into your *job account,* but since you are doing it at the cost of family time, you are withdrawing from your *family* account.

What happens when we withdraw from our actual financial account without making any deposits? We go in debt. The same thing happens with your life priorities. If you stop acting upon any of your priority, you will start losing the connection and will also go in debt. In the above example, not spending time with your family will lead to losing the relationship with your family.

Balancing our priorities is exactly like balancing a checkbook. Very often we appear to be torn between work and family and also other things that we need to do. But before we withdraw from any of the "account," we have to make some deposits. This is a very apparent rule to make all "accounts" grow together. Making appropriate deposits to each of our priority is a wise way of balancing our life.

Very often, when trying to provide for their family, people work extremely long hours. They think that their financial security will help them build stronger relationships and happier lives. But because they don't spend enough time to actually work on those relationships, they often lose them, and those relationships fall apart regardless of how great the financial security of that family is. But people, being blinded by one-way success and being afraid to lose the momentum of that success, may decide to completely stop working on other priorities in life, thus becoming lopsided and losing the grip to balance in life. There are millions of extremely financially successful people who still feel very insecure in every day's life due to that imbalance. Many of them understand what needs to be done to change their lives, but their possessed habits don't allow them to do so.

It also happens how spending too much time together that couples or families lose track and responsibility for the financial support of their families. Then financial difficulties destroy their relationships regardless of how much time they may have spent together.

These are just few examples how to balance the priorities, and it works the same for others.

Let's look at exercising as another example. Before we start thinking about taking fitness resolutions, we need to realize that exercising will take time out of our schedules. If our other priorities in life do not allow us to exercise regularly, we will give up. Of course, we can go and join the gym next January because this is the time when everybody is talking about it, but we also have to think of what will happen in March when this rush is gone. Will we be gone too? Will we still have enough time for our workouts or was this a temporary solution to make us feel better for a while?

Integrating fitness into your life is adding an equal priority and is like opening a "fitness account." It will require making some regular "deposits" before you can actually take advantage of that "account."

How much time to dedicate to each of your priority is totally up to you, and it depends how much value you give to one or another.

10. Do little things every day

When we make big plans, we all should be able to recognize that they all consist of small efforts. How otherwise would we get to where we are right now? Graduating from school, for example, is a big thing. How many small projects do you do to get to your graduation? Each and every of them is a small link.

When we give up on our big plans, we don't give up because we suddenly stop being attracted to the idea. We often give up because we don't like repetitively doing small efforts. But the ability to see the value of little things is the key in accomplishing all big goals. Regardless of how useless these little things may look sometimes, they all have tremendous value, and each of them is a next step forward.

A book is written in chapters, pages, paragraphs, sentences, words, and then letters. If we reverse this sequence and see any of our goals as a book, then we can easily climb up from letters to words, from words to sentences, from sentences to paragraphs, then from paragraphs to chapters, and ultimately, we will achieve our goal. Once we visualize this pattern, we can clearly understand the importance of every little step that we do when trying to accomplish our plans.

We always feel more insecure about big plans. They look sometimes like a big complex thing and often scare us away from pursuing them. This usually happens because we don't break down big goals into the small ones. If we are consistent with our actions and do little things every day, we will eventually achieve any big goal. There is no other way. Brick by brick, houses can get built, and little thing by little thing, any of our goals can eventually get accomplished.

If your goal is big, don't always concentrate on the final result. Realize that all small things get you to that final result. To help see it better, visualize your goal as Lego or a puzzle. This will always remind you how important small things are. Without each little part, your puzzle or Lego will never be complete.

11. *Don't despair because of setbacks*

Nobody likes redoing things or going back when the need is to go forward. But setbacks are natural, and they are part of any progress. We cannot expect everything in life to go smooth and always as planned. There are usually a lot of back and forth movements. Artists use up a lot of materials and waste a lot of time before they are happy with the final product of their creation. Photographers take hundreds of shots until they get the ones that are right. We, humans, can only predict so much.

Some days you will do more, some less, and some you may not be able to do anything. But never despair because of the setbacks.

Have you ever got stuck with your car in the snow, sand, or mud? Did you notice that trying to drive only forward does not always help you get out? You need to go back and forth few times until the tires of your car find the right grip. When we pursue our goals, we all look for that tight and perfect grip to move ahead. But sometimes we get stuck and need those back and forth movements to get ourselves going ahead again. We have to believe and understand that sometimes our moves back are just our attempts to move forward faster.

12. Use momentum

When we drive our cars, we don't always press on the accelerator pedal. Sometimes we let it go, but our car is still going. This is the momentum. When we use momentum while driving, we spend less gas and also save the car from overload. To move from standing position always takes more energy. Driving down the hill is easier because of the momentum too.

Life works the same way. When we do things more often, we get better at them, and then doing those things takes less effort for us. This is also a momentum. But when we stop doing those things for a while, we lose the momentum. We forget how to do some things or lose some skills, and in some cases, we may even need to start from the beginning.

This applies to everything we do. Using momentum is a smarter and easier way in achieving our goals including fitness ones. Staying in shape is easier than getting into one. When our body is already rebuilt into a better working machine, all we have to do is maintain our results.

According to statistics, the breaking point when most people quit their fitness resolution is about six to eight weeks. This is when more than half of people quit exercising regularly. Those who continue after eight weeks start enjoying the exercise more because they see results. But if they get off track and their exercise becomes irregular, then they stop enjoying it because they never catch up with their momentum. Those who exercise irregularly may always feel like beginners.

Of course, to get to the momentum, we need to put our initial effort, but as we go along, it gets easier and easier. The more often we practice, the more we enjoy it.

Successful people and athletes always use momentum. They understand the value of it and realize that it is much easier to maintain the momentum than to build it from scratch.

13. *Activity is not always about productivity*

I like learning this lesson from watching sports games when one of the playing teams plays better technically but another team scores more and wins the game. The end result in games always comes down to the number of goals scored. How good teams played will be forgotten very soon, but what will always be remembered is who won that game.

Productivity is the most important when you are trying to achieve your goals. You could be trying to do lots of different things, but if those things don't bring visible results, you simply will be wasting your time and efforts.

In every period of our life, we only have certain time for success. This applies to sports, education, entertainment, and some other things. If you, for example, want to become a gymnast, you have to start doing this at a very early age—when your body is prepared for it. Chances that you achieve the same results after you get older are reducing with every year of your life.

Activity itself does not automatically set you for your success. You have to try doing things that bring you closer to results. Otherwise you will be like a hamster running in a spinning wheel, burning his efforts for nothing.

People can last only for so long without seeing results of their efforts. Then they give up. Very often they assume that they are simply not capable. But in most cases, this is not true. Doing something in a productive way always takes knowledge, willpower, self-discipline, and patience. If those people take time to learn how to actually achieve their goals by going into the details, they will soon realize how easy it can be. Then every day will not only be active, but also productive.

14. Stay "hungry"

When I was a teenager, I noticed very interesting patterns in rock music. Some rock groups as soon as they become popular immediately "disappear from the stage." I could not understand what was going on: "Hey, you guys are so great! Just keep giving us good music!"

Later I realized what may happen to you when you get what you want—you get too comfortable, and then you stop producing. Notice how you feel after you have eaten really well—you want to lie down on your couch and do nothing. Right? The same thing may happen to you when you achieve your goal. You may get too comfortable and stop thinking of any further successes.

As I grew older, I learned that as soon as you get too comfortable in life, you may start losing what you have achieved, and all your successes start going backward. This has nothing to do with being unhappy or never appreciating things that you have. I like viewing it differently. Everything in life requires maintenance—you buy a beautiful house, but if you don't clean it, soon enough it will turn into a garbage dump; you buy nice clothes, but if you don't wash it, soon enough it will have a rotten smell. Success requires maintenance too, and the best way to achieve that is wanting for more of the success and always "staying hungry" for it.

15. Don't get attached to things; learn to let go

Back in former USSR when I returned from serving the Russian Navy, I was twenty-two years old. I got into the university and then started working as a physical education teacher in one of the local high schools. When I was twenty-five, two of my friends and I opened our first gym.

Everything was absolutely amazing—success, money, lots of free time, vacations anytime, etc. But about four years later, civil war in our state began, and my gym was taken over by the Russian army. We had invested in that gym not only our money, but also our souls and all our passion. We were hoping that this paradise will last forever. But . . . we lost it all in one day. Because of the new currency exchange, we also lost most of our money.

Was it regretful? Absolutely! But nothing was more regretful than the war itself between people who yesterday were friends, coworkers, or students in same schools.

"Sometimes when you lose, you win," I said to myself and left for Canada. My fully paid condominium, nice car, financial stability, and future security—all went down the drain.

I landed in Canada with $1,300 in my pocket and two bags of clothes for my kids.

Do I regret what I lost? Not a single thing! Everything I've let go I found in Canada, and I found even more—besides financial security I also found emotional and spiritual comfort.

Throughout almost twenty years of living in Canada and trying hard to build my future, I have lost a lot of things again and not once. But I've learned that things are just things, and no matter how valuable they may seem, sometimes you just have to let them go. If you feel like you are on the ship headed nowhere and you need to make a greater step in your life, drop all the things holding you from doing that, and move on. Until your heart is beating and your soul desires, you can get those things again.

16. Do it your own way

When I was very young, I often looked at other people who achieved great successes in life and tried to copy what they did to get the same results. Some time along the way I got disappointed with such attempts because they often failed. I couldn't understand why.

As I grew up, I slowly began to realize that somebody else's ways don't always work for you. You cannot reapply somebody else's skills to yourself because getting those skills requires a process, and that process is very personal and unique. You can try to learn some tricks that other people do, but for the most part, you still have to go to your success your own way.

Going your own way in most cases is even faster. It's almost like handwriting—you can try to copy somebody else's handwriting, but will you be able to write faster?

17. Reverse your thinking

People don't like to lose. Even when losing something is beneficial to you, such as losing weight or giving up on some of your bad habits, still reverse your thinking, and don't put it this way in your mind because psychologically you may appear to be against yourself. Remember, that if you want to overpower your subconscious mind, you cannot use negative approach, and your subconscious mind doesn't like the idea of losing anything. It always likes to gain.

Rewire your thoughts and perceive whatever you want to lose as a gain—a better body by losing weight, better health by quitting bad habits, etc.

People succeed on giving up or losing something much better if they gain something instead. This is just human nature.

18. Stay organized

Many people think of organizing as something that could always be done later. As time goes by and more things get disorganized, these people start spending enormous amount of time on looking for what they need. This brings frustration, nervousness, and disappointments. Many important life goals get drawn in useless routines of looking for things.

If you often feel that you are behind your schedules and cannot achieve your goals because of constant lack of time, maybe this is the sign that your life is not as organized as it should be. Make everything easily accessible for you, especially things that you use every day, and always remember that every minute you spend organizing yourself always saves your time in the future.

19. *Learn how to clear your mind*

One research has been found that approximately 60,000 thoughts go through our mind every day. Some of these thoughts pass through without affecting us, but some get stuck and bother us. It feels like someone is purposely vibrating your head or trying to distract your attention by telling you something. If we get possessed by these emotions, we will never be able to move on with the progress of our goals and things that we need to do. Sometimes even a small distraction can prevent you from achieving your goal.

Clearing your mind is like starting fresh or muting all the voices in order to do something else. This doesn't mean ignoring or forgetting those things. It just means this: "Everything is on hold until I am done!" Learn how to clear your mind when you need that total concentration.

20. *No time is a waste of time*

In my twenties and even in my early thirties I often got so frustrated when I was unsuccessful in performing some of my tasks. They often felt like a total waste of time. "Why did I do this? Why did I go one route when I could have tried the other?" For quite few years those things still bothered me.

But later I started to notice that all that experience that I received from doing "waste of time" things, somehow, one way or another, always came back to me. I felt like I was completing the puzzles that I started years ago.

Now I strongly believe that whatever you do trying to achieve your goals is never a waste of time, even if it feels that way sometimes. We are all choosing different paths to reach our goals, so don't waste your time on thinking that whatever you did was a waste of time. Because it is not! Whatever you do to get to your goal are unique and the only steps that you can take. And if your way is to reach your goals later rather than sooner, don't get too frustrated. It feels the same. As long as you reach them!

CHAPTER 7

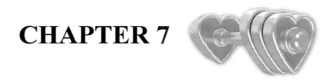

WILLPOWER

Many people confuse willpower with passion in pursuing goals and think that willpower is only applicable to the things that we love to do. Some say, "Oh yeah! When I find what I love to do, I will use my willpower."

But willpower is something quite different.

When we are passionate about doing something, we do it because we love it. Our mind agrees with us, and everything goes fine. But what happens when we get to something unpleasant? What do we do when pursuing what we love requires doing things that we don't like?

I am very passionate about my profession. I love fitness, energy, dynamics, and everything what comes with it. But to continue what I love and be successful at it, I have to do a lot of things that are not dynamic at all and have nothing to do with fitness or energy. They are the following: paperwork, accounting, planning, negotiations, etc. Sometimes I have to seat in front of my computer for days. I don't like those things. But what can I do? Without them I cannot continue what I love. Here is where the willpower comes in handy. Willpower allows us to pursue our goals further than just doing things that we love. It helps to go through all the steps toward our goals regardless if they are difficult, uncomfortable, or unpleasant.

When we watch movies or read books about strong people who achieved great successes in their lives, we admire and respect those people. What attracts us the most is how those people overcome difficulties, deal with unpredictable situations, and overpower the hardships. We also have a high regard for them for the ability to withstand the pain, pressure, and sufferings.

How do they do that? What do strong people have that others don't?

They have the ability to do all the things regardless if they like them or not. They train themselves to resist the weak part of their mind despite the consequences of pain, inconvenience, danger or threat.

Were they born that way? Some of them were, but many have developed this quality throughout their lives.

But willpower is not about cutting down the pleasures or putting yourself under stress and suffering. It's about making your subconscious mind work for you. It is about learning how to agree with the strong part of yourself and how to "volume down" voices of your weak part. By using your willpower, you can reverse your thinking and make unpleasant things look and feel pleasant.

Anyone can do things that are easy, but anyone can also learn how to do things that are hard. Willpower is the inner strength that can be developed by certain exercises. Just like exercising our muscles, we can exercise our mind. With a strong mind, we can make decisions and then take actions upon our decisions.

Willpower broken down into two separate words stands for the following:

Will—*determination, strength of character, inner force or self control,*
    and
power—*ability or capacity to perform or act effectively.*

Willpower allows us to use our determination to be effective and achieve our goals faster.

Waking up very early in the morning was never my favorite thing to do. But once I convinced myself to try it for a month, I discovered how many more pleasures in life I was missing. Early mornings are amazingly energizing and very peaceful. For quite a while I considered myself not a morning person, but later I realized that conceptions "morning person" or "evening person" are nothing but misconceptions. This is nothing but choices. What type of person you are lies inside your minds, and you have the power to change it at any time of your life. All you have to do is to decide to change your perception.

Just few centuries ago, in some countries, their leaders controlled their people by not educating them. The country's laws prohibited people to learn how to read and write. These laws were publicly read, and those who did not obey were jailed or punished. Secrets of life's success were hidden from the majority and mainly associated with the elite of people from high society. For the rest of the population, learning how to succeed in life was not only forbidden but also out of reach.

Now most of us know how to read and write, and anyone can become successful. We have access to millions of books; we also have Internet, phones, TV, and radio. Any information is now available to us at a snap of our fingers. But still, instant gratification and comfortable laziness destroys people's spirits and makes them immobile and impassionate about practically anything but immediate pleasures.

We all want our life to be enjoyable. But in order to achieve something, we need to learn how to enjoy doing not only easy things but also difficult ones. Sometimes taking an action requires getting out of comfort zones and experiencing unpleasant things. The willpower gives us the ability to carry out these actions, go against habits, persevere, and be firm on our decisions. Willpower allows us to stop procrastinating and act *now*, executing our life plans and achieving all the resolutions.

When you accomplish something big and difficult, the pleasure of this accomplishment is not just for a moment. It stays with you forever, and it becomes something to hold on to, when you are feeling down; something to be proud of regardless of failures, mistakes, or disappointments; something that gives you a value as a human being.

If the movies we watch or books we read are not filled with difficulties, we consider them boring. Why then should our life be boring? Let's fill it up with difficult things and have fun overcoming them. Let our lives be like those on the TV screen or in the best novel. Let's make our life an interesting story.

How willpower works?

The significance of the human brain's capability allows us to make choices in life. Even though our mind sometimes controls our behavior, we have the power to control our mind, and as a result, control our behavior. The power of our mind is tremendous.

When we achieve something in life, we start enjoying more things, and as we enjoy those new things, we want to achieve more. Once we taste the rewards, the difficulties don't scare us anymore.

The level of our achievements and success directly depends on how much of the willpower we have. If we push far, we get far. Willpower is our inner force that we apply in our minds every time it requires doing things that are unpleasant or difficult. But willpower is not something negative or something that always goes against us and forces us like a bully. The control of perceiving things is given to us, humans, through our self-awareness. We can accept any process as positive no matter how unpleasant it may be. Then our mind keeps working constructively regardless of any inconveniences that we experience during that process.

Ability to enjoy achieving things gives us ability to have the power. If we are suffering throughout the process, our mind can eventually "jump" on us with irresistible statements: "See! I told you it wasn't worth it! Why did you have to put yourself through this?" And then we give up, get lazy, or procrastinate. But if we enjoy difficult tasks, then we stop contradicting ourselves.

Ability to alter our thoughts is the ultimate skill that we develop with willpower. There is nothing hard and nothing easy, accomplishable or not accomplishable, reasonable or not, achievable or not. These are the choices that we make in our minds. Drinking a cup of tea without sugar can be just as enjoyable as with it, swimming in cold water can give just as much pleasure as swimming in the warm, and even the pain can go away if we decide not to let it control us. People do these things all the time.

When we make those choices, we decide to stay in control. Willpower is not about making ourselves suffer for the cause of learning how to take difficulties. It is a learning process that hardens your character. This process has to be accepted in your mind voluntarily and positively because when you force yourself to do things, one side of your mind will always tell you "do it" while the other says "don't." Physiologically, you will appear to be torn between two decisions to make, to do and not to do, and eventually may give up. They say, "Diets don't work." Why don't they work? For exactly the same reason—people get tired of being torn between two decisions. Living like this is not only psychologically difficult and confusing, but also unhealthy.

Every time you are torn between two decisions to make, you will always be applying your halfway efforts to your goals because the part of you that tells you "don't do it!" will always be holding you back, and you will never be able to realize your full potential.

Strong people can withstand the pain not because they have bodies with high level of pain tolerance, but because their minds are trained to do that. *Pain is in our mind*, and the level of it very much depends on how we perceive it. An athlete wins the race for the same reason.

*Most importantly is to realize that willpower is **not for you to feel forced by it** but for you to feel that <u>**you can force things to make them happen the way you want**</u>.*

How do you know what you want out of your life? Some people tell me, "I don't know what I want! How do I figure that out? Who can teach me?"

No one can teach you that. You have to feel it. It's like being in love. When you love somebody, no one can reconvince you not to love. Even if people tell you that love doesn't exist and what you are doing is wrong, it doesn't make you stop. Something inside of you is telling you otherwise—"It feels right for me!"

Some people are just afraid to make steps toward what they want. It's like always being on opposite sides of the same river with your dream. That dream is following you, but still on the other side. Willpower allows you to cross that river and become one. Once you learn how to do that, you start noticing different things in life. You pick pieces from your life that help you to move forward. You start seeing your life differently and in a totally different perspective. What attracted you before start losing its value, and what previously did not matter starts making sense. And then no one can reconvince otherwise, and nothing can influence you. Because it just feels right for you!

Three-Dimensional Thinking

When we make our decisions in life, we either enjoy or suffer the consequences of our decisions. Some of our decisions are irrational and spontaneous, and some are well thought of. But they all have consequences. Whether we want to enjoy those consequences or suffer through them depends on how we think and how then we act.

Sometimes we can act and behave ourselves without assuming the consequences. We can also make decisions or create situations in life that we regret about. Later we wish that we could rewind and change everything, but that is not always possible. When we act, behave, or make decisions without thinking of the consequences, we are thinking in "two dimensions." In this case, we are limited to a straight connection between ourselves and our actions. For example, smoking is two-dimensional thinking because when we start smoking, we do not think about the consequences and how hard it will be to quit.

Our mind has ability to expand our thinking. With willpower, our mind opens up to think wider. When our actions are based not only on immediate pleasures but also *on results of our actions*, then we are thinking "three dimensional."

Three-dimensional thinking is thinking preventively. It allows us to "filter" our life and protect ourselves from appearing in unwanted situations. This, in the end, speeds up the process of achieving our goals.

Self-Discipline

Our life now is much more comfortable than it was a hundred years ago, and we should be having more time for fun and achieving what we want. We should be more successful, healthy, and happy. But our researchers say opposite. With the growth of instant gratification (being inclined to only immediate pleasures), we did not get any happier or healthier or more successful. Sixty-five percent of us are now overweight and have various physical conditions and problems.

What are we lacking? Why don't we get better as our life gets more comfortable? It looks like comfort does not improve us as humans and doesn't change our mental state for the better.

I am not against making life more comfortable and convenient. I like comfort myself. We should have everything we want in life and enjoy every minute of it. But the comfort can deceive us and turn our life in the wrong direction. We all need to learn how to control it.

Self-discipline gives us that ability. When we aim to achieve something in life and instant gratification comes on the way to influence us, self-discipline helps us not to get distracted.

Many people unfortunately understand self-discipline wrong and perceive it as something hard and forcefully applied or something that belongs to only strong people. But self-discipline is a skill that can be learned by anyone. It gives you ability to become aware of your subconscious resistance and then learn how to overcome it. Sometimes what we want at the moment can totally contradict with

95

what we want in our future. That's because we are humans and have emotions. Sometimes these emotions can pull us away from our desires to be successful.

Learning self-discipline helps us to understand our own individual system and to coordinate our emotions with our desires to succeed.

Self-discipline does not create conflicts between our pleasures and our successes. On contrary, it resolves these conflicts, harmonizes them, and guides in one direction—toward our goals.

Self-discipline is not about forcing yourself to do things or feeling like a victim. It's the other way around—to be in total control. When we apply self-discipline, we do it because we want to do it and not because somebody or something is forcing us.

While growing up, we were taught discipline by our parents, teachers, university professors, or other adults. At work we are directed by the rules and regulations and that disciplines us too. But there is a big difference between discipline and self-discipline. With self-discipline, you are not directed by anyone but yourself. When you are in control, you possess your thoughts, and you can reject instant gratification without regrets or intimidation; you can ignore excuses and procrastinations in order to achieve your goals.

Self-discipline helps to stick to our actions and keep promises. With self-discipline, we carry out our decisions for as long as it is necessary to accomplish what we want.

Self-discipline is not a punishment or a restriction. It is a type of self-control that allows us to do what's more important without feelings of discomfort. No one is born with self-discipline, but anyone can acquire this skill.

Unfortunately, self-discipline is not being taught in our schools or universities as a subject so we can completely understand it. Without self-discipline, we lose track of progress, and without progress, there is no success.

Patience

Once I was in an elevator going up to the top floor of a high-rise building, visiting my friend in his office. The elevator stopped on the third floor, and one lady got in. She pressed number 17. The elevator closed and started moving. She pressed that button again, then again, and again, and again. Before she reached the seventeenth floor, she pressed it quite few more times, and I was thinking to myself, "What impatience! How does that help to move the elevator faster?"

On the way back from my friend's office and driving from downtown, I got into a traffic jam. "I hate traffic!" I said to myself and started changing lanes trying to win some distance. That did not help much because I kept seeing the same red truck ahead of me. Then I decided to go around by taking the shortcut through the road that I knew from before. This was a relief for me—that road was almost empty. Fifteen minutes later I was merging back to the previous road thinking of how many cars I might have passed and how much time I have saved. Driving happily and being proud of my decision, I suddenly noticed that the same red truck that was in my view fifteen minutes ago was still ahead of me. "How did that help me to move faster?" I thought to myself.

Our first invented cars were moving with speed of 20 kilometers an hour, fax machines were transmitting each page for several minutes, and first computers were starting up to 10 minutes and longer. We were impatient then. Now cars drive with speed over 240 kilometers per hour, fax machines transmit a page in few seconds, and our computers start up almost immediately. Did we get any less impatient? Not really. All these inventions did not change anything, and we will probably be even more impatient in the future. We will find our ways to express our impatience. It's just a human nature.

How many times a day do we need our patience? Waiting for a bus, dealing with people, handling problems, etc. When we are impatient, we use our emotions. We get angry or frustrated. This, in the end, may affect not only us but also the people around us and our relationships. Many times we regret about our impatient actions.

Our precious time!

We work, study, do our duties, take care of our family, etc. All these responsibilities take most of our time, and there is not enough time left for pleasures. That's why we sometimes get frustrated and impatient. But does acting irrational help us to get to our goals faster? In many cases it does not. Those decisions often take us to more mistakes, unnecessary efforts, disappointments, and failures. By acting impatiently, we sometimes wipe out many of our achievements. Patience allows us to base our actions on values and facts instead of emotional bursts.

No matter how paradoxical it may sound, but slowing down sometimes makes everything move faster. If you look back to your past, you can probably remember many times when stopping at the right time brought you better and faster results.

Patience is power, and it allows us to be effective in everything we do. When we use it wisely, we achieve our goals faster, with less effort and frustration. Some people have higher level of patience and some lower but anybody can train and strengthen this quality. We all learn how to be patient from school, work, sports and other activities, and also from our relationships. We are just not always aware of how to apply patience in different situations of life and also don't always give patience enough significance and appreciation. Being impatient and trying to win some time, we often lose it instead, and our goals go behind the schedule. It takes courage to withstand the pressure of being impatient.

Patience is strength and not a weakness. All successful people are associated with having a great level of patience.

Patience helps us to act reasonably in many stressful situations. Many times we wish that somebody stopped us when we act irrational or make impractical decisions. When we are patient, we take logical approaches. Patience allows us to *stop so we can have some time to think, analyze, and make right decisions.*

The sun needs time to rise up, music needs time to reach our ears, and there is time needed for every beat of our heart. So be patient. If you are persistent, you will always get what you want, but . . . it will take some time.

CHAPTER 8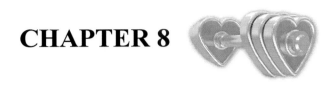

WILLPOWER TRAINING

Willpower, self-discipline, and patience are three most powerful tools in achieving goals. There are many talented and educated people who stay unsuccessful because they simply don't possess these important qualities, and there are also those who are less talented, but they have tremendous willpower, self-discipline, and a lot of patience. They usually get what they want. These people have great control over their habits. They know how to overcome laziness and also have the ability to reject instant gratification for a better cause.

Throughout my life I haven't had many problems prevailing over the circumstances and other people, but until a certain age, I've always had problems with dealing with myself. My inside logic often contradicted, and I wanted to find the key to myself so I can operate my own thoughts. Many projects that I started took me too long to finish, and some of them have failed. I knew that this happened because I didn't have the right tools in my mind. I wanted to be able to reach my goals quickly and with minimum effort.

I've known about willpower, self-discipline, and patience before, but until I started to use these three powers as one I could not find that golden key to my successes. I've realized that separately from each other or in random order—willpower, self-discipline, and patience may not bring you results that you want, and sometimes they can even confuse you. It is only together that they provide that super force, taking you to all your dreams.

People with willpower, self-discipline, and patience are doers and are willing to work toward their goals day after day for as long as it takes. They stay focused and alert until they accomplish their goal. Their effort is not based on their emotions. It is sustained and always maximal to their ability.

Being in control does not mean being restrictive to pleasures. There is tremendous reward and exhilarating pleasure following after achieving your goals. This type of pleasure is not just temporary or for a particular moment. It can last your lifetime and make your life feel worthwhile. It fulfills every minute of it with a sense and follows you anywhere you go.

Willpower, self-discipline, and patience complement each other when they work together. In order to make a decision and start working toward your goals, you need your willpower. To stick to the process, you need your self-discipline. And when that process gets boring or things don't work out as fast as you want, you need your patience.

Willpower tells us, *Act now*; self-discipline, *Stay and finish*; and patience, *Stop and think*.

Willpower, self-discipline, and patience are so tightly connected with each other that sometimes they can be viewed as one. In different people, these three disciplines can be developed differently. Some people can have a lot of willpower to initiate their actions but easily get distracted by other things and don't have enough self-discipline to stick to repetitive things. Some people have willpower and self-discipline but don't have enough patience to continue doing these repetitive things for a long time.

I could never say that I ever had a lot of patience. But the self-discipline that I possessed from the army and my willpower always help me to stay on top of things that I need to do. Every time I get impatient, I use my willpower and self-discipline to get my patience back.

Some people who have a lot of patience may be lacking the willpower or self-discipline. Just waiting for things is not enough, and our ability to initiate our actions is our initial success.

What willpower, self-discipline, and patience can do for you

- Help you to succeed in whatever you do
- Help you to make decisions and speak up your mind
- Enjoy more pleasures in life
- Break bad habits
- Look and feel better
- Make more money
- Be respected and loved
- Live longer and happier life

Willpower, self-discipline, and patience need to be understood before practicing them in real life. If we don't understand how they work, we will not be able to benefit from them. Here are some principles that we need to understand:

1. Mind-set
2. Inner resistance
3. Attention and concentration
4. Self-talk
5. Exercises

1. Mind-set

Before you go ahead and start doing things toward your goals, you need to prepare your mind and make some firm decisions. Without these decisions, you will always feel uncertain, lost, and insecure.

Figure out what is it exactly you want. Don't move any further until you know that for sure. Otherwise you will end up wasting time on the things that you shouldn't be doing.

Don't try to wonder how you are going to accomplish it. At this point, it is not important. Life will show it to you.

Decide that acquiring the inner strengths is important to you, and you will use your willpower, self-discipline, and patience to prevail over your weaknesses. Forget about your previous mistakes and failures and remember only accomplishments and successes. Decide that from now on everything will be different—you will be able to make your own decisions and act upon them. Feel firm on that; this is very important.

Think of how many advantages these changes will bring into your life and how much more power you will attain. Be willing to do all necessary steps and perform essential exercises. Stay firm on these decisions. Expect that things may not go as perfect as you picture them. Be willing to learn from mistakes and keep moving forward toward your goal regardless of how many of those mistakes it may be.

Put an end on only dreaming about what you want. Decide that from now on you will be in charge of all your dreams.

2. Inner resistance

During our life we acquire some habits. Later many of these habits control us and structure our everyday routines. When we want to change our life, habits often interfere and don't allow us to make that change.

Once we acquire a strong habit, our subconscious mind will always try to resist any change. This is called the *inner resistance*. Expect that resistance. When you have to perform the exercises to train your willpower, your mind may find these exercises ridiculous, uncomfortable, unpleasant, or simply not necessary to perform. Subconscious mind is not your enemy but also not your boss. Start believing that and also believe that you can overcome that inner resistance. From now on, you will be telling your subconscious mind what to do.

But let's think about it first.

Straighten both of your arms in front of you. Turn the palms of both hands down and place one hand on top of another. Give your hands names: the one on the *top* will be your *"pressure"* and one on **bottom**, your *"inner resistance."* Press with your both hands against each other with equal pressure. Your hands are not moving, right? You feel that great tension, but your hands are still in one place. Keep pressing, and you will notice how this position starts exhausting you up and you want to quit. This is what happens when you force yourself on doing things in life while your inner resistance is still high—you quit.

Keep pressing hard with your "pressure" (top) hand but reduce the pressure in your "resistance" (bottom) hand. You will not only notice how both hands are moving down but also how with the amount of resistance reduced in your bottom hand, the amount of pressure in your top hand reduced too. You don't have to press as hard with your top hand if the pressure in your bottom hand is reduced. This is exactly what happens when you reduce your inner resistance: you don't need to push yourself anymore, and achieving your goals becomes easier and gives you more pleasure.

Let's say you need to study a very difficult subject. But you don't like that subject, and one part of you is pushing you to do it, while the other part is resisting to it. If you keep studying this way, you won't learn much no matter how hard you try. Eventually you will give up or fall asleep being exhausted from both—your pressure and your resistance. But if you just reverse your thinking and pretend to like this subject, you will immediately reduce your inner resistance. Your pressure will be reduced too because you simply wouldn't need to push yourself, and your speed of studying will increase dramatically.

Willpower is not the ability to push yourself hard, but the ability to reduce your inner resistance. The higher resistance you feel, the less willpower you possess.

Powerful people are not the ones who know how to push themselves to their limits but those who know how to control their inner resistance, because no matter how great is your push, it will still be your half effort if your inner resistance is just as great.

To help yourself deal with your subconscious mind, create a statement—something that you will tell yourself to overpower your mind. Every time you feel weak or overwhelmed by your habits, read that statement. Your subconscious mind will learn your new commands and will eventually obey your new habits. Feel strong and believe your statement.

Sample statement:

From now on, I am in charge of my life, my habits and my thoughts. My subconscious mind has no longer control over me. I may fail and make mistakes as any human. But this will not stop me from getting what I want. I will pursue my goals regardless of my inner resistance and will eventually prevail.

3.   *Attention and concentration*

Have you noticed how fast time goes by when you are having fun and how boring and how long the minutes feel when you are doing something not interesting? Why is that? Because when we are involved in something interesting, our attention and concentration are grabbed by those things, and we focus on them. This does not happen when we do things that we don't like because we can't put our attention and concentration together with it. It feels like our attention goes someplace else. You may notice how your mind takes you away from doing things that you don't like. You may do one thing but think of completely another.

But what if things that look boring or not interesting can help us to achieve our goals, and we are, being ignorant to those things, simply not aware of those benefits?

I remember the time when I brought my first computer home. That computer was mainly for the use of my kids, and I myself had no interest in learning it. "Boring," I thought to myself every time my kids were trying to show me something on it.

But one day I decided to try it. My kids went outside and left the computer running with Microsoft Word on it. I started to type. My English wasn't that great at that time, and I knew that I was making a lot of mistakes. After I finished typing few sentences without looking at the screen, I looked up and noticed that there were no mistakes in my typing. "Cool!" I said to myself. "The computer corrected all my mistakes!" I was so thrilled about this because I had a pile of business letters that I needed to send, but they were handwritten and possibly with a lot of mistakes.

When my kids returned home, they stopped right next to me and stared at me for a while. "Dad, are you OK? What are you doing on the computer?" I shared with them what I've discovered, and since then, the computer became my friend. It often helps me to stay organized and be more productive.

When we are willing to open up our mind and get out of the box, pay attention to things that we don't know and then try them. Very often we find those things useful and interesting for us. Willpower, self-discipline, and patience help us in many ways to keep our concentration on a higher level and also give us the ability to pay attention to the things that at our first glance may look useless or boring.

4.   Self-talk

Our family always had pets in our house when I was a child, and I was the one to take care and train them. At the beginning, pets always resist you, but slowly they learn to obey, and one day, you don't have to say twice to get what you want them to do.

Remembering that makes me realize that our subconscious mind is just like those pets. When we develop our habits, we train our subconscious mind to obey and do things for us.

Once you've trained your pets to do certain things, it becomes very hard to retrain them back to stop doing those things. Same thing happens with our subconscious mind—it often resists our conscious thinking. When we want to give up some bad habits, our subconscious mind does not see those habits as bad and keeps doing what "was told".

But if we are persistent, through our *self-talk* we can retrain our subconscious mind to learn new habits. Habits can be relearned, and any of our behavior or attitude can be changed.

How do you use your self-talk?

Repetition is the key to success. The more you repeat your message, the harder your subconscious mind will work toward your desires.

The subconscious mind is a quick learner and will listen to you immediately as long as you apply the three rules that was described in chapter 3 "Mind Works"—*your commands must be in present tense, positive, and specific.* You will immediately notice how your subconscious mind will respond to you by helping you to get into your new action.

Use power words: "I choose to" or "I am." This indicates that you are in control. Using "I must," "I should," or "I have to" show that you are weak and you are under that control. When we have choices, we remain in power. "I must," "I should," or "I have to" words limit you, and they mean that you don't have that choice.

Minimize the use of "maybe" or "I am not sure" or "I'll see" or "What if?" They represent weakness and uncertainty.

Eliminate "not," "don't," or "won't." When we express what we want in a negative form, we often contradict ourselves and create conflicts. "I don't want to be overweight" will never work for you if you are already overweight, because with this type of self-talk, you are going against what you are at the moment. Use "I want to look great" instead. This way you are setting up your goal and saying what you want. With "I don't want to be overweight," your subconscious would not be able to take a direction where to go.

Your self-talk is your *inner reality*. Inside of your mind, you can create whatever you want. If you practice, your inner reality will eventually become your *outer reality*—you will become what you want. You will be amazed at what happens when you repeatedly, forcefully, and positively tell your subconscious mind what you want to be, do, or have.

5. *Exercises*

To get any skill requires performing some exercises, whether it is learning how read, write, doing something at work or at school. Just by looking at things we will never learn how to do them. We need to practice to develop those skills.

Exercises described further are to train your willpower, self-discipline, and patience. If you think you are lacking those skills but limit yourself by only reading about those exercises, you will end up changing nothing. Theory without practice is dead. A weight lifter needs to lift weights, a shooter needs to shoot, and a writer needs to write. Every new skill requires time, effort, and dedication. Only with performing exercises, specifically developing the willpower, can we actually understand what the willpower is. Same goes for self-discipline and patience.

The exercises are placed in progressive order and integrated with everyday life. With most of them you don't need to dedicate a specific time for it. If you practice continuously, they will slowly start putting you in charge of your behaviors and your life. At the beginning, when you try to do them, your subconscious mind will be forcing you to skip some of the exercises, delay them for later, or avoid at all. Some days you may feel lazy; some days you may forget to do those exercises. You may also find some of them too awkward or uncomfortable. You know what's happening—your subconscious mind is trying to control you and doesn't want the change.

Always remember the benefits of this training and the end results. Use your willpower to overcome the inner resistance. Soon enough you will gain more confidence. You will acquire new habits that you will be proud of, and you will believe in yourself more. Eventually your subconscious mind will become your friend and will help you in achieving your goals instead of being against.

Test yourself with these exercises before you start investing money and time into your big goals. See if you are ready. You may not need some of these exercises directly in your life, but by performing them, you will have a chance to experience exactly what you will be going through when trying to achieve your real-life goals. If you succeed in most of these exercises, you will learn the patterns how to get successful, and you will feel the power of becoming in charge of your life.

Take one day at a time. Do not devour all the exercises at once, and do not skip them. Follow the instructions! Do the exercises in order. If there is an exercise that you don't like, this is the one you need to perform the most. How else will you learn how to overpower your subconscious mind? If you do only exercises that you like, you will never be able to acquire the inner strength. Each exercise has its own purpose.

Keep in mind that the intention of each exercise is not to teach you the actual things that you are going to perform, but only *to be able to put yourself into action to overpower your subconscious mind.*

Remember that even though each exercise may be purposely selected to be against one of your habits, it is not selected to be against you; neither is it selected to be forcing you to perform. *Your positive attitude toward these exercises is far more important than your ability to obligate yourself to perform them.*

Exercise 1. Drinking with your other hand

Hold your cup or a bottle in your other hand when you drink. Pretend as if this was your normal way of drinking. Your subconscious mind may find this exercise uncomfortable, unnecessary, or having nothing to do with your real-life goals. Remain in control and try perceiving this exercise as fun.

For some of you, this exercise may look too easy, but the idea is not to perform it only once. Most important is to remember to hold your cup or a bottle in your other hand every time you drink and practice this exercise for at least one week. If you forget even once, your week starts from beginning. Move to the second exercise only when you are completely comfortable with this one. If you are still getting nervous about it or having negative feelings every time you do it, your subconscious mind is still controlling you, and you need more time.

Exercise 2. Holding spoon in your other hand

Hold your spoon or fork in your other hand every time you eat. If you are using knife too, your hands have to be switched.

This exercise is very similar to the first one but more challenging. The idea is the same, practice it for at least one week.

Exercise 3. Drinking coffee or tea without sugar

When having your coffee or tea, do not add any sugar. If you are one of those who do it anyway, move to the next exercise.

Practice this exercise until the presence of sugar in your coffee or tea makes no difference to you, and you are enjoying your drink as it is.

Exercise 4. Reading boring material

Grab a book, a magazine, or start reading a newspaper article about the subject that you are not interested in at all. Read it slowly and try to understand. Your mind will try to take your attention away and refocus you on doing something else. You may even start falling asleep. You know what's happening? This is your *inner resistance* kicking in. Stay focused and keep reading. Try to understand why some people like this subject. If you perceive your reading positively, your mind will eventually obey you, and you will get occupied.

This exercise helps you to keep your mind open for new things that at first glance may look boring, but later may become useful tools in achieving your goals.

Throughout our life, our subconscious mind gets "customized" for us to do only things that are comfortable and make sense for us at the moment, and we, often being judgmental or simply ignorant, find some other things being ridiculous, stupid, or useless. But whatever feels ridiculous, awkward, or uncomfortable may be eventually very helpful in achieving our goals. If our subconscious mind continues controlling us, we will always be living within the box or within invisible bubbles around us, and we will never have a chance to experience anything new.

Practice this exercise every day. Your reading doesn't have to be long. You will be amazed how many interesting things you may find. But always remember that whatever you choose to read has to be something that looks not interesting for you at first.

Exercise 5. Counting backward

Count from 1 to 10 as fast as you can. Now count backward from 10 to 1. Is it slower? If it is, practice until you get into the same speed. Advance this exercise by counting to 20, then to 30, and further up to 100.

Once you do well with counting numbers backward, try reading the alphabet forward and backward with the same speed.

Some people find this exercise very challenging and experience a great inner resistance to perform it. "Ah, who needs it?" "This is so boring?" "What has this got to do with anything?" "If I want, I can do it, but I don't have the time for this stuff!" If your subconscious mind "delivers" any of these messages to you, you need this exercise. Practice it until you feel absolutely no discomfort thinking about and can start performing it at any time.

Exercise 6. Listening to music that you don't like

Turn on the music that you don't like and notice how your subconscious mind may immediately try to resist you to listening to it. But this is only your first and immediate reaction. If you try to stay positive about it, you may notice how you are getting less and less irritated.

The purpose of this exercise is not to make you like this music, but only not to get irritated by it, and the music is just as an example. In life we are surrounded by many things that irritate us, and they irritate us because we allow them to.

Practice this exercise until you feel completely comfortable with listening to any kind of music and it has no affect on your feelings or performance at that moment. You will eventually notice how you will build tolerance not only to any music, but also to different things, the circumstances around you, and other people.

Exercise 7. Writing in the dark

Close yourself in your bathroom and turn off the light. Take lined paper and a pen and start writing sentences, trying to fit it in the paper lines. Turn on the light after completing a few sentences and review your writing. Rewrite same sentences with a presence of light and then try in the dark again. Practice until you make no mistakes, and your handwriting in the dark is very similar to your normal.

Exercise 8. Waking up fifteen minutes early

You may think that with giving up of fifteen minutes of your sleep, you will lose a lot of pleasures, but you will gain many of them too. This will be your time for a better breakfast or a relaxing cup of coffee, walk around the block, or simply better preparation for work or school.

This exercise trains your willpower and self-discipline. When you wake up, do not use this time to cuddle up in your bed.

Exercise 9. Organizing your documents

I used to hate organizing documents, just like probably many people, and every time I would start doing it, I would always end up doing something else, and my documents were always in halfway organizing position and never really had their own place. When time came to find something, I spent enormous amount of effort to look for things. I knew that I had to get organized, but I always felt like organizing was a waste of time. "Who cares, I will find it when I need it, but now I have to do something more important."

Staying organized helps us to save time when we are trying to achieve our goals. When everything is at your hands, you don't need to spend time looking for it. Everything goes smooth, and time spent feels enjoyable.

This exercise requires a lot of patience, self-discipline, and also willpower. But as soon as you complete it, you feel your own power. Perform it at least once a month and try to maintain your documents every day. You will enjoy the products of your efforts.

Exercise 10. Watching TV while doing something important

Turn on your favorite show or TV program and turn off the sound. Find something important to do while being beside your TV—going over your bills, bank statements, organizing receipts—something that requires a lot of concentration. Do not look at the TV and try to keep your attention on important things. Your mind will try to refocus you on the TV, but do not let it interrupt your work or decrease your productivity.

This exercise requires a lot of self-discipline and patience, but when you succeed, it will immediately put you in charge of many of your habits.

Once you get better with this exercise, you can take it to another level: set the alarm clock for 15-20 minutes after you start watching your favorite show, and stop watching it immediately after the alarm goes off. Plan on doing something important at that time, and switch to that activity promptly without delay.

Exercise 11. Standing still

Take your most comfortable standing pose. Reconfirm with yourself again and again that this *is* your most comfortable way to stand. Now freeze your body in that position and imagine yourself being a statue. Do not move any of your body parts, breathe shallow, and try not to blink your eyes. Do not feel threatened by looking ridiculous or silly.

In few minutes you will feel that standing in this position is no longer comfortable. You may start feeling body itches. Do not pay attention;

these are just tiny muscle contractions. If you ignore them, you will notice how they will slowly go away.

This exercise develops great level of patience and willpower.

Exercise 12. Being stuck in traffic

A very common situation that almost everyone experiences is being stuck in a traffic jam. Don't we all hate when a highway freezes and we are getting late for work, school, or some occasion?

Do these frustrations help? They only destroy our mood, attitude, and sometimes health.

Don't get me wrong. We are all allowed to get emotional when things don't go our way. But some emotions can get easily overboard and start physically killing us. Traffic jams are not going to get any better in the future. If we don't want to turn ourselves into nervous wreck machines, we need to learn how to handle these situations.

Three powerful tools—willpower, self-discipline, patience and a little bit of imagination can turn your exhausting experience into a fun game:

- Look at the cars around and view them as something a little bit different than they are—for example as your personal escort. Relax behind your steering wheel and feel protected. Smile. Turn on your favorite radio station and enjoy the ride.

  Or

- Read the license plates on cars in front of you and try getting some ideas how to make sentences out of the letters or create arithmetic combinations out of numbers that would make sense to you.

Of course this exercise will not help you to get any faster where you are going, but it definitely will help you arrive alive, a bit healthier, and in much better mood.

Exercise 13. Holding your sneeze or yawn

Have you noticed how sometimes you start yawning because someone else does it? It can even happen when you watch it on TV or hear it on the radio. This simple reflex is not unusual and happens to everyone. It can even get initialized just by thinking about it.

Notice also when you are trying to sneeze and someone interrupts you, you may lose it. What happens? Your mind gets occupied with something else and refocuses.

Try controlling your sneeze or yawn. This exercise will teach you how to play with your thoughts and control them. Dramatize a little and use your imagination. For example, when you want to sneeze, imagine that you are hiding from someone and don't want to get noticed, or when you want to yawn, imagine that you are on TV and hosting a popular show.

Exercise 14. Eating lemon

Cut a lemon in slices and try chewing them slowly without any sweeteners. Look at yourself in the mirror while doing that and make sure that the expression on your face demonstrates pleasure. Once you master eating slices, try eating a whole lemon, biting it like an apple. But remember, the expression on your face must demonstrate pleasure.

Exercise 15. Dealing with fears

Close yourself in your bathroom or closet. Turn off the light. Imagine something that always scares you in the dark—spiders, mice, snakes, etc. Imagine that with every second those scary things are getting closer and closer at you. Turn on the light when you reach your limit.

Now turn off the light again, but this time reverse the situation. Imagine that the darkness saves you from things that you are scared of, and with every second, those things are going farther and farther away from you, and if you turn the light on, they will turn back on you. Suddenly darkness becomes your friend.

This exercise helps to realize that most of our fears are imaginary, and the same situation can be viewed totally different. The power of our mind is so great that most of our fears can be eliminated or turned into something positive instead of blocking us from pursuing our goals.

Exercise 16. Organizing your kitchen

The purpose of this exercise is not to make your kitchen look tidy or clean. Through this work, you will learn how to organize your thoughts, pay attention, and be detailed—all major components in achieving any life goal.

- Open all your all kitchen cabinets and take everything out. Place everything in one place.
- Look at everything you took out and think carefully how you can put it back in the way that makes most sense. Do not rush with this task. Use a piece of paper to write down your ideas.
- Clean all the cabinets and start putting everything back based on your plan. You will find out how well you've organized your kitchen when you start using things.

Exercise 17. Going to an all-you-can-eat buffet

Go to your favorite all-you-can-eat buffet, but when selecting foods, make only the healthiest choices, and your plate should not contain more than 500 calories. Sit down, eat slowly, and enjoy every bite. After you finish your meal and before you pay, walk around food stations again to test your willpower. Go to the cashier, pay your bill, and don't feel that you did not get your monies worth. Feel proud instead.

Exercise 18. Eating half and half

Put on the plate your most favorite meal, for example, ice cream. Make sure that your portion size is the same as usual.

Cut your portion in half and leave both parts on your plate. Move the second part to the side of your plate and start eating the first one. Eat slowly, and after you finish it, put the second part back in your fridge or throw it away. Your subconscious mind will try to resist you, forcing you to eat the second half, but stay in control. Remember your statement. Train yourself with this exercise until you feel completely comfortable (without pressuring yourself) eating as little as a quarter of your regular portion.

Exercise 19. Keeping it clean

Choose one room in your household where the most traffic is, for example, kitchen, or family car, and promise yourself to keep it amazingly clean for one month. Regardless how busy or tired you are, keep an eye on that room or car throughout the day, and make sure that it always stays in the same clean condition. Do not tell anyone in your family about your intentions because your main motivation is not to show off or do it for any kind of reward or appreciation but to train your willpower.

Exercise 20. Resisting the influence

Think of someone whom you are in a strained relationship with and search for contact with him/her. This person *should be* someone who always intimidates you when thinking about him/her.

Call, or better yet, meet with that person. It shouldn't matter to you how he/she will react to your call or the meeting. What is more important is to how you will react.

Control your emotions and use detachment to stay calm on that meeting. Use your self-talk, and remember that what is happening to you is mostly your imagination creating your fears. Your subconscious mind possesses those fears. You can reverse your thinking to eliminate your fears by bringing your subconscious feelings into your conscious, and then analyzing them. You might not succeed from the first time, but if you practice, through this exercises you will learn a very valuable skill. This skill will help not to be affected by anyone or anything when pursuing your life goals. If there is no real physical threat to see that person, dismiss your fears. No matter what that person says or does, you cannot allow this affect you. Don't bring any negativity with you by thinking of the past. Stay in the present.

You don't have to make any conclusions of this meeting. The purpose of it is not to fix your relationship or to break it more, but only to test your willpower.

CHAPTER 9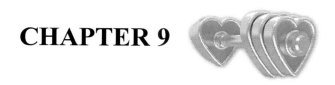

DEALING WITH EMOTIONS

Not only **do** we need our willpower to push us forward, but also we need it to hold us back from our emotion overflows and overreactions. Many times when we overreact, we lose what we gain. There are also times when our emotions produce fear, and this, as a result, does not allow us to get what we want. Our ability to control our emotions helps us to minimize mistakes, make the processes of achieving our goals less painful and more consistent.

All our emotions are very tightly connected with all our goals. We may know exactly how to achieve our goals, but if we don't know how to control our emotions, all this knowledge about our goals can become useless—being frustrated or angry, we will give up for no valid reason.

Ego

Among all the emotions that people go through when interacting between each other, ego is the most difficult to overcome. Many people as soon as they identify their status related to learning, work, money, fame, or public acceptance, completely forget their real identity as human beings. If this identity stops dictating their actions, it is very easy to become materialistic and lose sense of spirituality. As the material power boosts people's ego, they become nonsensitive to each other and subconsciously give in to the power of materialism. The materialism itself then dictates its rules further, making people greedy and forcing them to look for more ways to expand their "territory." Greed and ego develop resentment and hatred and make people view each other in a rather competitive perspective than in an equal one.

How can we guard ourselves from surrendering to ego and greed so we can still remain spiritual and human?

Let's first define what *ego* is.

Ego is essentially a feeling of being separate from the rest of the universe. Ego always claims special abilities and takes credit for accomplishments. It also always blames others for everything that goes wrong. Ego can be just as sensitive as the feeling of being injured.

As ego separates from the rest of the world, it also limits us in our abilities to open our minds and chase our dreams freely without being afraid of getting judged or manipulated.

Below are some strategies that can help avoid getting trapped by ego:

a. Avoid regret and pride

Do not feel sorry for anything you discover about yourself. Feeling sorry for a deficiency also reinforces feeling proud of your good qualities. While there is nothing wrong with feeling proud of your good qualities, be careful how you perceive it. If you give too much value to these qualities, you can easily get hunted by your ego. Be grateful for what you have and what life gives you and always aspire to be better.

b. Take others' point of view

If there are people who are always right and others who are always wrong, we probably wouldn't have laws, lawyers, or courts. Every point of view has a truth in it. Recognize that and try to understand the opposite point of view. Learn how to see the truth from the other side and appreciate it. Truth is never about being right or wrong. Truth is about the reconciling of opposing views. It is not even about a compromise, but more like seeing viewpoints of both sides. When you take a genuine effort to recognize *somebody else's truth*, you come out of ego and stop defending yourself just for the cause of the feeling of being in control. In most cases, the other person immediately becomes much more open-minded and reasonable to you too.

Sometimes when we think of how other people perceive us, we don't realize that the way we see it is only our own way. Many times we are being wrong in those prejudgments and later realize that people did not really think about us that way. You have to always remember that what you think about how people think of you and how they perceive you is only your opinion. You may realize later that what you were thinking was totally wrong. If you fall into such series of prejudgments, your mind may create strong feelings toward those people including jealousy, resentment, or hatred. To get out of these feelings later can become very difficult because they will become your new habits and settle in your mind subconsciously.

c. Practice silent will

According to *The Secret*, when we formulate a clear and powerful intention, the universe will respond and create the conditions for us to fulfill it.

Silent will is based on a similar principle. It is a method to overcome the generated opposition when we do not say our ideas or intentions to others, but only formulate a clear thought or will, without expressing it. Later we find how other people respond to our intentions in ways we want.

Silent will works because thoughts are universal. When we refrain from expressing our thoughts in words, the vibrations of our thoughts reach other people. Often they receive it as their own thoughts.

All of us have a tendency to give more value and credibility to our own thoughts than thoughts of others. In many situations we think that we know exactly what should be done, but when we express our ideas to other people, they may immediately disagree with us. This negative response is natural to the human mind, and especially the ego, which feels the urge to dominate over others and does not enjoy submitting to the views of other people.

Ego always seeks to dominate or control others.

d. Recognize the truth of inner-outer correspondences

Our attitude affects our well-being, and everything else is shaped around us based on that attitude. This phenomenon also was very widely explored in *The Secret* and now has a scientific proof based on quantum physics: two particles of a substance can affect each other even if they are placed on opposite sides of the globe, or even the universe. If an electron of a single atom shifts, the other electron of the same atom shifts too even if they are thousand miles away from each other.

People who consciously create positive intentions from within themselves attract positive circumstances immediately from anywhere in the world. Negative intentions and emotions attract negative circumstances and conditions.

We sometimes attempt to be having positive emotions on the *outside* while being deeply negative *inside*. These attempts to better the circumstances are nothing but putting patches on infected wounds. Only when we make a positive *inner change* can we affect the positive conditions and attract similar circumstances. Then our life starts bringing us everything what we deserve—trustful relationships, real friends, financial security, and emotional comfort.

In order to become a better person, we need to make some progress, believe, and truly recognize the affect of *inner-outer correspondences*.

Ego separates us from the universe and the people. Our achievements and successes wouldn't mean anything if we are not sincerely happy with ourselves and fulfilled with joy and true celebration of being a real human. Life then becomes a wonderful mirror for self-knowledge and a powerful support for our spiritual progress.

Once we accept the spiritual truth, we stop condemning other people, and instead of reacting to their behavior, we try to become more conscious of the corresponding aspects of our own personality. Very often, things that bother us in other people are characteristics that we possess ourselves but are trying to hide from them by blaming it on other people.

Hatred

Hatred by the definition is a feeling of intense hostility toward somebody or something. Hatred, just like ego, can also create a feeling of being restricted. Some people may feel very insecure in front of those who they hate, and some can feel very intimidated by certain circumstances. As such, hatred is not a power but a limitation of freedom and emotional weakness. If we allow ourselves to get influenced by it, hatred can interfere with all our dreams and become an obstacle when we pursue those dreams. All our efforts can be easily zeroed down when we meet with certain people or when it appears in some circumstances.

When someone hates someone or a group or people, he/she usually does the following:

- Tries to ignore and avoid those people
- Gets easily aggravated by their behavior, looks, or attitudes
- Gets agitated when thinking about them
- Has an antagonistic attitude
- Finds being cruel, vicious, vindictive, or revengeful toward them
- Becomes rude, aggressive, and intolerant

All these feelings can intoxicate one and completely take his/her attention away from pursuing goals. Willpower, self-discipline, and patience help us to focus our attention on those goals. When we understand our subconscious mind, we also understand why we are getting so irritated and agitated by other people, and when we stop being *reactive* and will not allow anyone or anything control our behavior, only then will we be able to be in charge of our life.

Resentment

Resentment is an emotionally devastating condition. When unresolved, it can have a variety of negative results on the person experiencing it, including bad temper, nervousness, impatience, and anxiety when thinking of the person whom they are resenting. If the person being resented gets positively recognized by somebody else or a group of people, the one who resents may experience anger or even hatred. In the long run, resentment can develop a hostile, cynical, sarcastic attitude that can become a barrier against not only other healthy relationships but also personal goals.

Resentment builds up lack of personal and emotional growth, difficulty in self-recognition, trouble trusting people, loss of self-confidence, and a feeling that "everyone owes you."

Resentment is most powerful when it's toward someone in a close or intimate relationship. Resentful feelings can cut off the communication between those people, and further miscommunications may develop even more resentment, making fixing those relationships very difficult.

Because of the consequences they carry, resentful feelings are dangerous to those who resent. They can cause not only emotional but also physical and neurological problems and even diseases.

But despite of complex feelings that resentment develops, it can still be gradually overcome through a detailed self mental examination and forgiveness. Resentment, in a way, is similar to our fears and also like our fears controlled by our subconscious mind. As such it can be dealt in a similar way.

First, one needs to identify the source of such feelings.

Second, analyze the significance of the cause of the resentment. Then do a detailed examination of everything that caused that resentment and try to see the other point of view.

Third, realize the benefits of letting go for the present and for the future.

And fourth, be able to forgive and forget.

"Forgiveness liberates the soul"—Nelson Mandela

CHAPTER 10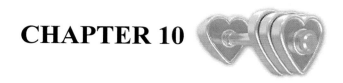

DETACHMENT

Our personality and environment where we grow up create our attachments to act and live in a certain way. We develop some strong habits and carry them out through our life. We are not always proud of them, but emotional attachments keep us linked and often do not allow us to change the direction of our lives.

Smoking, drinking, using drugs, overeating are all attachments. Everyone understands the downside of it, but the temporary emotional and physical comfort that these things provide does not let many people quit. After every next cigarette or late eating at night, one may feel terribly guilty, but this does not help when the next urge rises. As this keeps happening over and over again, the bad habit gets stronger and stronger.

Some of the bad habits can be also our overreactions upon somebody's behavior or certain actions. We may later regret how we use our emotions, but just like with any other bad habit, these regrets don't help when we appear in a similar situation next time.

The ability to stay calm when these emotional urges arise is called detachment. Ability to stay detached helps us to be independent from influences of the circumstances and other people.

If we think about it, we can clearly understand that our habits and other influences are not part of us, and at some point in life, we lived without them. We can change this again if we really want to. These attachments are our emotional weaknesses, and if we continue living ruled by them, we may eventually lose our own identity.

Other people, possessions, circumstances, and bad habits often bother us and prevent from achieving our own goals, make our own choices in life, and live the way we really want. Detachment helps us to prevent appearing in many of those unpleasant situations.

Being detached does not mean being indifferent, cold, and with a lack of energy. While respecting opinions of others and varieties of other choices, we can still choose our own and live the way we want.

Commercials that we watch on TV, fliers we receive in the mail, many websites that we browse through the Internet, or advertisements that we hear on the radio, all have a purpose to sell us something. People who are selling those things have to make their products look attractive regardless of the nature of it. Even cigarettes must look nice to make us buy them—a beautiful girl or a handsome cowboy on the background dressed up nice and well groomed—are usually the upbringing selling features of the cigarettes. Who cares if millions of smokers die from cancer? They have to sell and make their product look attractive. When we watch or hear those commercials very often, we emotionally fall for them without thinking of the consequences: "Ah, enjoy life to the fullest!" And then slowly but surely we get more and more emotionally attached to the bad habits. The subconscious mind, controlled by these emotions, receives these messages and accepts them as good. Later it becomes very hard to re-convince your subconscious mind that what was considered to be good before is bad now.

People are people, and we all fall for what looks good, sounds or feels great, even if it's bad for us. How many times do we buy something we don't even need? We hear nice music on the background in the shopping mall, watch other people shopping, and start buying ourselves. This is how we get influenced. The same happens when we get hungry. Many times we eat emotionally without even being hungry. Our fears, worries, and insecurities reinforce these types of actions.

We have to know how to protect ourselves from influences that are not good for us, and detachment here comes in handy.

Here are some suggestions on how you can facilitate the display of detachment:

- Refuse to let your fears and worries occupy your mind. When you lose them, you will also lose the attachments to bad habits, circumstances, and other people.
- Never give value to the things that prevent you from reaching your goals regardless of how attractive they may look or be advertised.
- Delay your reactions that are aroused by your emotions. Take a few seconds' pause before reacting, and try to calm yourself down. Taking few deep breaths during that pause may be sufficient enough to facilitate the detachment.
- Always remind yourself about staying calm in situations when you need to stay detached. This will help you to be prepared.

When you argue with someone, notice how sometimes you can get easily irritated by somebody else's words, body language, or actions. You may react doing the same without even realizing that your reaction is nothing but mirroring that person's emotions.

Whatever we focus our attention on usually grows in our mind. The more we think about it, the bigger it gets. But we, as humans, through our self-awareness have the ability to keep our emotions under control and, as such, choose our ways to react in different situations of life. We can either let our emotions grow bigger and control us, or we can take that control in our own hands.

Willpower, self-discipline, and patience allow us to have that control. When we are not blinded by our emotions and are able to recognize the consequences of reacting one or another way, we will be able to get the most benefits out of every situation in life.

The elevator broke, your car doesn't start, reckless driver, friend who betrayed you—these are only few things that can trigger our emotions, get us angry and out of control. But when we lose that control, we may completely lose track of pursuing our life goals. Then we slow down or sometimes even give up.

CHAPTER 11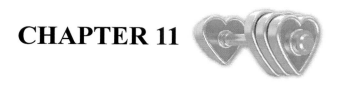

FINISH WHAT YOU STARTED

The ability to go on until the end regardless of the inner resistance makes winners stand out. Imagine a marathon runner who doesn't finish his race. What would our life be if we all just gave up whenever we felt like it or when things get hard?

"Life gets in the way!" say those who quit gyms. "Lack of time, family problems, motivation is lost"—all sorts of reasons. But look at this! By the statistics, those who don't quit are actually much busier in life than those who give up. It appears that the reasons for giving up are not life problems or people's busyness.

Anyone can train himself to last until the end. This is not something that only special people have. This ability can be developed at any age and any moment in life. There are thousands of stories and movies about those who became winners from being losers.

If we see the results of our work, we get motivated; if we don't, we give up. But to see results, we need to put our initial efforts, and then only if that effort is sustained do we see results. Then the more results we see, the more motivated we get to continue.

In order to motivate us, results don't always have to be big. The biggest achievements consist of many small ones within. As long as there is progress, we usually stay motivated.

When my kids were little, I was very concerned about them spending a lot of time playing computer games. I wanted them to learn the real life and how to achieve their goals outside of their computers too. But what I did not realize then was that besides all my lessons, my kids were already learning how to go until the end through their computer games. I tried some of those games myself and can tell you that to finish even the easiest one is a difficult task. You need a lot of patience, self-discipline, and even willpower. The only problem with computer games is that they are addictive, and many people get attached to them, completely losing track of their other life goals.

The more we practice, the better we get at it—a simple formula of life. You don't need to run a marathon or do something significant to learn how to last until the end. Do something small first—something that doesn't require much time and effort, and then gradually something bigger and bigger. But always finish what you start. Once you learn how to finish something, you will be able to finish anything. Progress to harder tasks only when you feel ready. Don't look at someone else's progress—you might get discouraged.

CHAPTER 12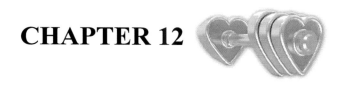

SEEING THE OTHER SIDE OF A COIN

Almost every situation in life can be viewed as negative or as positive, and not the situation itself usually is bad or good but our perception of it.

I don't like flying. Being on the plane makes me so nervous that in order to calm myself down, I have to put my brain into 100 percent working capacity. I understand that flying is still the safest way of transportation, but when I am in the air, something inside of me tells me the opposite. I look around the seats and wonder how some people can feel so relaxed when I am so nervous—they are reading books, watching TV, or just sleeping. At that moment I wish that somebody would knock me out until the end of flight and wake me up when it's over.

Some situations can be bad, but it only gets worse if we perceive it as bad in our minds. In most cases there is another way of seeing it. We always have a choice to improve our vision of every situation in life. What we create in our minds does not always reflect the reality, and we, as humans, have the ability to control how to accept our surroundings and see "the other side of a coin" so we can stay more

MIND

productive and be spiritually up because the way we think always influences the way we act. Situations are never one way or the other; they are always the way we choose to perceive it.

When we think constructively and positively, the puzzle of life comes together. We achieve our goals and see the results of our efforts. But if we go down and always see the bad instead of the good, our life breaks down because the way we think reflects what we do.

Often we are unreasonably harsh with ourselves or instinctively jump to wrong conclusions. This can send us into a downward spiral of negative thinking.

If we think negative, we always lack something and feel insecure. Even our successes don't keep us happy for too long. We always live in the future and view our life getting better only in the future, and we are never satisfied with what we have. If we don't learn how to enjoy today, our future is always going to be somewhere out there, in the future, and will never appear as today.

Negative thoughts move first into our consciousness, do their damage, and go further into our subconscious where our attitudes are being created. If we don't bring our negative thoughts back into our consciousness and start analyzing them in order to change our attitudes, these attitudes start dictating our life, which later can be very hard to break. Being aware of negative thoughts is the first step to change them to positive.

When we think positively, all our achievements make sense to us, and we always appreciate what we have. Regardless of what other people might say or think, we still feel good about ourselves.

Nothing can erode your powers more than negative attitude. As soon as you get negative, you are giving up your powers. Find inspiration everywhere and in everything. Life is inspiring. Try to be positive about everything you see, and never dwell on the past.

In the former USSR, where I grew up, many people have a mentality that if good things happen, expect something bad following after that.

"It's too good!" they say. "There must be something bad coming!" I don't even know why people decide to take that approach in life, but it comes from generation to generation—people being afraid of the good, and, for some reason, perceive it only as the "package" together with bad. Guess what? That's how it usually turns out to be—their bad things follow after the good ones, because by expecting them, those people subconsciously wish for those bad things to happen. In *The Secret*, this phenomenon is explained as *law of attraction*. So when people think about bad things coming, they are attracting them.

Already living in Canada I've heard another silly theory here: "Bad things come in threes." It looks like in Canada, people don't like *the good* either.

We should stop attracting the negativity to ourselves with all those baseless theories. There is no truth behind them except for experiences of those who attracted the negativity by thinking this way. Bad things don't have to come in "threes," and they don't have to come even in "ones" unless we accept that fact in our minds. Then our mind builds our attitude toward them, and everything bad gets attracted to us because how we think is usually what we do.

CHAPTER 13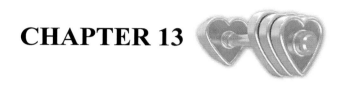

RESISTING TEMPTATIONS

Temptation, by definition, is an act that looks appealing to somebody, but often has negative consequences, and as such, tends to lead a person to regret his/her actions for various reasons. Temptation forces someone into committing such an act by *manipulation*, *curiosity*, *desire*, or *fear of loss*.

Some temptations are our first-time actions, and some are already our habits. First time actions are usually the ones that are easier to resist because we still don't know how exactly they will feel, taste or sense.

Once we get "the taste," we begin being attracted to the temptation also by our own senses. Then our consciousness starts losing control. Consciously we understand that giving in to our temptations is not good for us, but it still doesn't help us to avoid them. The more times we give in to a temptation from the start, the more it starts being controlled by our subconscious rather than conscious. Over time we develop a new habit that gets harder and harder to quit because *our subconscious is led by our emotions.* Every time we feel emotional, we immediately give in to our temptations, and it makes no difference whether we are emotionally happy or upset. Subconscious mind does its dirty job regardless of the source of our emotions.

The more often we "practice" giving in to our temptations, the harder it becomes to quit. For example, occasional drinking doesn't lead to alcoholism while everyday drinking does.

Once a new habit is developed, trying to resist temptations in most cases is useless because contradicting with the subconscious mind will only bring contradictions within ourselves. Then it develops stress, and eventually, we give up.

The best way of overcoming the temptations is finding an alternative for them. Since the subconscious mind is controlled by our emotions, *we need another emotion that would trigger the subconscious mind into a new action to quit a bad habit. The motive for that action has to be very strong.*

First five years of my fitness career I spent working as a gym teacher in elementary/high school. Dealing with kids made me realize that one of the best ways to make kids stop boisterous behavior is to give them something else to do instead. Then there is no need to tell them to stop that behavior. Their attention immediately was drawn to those new things, and we both avoided unnecessary arguments.

Our subconscious mind works the same way. What is the point of arguing with yourself and trying to prove that certain things are not good for you? "How can it be bad if it feels good?" your subconscious mind will respond to you. And then you are done.

Whatever you choose to replace your temptation, it has to be a substantial replacement. You will not be able to replace drinking alcohol with drinking water. Find something more powerful. Otherwise your temptation will eventually win.

CHAPTER 14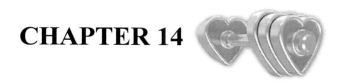

CHANGING "HAVE TO" TO "WANT TO"

People are generally motivated by *"what they want"* and not by *"what they have to"* do.

How many times in our childhood we were told "You have to do this," "You have to do that." How did it make you feel? Obligated? Forced? Maybe even distracted and confused.

"I have to go on a diet!" "I have to lose weight!" "I have to join the gym." "I have to quit smoking." We keep using that approach even when we are adults. Does it make us feel any better?

My parents put me in a technical college when I was only fifteen because I was badly influenced by heavy metal music, and I always wanted to be a rock star. I skipped a lot of school because of my rehearsals and listening to music. Four years later, after I finished college, I went to work. Every day going to work was a struggle for me. I hated it and worked because I "had to" and not because I "wanted to." I lasted like this approximately six months and eventually quit.

MIND

Can "have to" be effective in terms of bringing us results? Of course, but life works out much better on "want to" rather than "have to." When we say "I have to," something just does not align with our energy inside. Then we get demotivated, give up on the things that we *"have to"* do, and start doing things that we *"want to"* do instead.

When we say "have to," our subconscious mind picks up that message and learns that with everything we do in life, we have to obey, be forced, or be ruled. As we practice "have to" more and more, our mind slowly shuts down on our "want to."

With "want to," we don't need anybody to force us because we are getting that force from inside of ourselves and enjoying the process.

What we say has a tremendous power and influence on us and our subconscious mind.

With *"have to,"* we may still do things, but we wait for them to be over, so we can go and do things that we *want to*.

The more we practice saying "I have to," the more we learn to obey, and the less we feel in control. Even in our everyday life, we say, "I have to" when we can actually say, "I want to."

"I have to pay my telephone bill!" Why don't we say, *"I want to pay my phone bill"*? Probably, because we are not really thrilled about paying our bill? But we still "want to" have the phone, huh?

Of course the amount on the phone bill does not change whether we say, "I have to pay my bill" or "I want to pay my bill." But what does change is our perception about the things that we do, and with every "want to" instead of "have to," we get more powerful.

Selecting words in our language helps us to retrain our subconscious mind. When our subconscious mind hears "want," it senses the pleasure and obeys us better. We can easily turn things that we "have to" do into things that we "want to" *so then we no longer have to do them*.

*   *   *

Put your goals into action today. Take one day at a time. Be patient but be persistent. If you apply your willpower, self-discipline, and patience to your life goals, you will eventually prevail, not only over yourself but also over anything your heart will desire. Don't be afraid of difficulties and challenges. They will open up so much power inside of you, so you will be amazed how far you can really go with your dreams. You will never quit again. Take the knowledge you acquired so far and apply when you do your physical exercises. You will notice how much easier it will be for you to operate your body when you know how to operate your mind. Physical exercises are great, but your mental state will always define your physical state. The way you think—the way you will always look and feel.

Part 2

Body

CHAPTER 15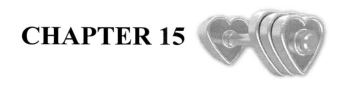

STAYING ALIVE

I have watched my parents going through different stages of their lives and have witnessed an example of how our minds can give up when we get older and how our bodies get weak. When my mom and my dad were in a good physical shape, they were always the most successful at what they did. My mom was a top chief in the city, and my dad was the most skilled welder. He was awarded with many medals and certificates for his outstanding achievements, and his huge portrait was always hanging in the center of our city under the title: "Our city is proud to have them as citizens."

But time went by, and when my parents reached late fifties, their bodies started to give up on them. My attempts to convince them to exercise were unsuccessful. My dad would laugh at me and say, "I do enough of physical activity at work, and I am not stupid to strain my muscles without getting paid for it." My physiological explanations about how good regular exercise is, did not work on him. My mom's philosophy was this: "To stay strong and healthy, you have to eat a lot."

When my parents were making parties, our tables were always loaded with food. Very often fried and with lots of sauces and spices and nicely designed dishes—they always tasted really good. My mom knew how to impress people with deliciousness. But what all this food and physical inactivity did to my parents was very unfortunate. With my mom, it started with her knee problems. Because of weak leg muscles, her kneecaps became loose and wobbly leading to bone damage. Living with constant pain, my mom was still inconvincible when I tried to explain to her that if she would make her legs strong, the muscles would hold her kneecaps in proper position, and then the pain would go away. She used to put warm patches or take painkillers, and that was her treatment.

Eight years before she died, she almost completely stopped walking. Not only had her leg muscles got weak, but all the others too, including her stomach muscles. Her internal organs were pulling her stomach down and developed hernia as a result from a congenital weakness in the cavity wall. She had two unsuccessful surgeries to fix her hernia, and this made her situation even worse because she had to spend most of her time in bed. That was the time when she completely gave up on herself. She often cried to me about how she wouldn't wish to anybody to be sick like her and how valuable our health and ability to walk is.

I really wish I could have found my way to convince my mom to exercise before it was too late. But there is nothing I can do right now except to pass this experience to those who are still reluctant to get physically active and to those who think that our muscles are there just to be taken advantage of.

All my life I have been trying to recruit people into thinking of their bodies in order to prevent many physical illnesses and health problems. To look good is great, but to feel good is a necessity to enjoy life. When you lose health—you don't want anything. There were times in my life when I was taking my health for granted, and every time, sooner or later, my body would let me know that I was wrong by making me either sick or emotionally drained.

Our body can handle a lot, but it has a limit. We, as humans, should to be able to realize when that limit is and try working preventively instead of fixing problems later because it can quickly get to the point where it will be too late to fix.

Going Naturally
(inspired by the movie *Bigger Stronger Faster*)

Everybody wants to look good. There is no doubt about that. We all want to have nice bodies to fit into those beautiful dresses or jeans or just walk in our bikinis on the beach. Being in good shape makes you feel better—you are surer of yourself and feel comfortable in any clothes anywhere you go.

But this is only good if your body is in a good shape on the inside too. Some people risk too much for their looks. It does not make sense when you look good but don't feel well. The price of having a nice body this way is too high.

Many pills, steroid injections, suspicious supplements to speed up the process of looking good, unfortunately, speed up the process of getting sick too.

Throughout my life I've seen quite a few people getting very seriously ill. Those were my mom, two of my uncles, some of my friends, and also very young people—my students. I've witnessed how being on the death row these people were reevaluating their lives. All I could read in their eyes was this: "I want to live!" "I just want to live!" "A little bit longer!" "As long as it's possible! And with minimum pain!" They were not talking about having nice bodies. They were not even talking about being healthy. They just wanted to breathe, hear, and see.

They were telling me how beautiful this world was and how they were noticing every day's simple things that they've never noticed before. I've learned from them to value those things and appreciate life as a chain of wonderful moments and not as some kind of long-term plan. I've also learned how to catch those moments inside of my mind, hold them there for as long as possible, and then take them with me into my tomorrow, so my every new day will be better and my life will feel worthwhile living.

Some of these people, including my mom and both of my uncles, unfortunately, never made it. But those who did completely changed their perception of life. While they do appreciate being in a good shape, feeling energized, and having a good health, what they still value the most is just staying alive.

If you are not in a good shape, you can change it. If you have health problems—many of them you can still fix. But if you are dead, there is nothing you can do—you are dead.

Thinking of my own experience, experiences of those who died and also those who survived deadly diseases, I realized that when people make plans to improve their lives, they don't always put priorities in a proper sequence.

A nineteen-year-old girl comes to me and says, "I want to lose weight faster. Can you recommend me some pills? I've heard of fat burners that bodybuilders take before their competitions. Which ones are best?"

I looked at her and figured, "She needs to lose ten pounds at most. She is young, and even if she doesn't take those pills, she can still lose those ten pounds in less than two months."

"Do you want to live?" I asked her with a smile.
"Yes," she said and smiled back at me.
"Do you like to live being sick?" I asked again.
"No," she said.
"Do you still want me to give you the name of those pills?" I continued.

She understood my sarcasm and realized that she had made a mistake.

It may sound banal to even talk that staying alive is what we all should be thinking about first. But many of us don't. There is an old saying, "You don't know what you've got until you've lost it," and most of those who have never been seriously ill don't know how it feels to be on the death row. They take life for granted and think, "Oh, cancer and heart attacks are something that other people get. It is not for me. Look, I am OK."

But everyone thought that way . . . until they've got it.

We go on unhealthy diets, take fat-burning pills, steroids, growth hormones, underdeveloped substances, and protein shakes, you name it. Without going into a research, we trust advices of uncertified personal trainers, suspicious commercials on TV, or local weight loss clinics that hire people who don't even know the anatomy of a human body. We know that people are dying every day from cancer, heart attacks, and other degenerative diseases. But what we don't know is what actually caused those deaths. Not everything deadly dangerous has immediate effect. Smoking, alcoholism, and drugs, for example, kill over time. So do steroids, fat-burning pills, and even some supplements if taken continuously.

Why should we be risking our precious lives for the cause of looking good? While striving for better looks, let's think about staying alive first. If we stay alive, we can change our bodies. Let it be a bit later, but let it be.

Don't get too frustrated if something doesn't work out as fast as you want, and don't fall right away for quick solutions because they can cost you your life. Enjoy other things. There is a lot to see in this life, and there are tons to experience at absolutely any age. You can do whatever you want to do and be whoever you want to be. But only on one condition—if you stay alive.

CHAPTER 16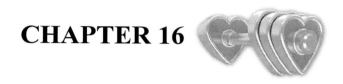

FEELING GOOD

A t least half of the time I don't really want to go do my workouts, and I could probably find something else more enjoyable to do rather than spinning my elliptical trainer, running the treadmill, or lifting weights over my head. But the feeling that I get after workouts doesn't let me stay home and give in to immediate pleasures.

Nothing can compare to the feeling after a good workout—it's like being on top of the world every time. Your body is light, your mind is relaxed, and every single inch in you is saying, "Thank you for your effort. I will now make sure that you are OK. I will pump your blood in the most efficient way. I will take care of all your organs and will also make you the smartest on earth." It feels like everything works perfect for you. There are no

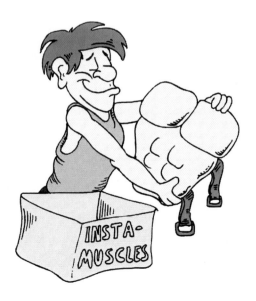

worries or problems. Exercise is my biggest addiction, and the more I exercise, the more I want.

I exercise every day, most days twice a day. I exercise even when I am tired, when I have sleepless nights, and even when I am sick. Some might disagree with me and say that this is too much, but every time I finish my workout, my body is telling me the opposite—it makes me feel better.

CHAPTER 17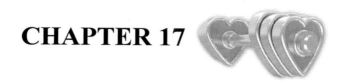

WHY DO WE GAIN WEIGHT?

I have been asked this question thousands of times. But the question I was asked even more was this: Why do some people gain weight and some stay slim even when they eat the same?

My mother and my father for the most of their lives stayed overweight even though they moved physically a lot. Their friends ate much more than they did but somehow managed to stay slim. And I started to wonder then why such a thing was happening. Is it only because of genetics or because of some kind of environmental influences?

Every one of us is different. Even though our bodies work the same in general, there are still some factors that affect one person more than the other.

The answer to the question, Why do we gain weight? splits into two segments:

- *In-body reactions*—something that happens inside of *some bodies* that cause them to gain weight

• *Outside-the-body causes*—things that we do to ourselves to cause weight gain.

Source: (Frances Sizer, 2006), p. 325-328. Some parts were rephrased for easier reading and expanded with additional information.

In-Body Reactions

These reactions are developed in some bodies due to some not fully known biological changes and referred further to as theories:

1. Set-point theory

The body may "choose" a weight it wants and defend that weight by regulating behaviors and metabolic activities. It starts working like a home thermostat that sets for a certain temperature and heats up when the house gets cold or cools down when it gets hot. Whenever some people lose or gain weight, their bodies will always try to bring it back to its "chosen" weight. Why the body does this is still unknown, but there are possible theories behind it:

a.   Brown fat theory

Lean people have more brown fat. White fat is more sluggish while brown fat cells actively metabolize fat, releasing its stored energy as heat. A person with more brown fat may stay leaner even if he consumes the same or more calories than the one with more white fat.

b.   Thermogenesis theory

In some people, their body tissues—muscles, spleen,* and bone marrow**—can convert stored energy into heat in response to various factors: cold temperature, physical conditioning, overeating,

---

* a ductless vascular organ in the left upper abdomen of humans and other vertebrates that helps destroy old red blood cells, form lymphocytes, and store blood

** a soft reddish substance inside some bones that is involved in the production of blood cells. New white and red blood cells are formed only in the marrow of the flat bones such as the ribs, breastbone, or pelvis in adults

starvation, trauma, and other stress. Heat can even be produced to "waste" fuel without any useful work—for example, when those people eat a lot. They burn more energy even at rest.

Some bodies can decide to conserve energy when people stop eating.

Let's look at this in terms of money. When do we spend more money? When we get them often or sometimes? The answer is obvious. The more often we get the money, the more secure we feel about spending them. If there is a delay, we tend to hold on to money, and this is what our bodies may do too. If we eat often, the body feels secure to release the energy out to burn, and if we don't supply food for a while, our body shuts down and holds on to that energy as we would hold on to our saving bank accounts when we don't receive money.

When some lean people eat, their metabolism may speed up for a while; while in overweight and obese people, no change in metabolism occur after eating.

Tip

People who exercise regularly and eat often may rebound this theory and make their bodies change the chemistry to use the energy more effectively in order to store less fat.

2.   *Fat cell number theory*

We are all born with a certain number of fat cells in our body. When we overeat, our body has the ability to fill available fat cells with fat from food and then to build more fat cells if needed. When someone is gaining fat, his body keeps generating more fat cells, but when someone is losing fat, his body only "deflates" generated fat cells, allowing the fat to go out, but the new number of fat cells remains unchanged.

The more fat cells is being generated, the more that person has a tendency to gain weight in the future because the emptied fat cells "sit and wait" to be filled with fat again. If someone was already obese or overweight before, it is much "easier" for him to gain fat again than for someone who has never built that many fat cells in his body.

Tip

We should always aim to prevent from generating more fat cells. With less fat cells, it will be easier to maintain weight in the future.

3.   *Bone density theory*

As we get older, we may start losing some bone density, and at some point in life, the body may decide that it is too dangerous to be lean. In case of an accident of falling, our bones will break more easily if they are not protected with special padding. The role of that padding is played by the body fat that our body generates to protect weak bones.

Tips

In order to avoid building padding (fat) as we get older, we should try aiming to save bone density and do the following:

1.   Balance your calcium/magnesium consumption
2.   Do resistance training
3.   Eat balanced meals
4.   Manage your stress
5.   Spend time under the sun

According to numerous studies and aging manuals, strength training with consumption of adequate amounts of calcium and magnesium is known to increase bone mass and thus decrease the possibility of extra fat gain.

Postmenopausal women are especially prone to bone density loss because they lack estrogen. Most women know this and begin to take calcium and magnesium supplements to ward off the debilitating disease. While these supplements can partially solve their problem, they are not enough. Balanced meals, resistance training, stress management, and adequate time spent outdoor under the sun is a more complete way of saving your bones.

a.   Balance your your calcium/magnesium consumption

Osteoporosis

Osteoporosis is a degenerative bone disease that primarily affects postmenopausal women. It is estimated that every second woman over fifty will have an osteoporosis-related fracture. Literally meaning "porous bone," osteoporosis is characterized by a decrease in normal bone density due to the loss of calcium and collagen. A loss of bone density causes bones to become brittle, and in turn, leads to frequent fractures and other serious effects. Osteoporosis is a threat to 28 million Americans and is currently one of the most underdiagnosed and undertreated disorders in medicine.

According to the National Osteoporosis Foundation, once a woman reaches sixty years of age, she has a one in four chances of breaking a bone due to osteoporosis. Elderly women who suffer from severe osteoporosis experience hip, wrist, spine, and other traumatic fractures from minor falls that would normally not occur in young adults. Hip fractures in elderly people can be difficult to treat and sometimes require prosthetic hip reconstruction and painful rehabilitation. Other serious effects of osteoporosis include loss of height, restricted mobility, and a humped back.

In 1997, the National Academy of Sciences increased its daily recommendation for calcium by 50 percent for older Americans. Sounds like good news for milk production companies and those who sell calcium supplementations: "Hey, people are busy. They don't have time to research what calcium overconsumption does. Let's just sell them!"

And here you go—milk is advertized everywhere. Most doctors recommend taking calcium supplementations. "Calcium, calcium, calcium." It's on the tip of every elderly woman's tongue, and every menopausal woman has something in her fridge with a calcium label on it.

But do we really need that much of calcium, or is this just another propaganda to get the money out of our pockets?

Let's first look at the rest of the world. Are all the countries so paranoid about calcium intake or is this just us—North Americans, who consume most of the milk in the world but still don't get enough calcium?

"In general," writes Emily Yoffe, "world dietary patterns show that countries where people consume large amounts of calcium are also countries where people eat extravagant amounts of animal protein, places such as the United States and northern Europe. These countries also suffer among the world's highest rate of fractures due to osteoporosis."

"The correlation between animal protein intake and fracture rates in different societies is as strong as that between lung cancer and smoking," says T. Colin Campbell, professor of nutritional biochemistry at Cornell University.

Our bodies contain two pounds to four pounds of calcium, 99 percent of which is in our bones and teeth. The rest circulates in the blood where it is necessary for nervous system function. Eating animal protein, which is high in sulfur-containing amino acids, requires the body to buffer the effects of those amino acids. It does so by releasing calcium from the bones, literally peeing them away. But this leaching of calcium should be offset if the balance of calcium to protein in the diet is within a reasonable range. Robert Heaney, professor of medicine at the Creighton University School of Medicine and a proponent of high dairy consumption, found in a study he coauthored that the "single most important determinate of the rate of bone gain in young women was not the amount of calcium consumed but **the ratio of calcium to protein**. But it is a difficult balance to strike when it is common for Americans to eat **double the protein** we need, with **70 percent of it coming from animal sources**."

Chinese (living in China) consume **less than half the calcium they're told is necessary**, mostly all of it from leafy green vegetables, and they have one-fifth the incidence of hip fracture of Americans. Although they consume more calories per day than we do, only about 10 percent of their diet is from animal sources.

The Japanese (living in Japan) get almost all their calcium from soy, the bones of small cooked fish, and vegetables. They also have about 40 percent the rate of hip fracture of the West. The British diet is similar to ours and so is their hip fracture rate.

It looks like we North Americans are mistreated, misinformed, and trapped again by our trustful foolishness by those who sell us their products, assuming that we just don't have the time to educate ourselves or are too busy watching our TVs—the place where they usually advertise their products.

Calcium deficiencies cannot be fixed just by increasing the intake of it. Our body works in balance. When we add something, we always take something away.

The risk factors for osteoporosis can be divided into two categories:

in-body reactions/changes—those that cannot be alternated, such as gender, race, and family history and

outside-the-body causes—those that can be changed by us, such as alcohol consumption, smoking, and calcium intake.

In-Body Reactions

Female gender. Because women have lighter, thinner bones than men, osteoporosis is much more frequent in women. At age thirty-five, men have 30 percent more bone mass than women. Bone loss also occurs much more slowly in men than women.

Advancing age, especially the onset of menopause. Before a woman reaches her midthirties, her body gains more bone than it loses. Around age thirty-five, this process balances out. When a woman reaches menopause (typically around age fifty), her body produces less of the female hormone estrogen. Since estrogen helps maintain body density, a decrease in the hormone will result in some bone loss. If bone loss is severe, a woman may experience an increase in bone fractures, loss of height, restricted mobility, or a humped back (also known as a dowager's hump). Women who experience menopause at an early age (forty-five or younger) are at even higher risk because their level of estrogen will be lowered at an earlier age.

Family history. Women whose family members have had osteoporosis are at increased risk for the disease. Body type is often similar among mothers or sisters.

Race. Asian and Caucasian women are at a greater risk for osteoporosis since their bone density is 5 percent to 10 percent lower than that of African American women or women of Mediterranean or aboriginal decent. Women with fair skin, freckles, or red or blond hair are also at higher risk.

Build. Women with thin or small frames have a higher risk for bone fractures.

Diseases. Women who have anorexia (an eating disorder), celiac disease (an inability to tolerate grain products), diabetes, chronic diarrhea, or kidney or liver diseases are at an increased risk for osteoporosis.

Outside-the-Body Causes

Smoking. Since smoking interferes with the body's processing of calcium, smokers experience vertebral fractures more frequently than nonsmokers. In addition, women who smoke usually experience menopause earlier than nonsmokers. Thus, their estrogen deficiency begins sooner than women who do not smoke.

Alcohol consumption. Studies show that consuming two or more alcoholic drinks daily decreases a woman's rate of calcium absorption, which may lead to bone loss. Alcohol also interferes with vitamin D synthesis, a process that helps bones absorb calcium.

Childlessness. Women who never had children are at higher risk for osteoporosis. During each pregnancy, women experience temporary surges of estrogen that helps protect them from osteoporosis.

High meat consumption. See above.

Too little exercise. A sedentary lifestyle with little physical activity can lead to osteoporosis. Bones can lose their mass during long periods of inactivity. Exercise helps maintain bone strength and growth. For women with low bone density, exercise stimulates bone growth.

Weight. Women who have poor muscle tone are at higher risk for osteoporosis.

Certain medications and steroids. Commonly prescribed steroids to treat asthma and arthritis (such as cortisone and prednisone) and high doses of thyroid hormone increase the chances of osteoporosis. Also, certain medications used to treat seizures (such as phenobarbital and phenytoin (trade name Dilantin) interfere with the body's ability to absorb calcium.

Symptoms/Indicators of Osteoporosis

Back pain. Vertebrae fractures are the most common bone fractures associated with osteoporosis. An early symptom of the disease is chronic lower back pain. Women may also experience sudden muscle spasms during periods of inactivity. This sudden back pain is caused by the spontaneous collapse of small, weak sections of the spine. The type of back pain associated with osteoporosis is confined to one area of the back and does not usually spread. Often, women who develop osteoporosis will begin to experience chronic lower back pain about nine and a half years after their last menstrual period or thirteen years after surgical menopause.

Height loss, curving spine. The loss of height indicates the collapse of a spinal vertebra. These collapses typically occur at the weakest point of the spinal column—the spinal curve. Women with osteoporosis may lose two and a half to eight inches in upper body height. Older women should routinely measure their height.

Chest x-ray showing osteopenia. Osteopenia is a condition in which a woman's bone mass is lower than normal. A decrease in bone mass will affect the strength of bones, causing them to break more easily.

Tooth loss. Tooth loss and the thinning of bones that support the teeth (periodontal bones) may indicate osteoporosis.

Hoping to have strong bones, we often fall for underresearched "calcium containing" substances, the absorption of which has been proven to be as low as 1 percent. The best sources for calcium are the ones that come from real food. No matter how great your supplementation may be, nobody will ever invent a better formula than Mother Nature did. Natural foods combine calcium tightly connected with other nutrients, which enhances calcium absorption. This cannot be achieved with supplements. Those who try convincing people into taking calcium supplements are usually the ones who sell them.

The recommended daily norm for calcium intake in United States is now 1,000 mg, which, in my opinion, is ridiculously overrated due to the Standard American Diet. If we balance everything else that leads to better calcium absorption, we will not only get better bones but also less fat and better health. Table 1 demonstrates how easily we can get required amount of calcium per day if we just eat right, avoid stress and bad habits, and balance our meals.

Table 1. Calcium-rich Foods

	FOODS	Serving Size	Calcium (mg)
EXCELLENT	Sesame seeds	¼ cup	351
	Firm Cheese	50 g	350
	Milk	1 Cup	300
	Plain yogurt	175g	300
	Almonds	¼ Cup	200
	Salmon, canned	107g	235
	Spinach, boiled	1 Cup	245
	Sardines, including bones, 8 small	45g	165
	Turnip Greens, cooked	1 Cup	197
	Soybeans, caned or boiled	1 Cup	175
	Tofu	½ Cup	110
	Bok Choy, cooked	½ Cup	84
	Broccoli, cooked	½ Cup	35
	Mustard Greens, boiled	1Cup	104
	Kale, cooked	½ Cup	103
VERY GOOD	Basil, dried, ground	2 tsp.	63
	Thyme, dried, ground	2 tsp.	54
	Cinnamon, ground	2 tsp.	56
	Blackstrap Molasses	2 tsp.	118
	Swiss Chard, boiled	1 Cup	102
GOOD	Dill Weed	2 tsp.	36
	Oregano, dried, ground	2 tsp.	47
	Kelp (sea vegetables)	¼ Cup	34
	Rosemary, dried	2 tsp.	28
	Romaine Lettuce	2 Cup	40
	Celery, raw	1 Cup	48
	Cabbage	1 cup	47
	Brussel sprouts	1 cup	56
	Oranges	1 each	52
	Asparagus	1 cup	36

Calcium builds better bones in combination with another important ingredient—magnesium. Approximately 70 percent of the magnesium in the body is found in the skeletal system. At least half of the magnesium in the body is combined with calcium and phosphorus in the bones. The remainder is in the muscles, red blood cells, and the other tissues of the body.

Magnesium ensures the strength and firmness of the bones, and it also makes the teeth harder.

The recommended daily norm for magnesium is 400 mg. Table 2 below displays that with proper meal plan, it is not hard at all to supply those amounts through regular food.

Table 2. Magnesium-rich Foods

	FOODS	Serving Size	Magnesium (mg)
EXCELLENT	Trail mix, nuts, seeds	1Cup	235
	Bulgur, dry	1 Cup	230
	Oat Bran, raw	1 Cup	221
	Fish, Halibut, Atlantic and Pacific	½ fillet	170
	Wheat flour, whole grain	1 Cup	166
	Spinach, canned, drained	1 Cup	163
	Barley, pearled, raw	1 Cup	158
	Spinach	1 Cup	156
	Soybeans	1 Cup	148
	Beans, White, mature seeds, canned	1 Cup	134
	Cornmeal, whole grain, yellow	1 Cup	110
	Tomato products	1 Cup	110
	Beet greens, cooked, boiled, no salt	1 Cup	98
	Okra, frozen, cooked, boiled, no salt	1 Cup	94
	Baking chocolate, unsweetened	1 square	93
VERY GOOD	Muffins, oat bran	1 muffin	89
	Rice, brown, long grain, cooked	1 Cup	84
	Milk, canned, condensed, sweetened	1 Cup	80
	Fish, flatfish (flounder and sole) cooked	1 fillet	74
GOOD	Sweet potato, canned, mashed	½ Cup	61
	Soymilk, original and vanilla, fortified	1 Cup	61
	Artichoke, cooked	1 medium	47
	Chocolate, Semi-sweet	¼ Cup	46
	Squash, acorn, baked	½ Cup	43
	Yogurt, low fat varieties	1 Cup	37
	Tofu, raw	4 oz	100
	Cabbage	1 cup	47
	Brussel sprouts	1 cup	56
	Oranges	1 each	52
	Asparagus	1 cup	36

Toxicity

Excessive intake of calcium (more than 3,000 mg per day) may result in elevated blood calcium levels, a condition known as *hypercalcemia,* which can lead to soft tissue *calcification.* This condition involves the unwanted accumulation of calcium in cells other than the bone. Dietary magnesium very rarely poses a health risk, but very high doses of magnesium supplements can promote adverse effects such as diarrhea.

Nutrient Interactions

- Vitamin D accelerates the absorption of calcium.
- High intakes of sodium, caffeine, or protein cause calcium to be removed through urine.

b. Do resistance training

Resistance training increases bone mass, especially spinal bone mass. According to Kathy Keeton, a research study by Ontario's McMaster University found that a year-long strength-training program increased the spinal bone mass of postmenopausal women by 9 percent. Furthermore, women who do not participate in strength training actually experience a decrease in bone density. Source: Natural News (naturalnews.com)

c. Eat balanced meals

Balanced meals, providing all other necessary nutrients, play a vital role in helping the body properly absorb dietary calcium and magnesium.

d. Manage stress

When stress triggers, the body puts out stress hormones, magnesium and calcium, among other things, into the bloodstream. Much study at the cellular, biochemical, and physiological levels have shown that the stress response vitally involves the influx of calcium into cells, resulting in a drastic change in the cells' internal magnesium to calcium ratio (Mg:Ca). Calcium ions, for the most part, are kept outside cells while magnesium ions are kept mainly inside cells. The stress response changes this. During stress response, calcium ions rush inside the cell, and this alters the internal Mg:Ca ratio.

Physical exercise not only promotes overall fitness, but it helps you to manage emotional stress and tension as well, thus helping manage a proper Mg:Ca balance.

e. Spend time under the sun

When I was a teenager, my friends and I spent most of our free time somewhere outside playing games under the sun being in shorts and topless. We didn't even know that there was such thing as sun protection. If somebody told us about it, we would probably laugh that person out. Protection from the sun? Why? Sun is good. It is natural, and it is given to us to enjoy.

But . . . here comes the business. Somebody who invented sun-protection lotions decided something else for us. Sun lotions are promoted so well that when we go on our beaches, we don't smell the ocean breeze anymore but all day inhale drops of those sun lotions or sprays.

Lately the sun is blamed for all dermatological problems. Sunscreen lotions are promoted to be used even when staying in the shade.

I was against sunscreen lotions from the first time I've heard about them, but now the research is finally coming out to prove it: sunscreens cause cancer (not only skin cancer), according to comprehensive new research published in the United Kingdom. It appears that it is not the sun that might be the main reason why people get skin cancer, but those lotions that they use to protect from it.

There are two primary reasons why sunscreen causes cancer. *First,* and most importantly, the use of sunscreen blocks the skin from absorbing the sun's rays. That's what it's supposed to do, right? Yes, but in doing so, it also blocks the creation of all-essential vitamin D, the nutrient that the human body desperately needs to prevent as many as twenty-five chronic diseases: prostate cancer, breast cancer, osteoporosis, schizophrenia, heart disease, and many others.

It turns out that most people living in the Northern Hemisphere are chronically deficient in vitamin D. By wearing sunscreen, they're depriving their bodies of perhaps the single most important nutrient they need to stay healthy.

The second reason sunscreen causes cancer is because it contains toxic chemicals in the form of artificial fragrance, chemical colors, and petroleum products used as fillers and stabilizers. These chemicals *are absorbed through the skin where they enter the bloodstream and wreak havoc on the immune system.* Artificial fragrances, just by themselves, may contain dozens of carcinogenic chemicals that damage the liver, the heart, and even promote systemic cancer.

Of course, the sunscreen manufacturers continue to deny all this while propagating the ridiculous myth that "there's no such thing as a healthy tan."

In reality, there's no such thing as a healthy pale person! A tan is a bona fide sign of good health, and a deep tan actually protects you from cancer.

Many of the researches supporting the theory that sun exposure leading to skin cancer are to indirectly promote sunscreen lotion manufacturers. There is some truth to what they find, but they have an annoying tendency *to generalize from limited to the infinite.*

All this has come out in this comprehensive new research report entitled "Sunlight Robbery." To summarize the findings of the report, "To ensure optimum levels of vitamin D and optimum health, people need to sunbathe whenever they can, wearing as few clothes as possible, *while taking care not to burn*. Vitamin D obtained from food provides only about 10 percent of our needs."

Well said. So much for the myth that sunshine is somehow bad for you. Enjoy it, and once again, trust Mother Nature. She expresses her love to you through the sun's warmth and its light. We are the creatures of the sunlight.

Source: naturalnews.com

Recommended Sunlight Exposure

Best time to sunbathe is before 11:00 a.m. and after 4:00-5:00 p.m. At this time, the sun is gentler, and chances that you will burn your skin are minimal. The paler your skin, the less time you should spend under the sun. As you get darker, your skin gets protected from burns, and you can spend more time enjoying the sunlight. At least one hour a day of open-air, unfiltered sunlight is recommended for health. The sun does not have to be shining directly on your skin. Indirect sunlight is acceptable, but it should not be filtered through glass or glasses that block UV rays.

4.   *Enzyme theory*

This disorder affects about 1 out of 1,000,000 people. The condition is usually first seen during infancy or childhood and is based on deficiency where a person lacks a protein needed to break down fat molecules. The disorder causes large amounts of fat to build up in the blood. It is usually caused by a defective gene that is passed down through families.

Persons with this condition do not have a substance called *lipoprotein lipase*. Without it, the body *cannot* break down fat from digested food. Fat particles called *chylomicrons* build up in the blood.

Tip

Regular exercise burns dietary and blood fat for energy, thus helping to fight this disorder.

5.   *Menopause and age theory*

As both men and women get older, the number of calories their bodies use declines. Partially this happens because of the reduction in the body's lean muscle mass and partially because of hormonal imbalance due to menopause in later years.

"I think menopause is a convenient thing to blame," says Howard whose research was published in the issue of the *Journal of the American Medical Association*. The research found that women who ate a low-fat, high-carbohydrate diet after menopause were less likely to gain weight than women who ate more fat. But diet probably is not the sole explanation for midlife weight gain. What seems to be the real problem is *people's tendency to turn down their level of physical activity as they get older.* As Howard puts it, "If you look at that stage of life—the kids leave, you may be less busy at home—it's likely you become more sedentary."

"Changing levels of hormones at menopause may have some effect on women's proportion of lean mass to fat," says Barbara Sternfeld, a senior research scientist at Kaiser Permanente of Northern California who has studied exercise and weight gain in women around the time of menopause. "Hormones may also affect where that fat settles on the body—around the waist rather than a more even distribution. Those changes," she says, "may give women the impression that menopause is the major cause of their newly padded bodies when, aging is a more likely explanation."

Tip

Most people think that gaining weight and getting older go hand in hand. Recent studies tell us opposite. While muscle loss is the main cause why people gain weight with age, the key reason for that muscle loss is that it is fun to sit around and watch TV and play on the computer. If we spend too much time doing it *when we are younger*, it's that **much harder to stop** when we get older. *Everyone gets old, but **some stay active and agile** and enjoy their bodies throughout any age, while **others fall apart** and deteriorate due to their bad habits and weak will.*

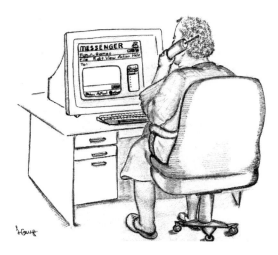

Being active helps to preserve your muscle and increase your bone density while maintaining a higher metabolism. To avoid weight gain or to lose some extra padding, I'm afraid our sitting-around days are over. Not only you have to stand up, but you also need to do the following:

- *Exercise aerobically.* Squeeze in at least thirty minutes of cardiovascular activity such as walking, running, swimming most days of the week.
- *Do weight-resistance training.* Have a structured program and switch it every 6-8 weeks.
- *Seek for any opportunity to use your body throughout the day.* Take the stairs instead of the elevator/escalator, park your car farther from entrances, do not sit around at your lunchtime, and try to get physically involved in your home duties.
- *Eat healthy.* Try eating 5-6 small meals throughout the day to boost your metabolism.
- *Reduce your calorie intake or increase physical activity by 0.5 percent to 1 percent every year after the age of 35-40.* Don't starve yourself, but recognize that your body will need less calories as you get older. Whether you like it or not, gradual loss of body cells with age leads to burning fewer calories at rest. Keep that in mind and remember that your metabolism with age is declining. Check your weight regularly, and if you notice that it is increasing every year, restructure your meals.

Cutting down calories doesn't necessarily mean reducing the amounts of food or avoiding your favorite meals. This can easily be achieved by replacing some foods, changing sauces and other additives, or eating calorie-rich foods in the afternoon instead of evenings when your metabolism is slower.

Ways to Speed Up Your Metabolism

- *Exercise regularly.*

After you finish your workout, your body continues working; it repairs muscle tissues that are broken down during training.

- *Eat small meals often throughout the day.*

Your body can only digest certain amounts of food at a given time, and you can only force it to digest more if you start spending more energy. Whatever is not digested within a certain time frame will be turned to body fat. When you eat small portions often, you are not only avoiding gaining extra fat but also forcing your body to spend more energy on digestion itself.

- *Build muscles. The more muscle tissue you have, the faster is your metabolism. Denser muscles require more energy.*

If there are two cars racing on a highway and one of them has bigger engine, that car will always burn more gas for the same racing distance. Two people who have the same body weight, but different muscle density, burn different amount of calories. Muscle *is the only tissue* that can burn fat.

- *Do not diet. Your metabolism can drop up to 30 percent.*

If you starve yourself or go on a low-calorie diet, your body starts releasing energy very economically. Not only will you not be able to perform good workouts but will also lose muscles instead of fat. You may also end up with overtraining or depression.

- *Expose yourself to heat or cold.*

Body temperature increase or drop of 0.5°C elevates metabolism by 7 percent. The chemical reactions in our bodies occur faster, which in return speeds up our metabolism. Sauna and steam room lovers, wintertime-outside joggers, or those who work outside can benefit from this fact of burning more calories because our body tends to always maintain a stable internal environment. Our brain's "thermostat" is set for approximately 37°C, and this is our normal body temperature. If we get exposed to cold or heat and our body temperature begins to change, our brain senses this change and triggers heat-generating and heat-conserving activities. Someone who experiences cold, for example, may start to feel shivery (first body-heat-generating reaction) or begin to actively move around. If we get overheated, our brain also senses this, but turns on a different mechanism that leads to increased loss of body heat, which stimulates sweat glands. As the water evaporates from our body, some heat gets carried away, and our body gets cooled. This process affects not only our skin but also deeper tissues and organs—our blood vessels widen, breathing rate and heartbeat increase, allowing the heat to be carried away faster.

- *Balance your diet.*

Essential fatty acids (EFAs), B-complex vitamins, and minerals including potassium, calcium, and manganese increase the efficiency of oxidation and raise metabolic rate, energy, and activity level.

What Slows Down the Metabolism?

- Aging
- Inactivity
- Depression
- Lack of sleep
- Low-calorie diets

6. *Thyroid activity theory*

Thyroid activity affects metabolic rate over a wide range, from hyperactive or increased metabolic rate, down to underactive or lowered rate. The slower the rate, the less calories are burned, and the easier it is to put on weight.

A worse problem is the lack of testing. An estimated 200 million people worldwide have thyroid disorders; thyroid function tests are rarely given unless the doctor suspects a thyroid disorder, and most doctors do not suspect it because the symptoms are subtle. Of the estimated 13 million Americans affected by thyroid disease, more than half are unaware of their condition.

Iodine is essential to the structure of thyroid hormone, and iodine deficiency can lead to underactivity of the thyroid. Symptoms include slowed metabolism, fatigue, mental problems, hypoglycemia, breathing problems, slow heartbeat, high cholesterol, and weight gain.

Resistance to produce the thyroid hormone can also be a genetic disorder. Patients with this disorder usually have an enlarged thyroid gland. Underactivity of the thyroid is called *hypothyroidism*.

Tips

- *Check your thyroid levels regularly.* If you discovered a thyroid problem and were prescribed a medication, remember that the thyroid function can change quite quickly and needs to be monitored at least every six months so your medication is kept at the correct dosage.
- *Get active.* Physical activity is especially important if you suffer from *hypothyroidism*. It is essential in order to help speed up your metabolism and increase weight loss.
- *Adjust your diet.* It is believed that selenium intake helps to increase the activity of the thyroid. This can be done by eating foods such as whole-wheat bread, bran, Brazil nuts, tuna, onions, tomatoes, and broccoli. Include some of these foods on a regular basis. Other foods that are helpful for the thyroid function are carrots, spinach, apricots, asparagus, olive oil, avocado, sunflower seeds, whole-grain cereals, bananas, oily fish, so choose meals that include these foods.

It is well documented that a diet low in iodine is associated with hypothyroidism or underactive thyroid. The best supply of iodine is from sea salt and seaweed.

Vitamin E has been found to help iodine be digested. Tests of 4 mg of iodine supplements and 600 units of vitamin E have shown to *take up* the thyroid gland activity "almost immediately and markedly."

Reduce the amounts of foods that interfere with iodine *uptake*: cabbage, kale, broccoli, kohlrabi, mustard, lima beans, linseed, sweet potato, peanuts, soy products. You don't need to cut these foods out completely but keep them to a minimum.

Avoid caffeine drinks: coffee, cola, etc.

Avoid smoking and alcohol.

- *Reduce stress.* Stress is thought to be a major contributor to the development of hypothyroidism. One of the best ways to reduce stress is to take regular exercises.

Source: ProQuest, www.csa.com. Rephrased for easier reading.

Outside-the-Body Causes of Gaining Weight

1.   **Technology influence**

People always seek ease; this is just a human nature. All the latest inventions prove that fact, and technology is slowly replacing all our physical labor.

Year by year we are getting used to the idea that we just don't need to move anymore, and it's no longer a surprise to notice how many people, when driving in, are looking for the closest parking spots beside the stores. Sometimes they sit in their cars for 10—15 minutes and wait for that "lucky" spot. I sometimes wonder, "Maybe those people were unloading bricks from trucks all day? Or maybe they are marathon runners coming from their races? Who knows?" What makes those people feel so tired? I have even witnessed two cars bump into each other trying to be first to get the closest parking spot at one grocery store.

I love technology myself, and I think it should help us to make our life better. But unfortunately, many of the technological inventions made our life worse and not better. What people could do physically fifty years ago now becomes a challenge for them.

Technology and latest inventions influence people to stop moving their bodies, and this became one of the main reasons why people are getting so overweight. By the latest research, most people are overweight not because of overeating but because of their lack of physical activity. This is very easy to prove. If we look at our history, we can see that in our past, people ate a lot too. But those people also moved around a lot. They didn't have cars, TVs, computers, remote controls, or home appliances. The absence of those things forced people to stay physically active. The technology "spoiled" us to the point that we became addicts of inactivity and cannot imagine ourselves anymore without phones or remote controls in our hands. People and all these things go together these days. But what is unfortunate is that with all these things, there are other things that go together—our fatness, chronic tiredness, and degenerative diseases.

2.   Emotional eating

Almost everyone had experienced walking into a food store, gas station, or convenience store, not feeling particularly hungry, and, after viewing vast variety of foods or snacks on displays, end up chewing something on the way out.

People are prone to overconsume when they are presented with lots of choices. Overeating occurs in response to many human sensations and emotions—loneliness, grief, depression, celebration, happiness, etc. Foods help people elevate their mood when they are feeling down and reinforce their happiness when they are celebrating.

Some people have a tendency to get attracted to overeating at certain times of the day, having formal lunches or dinners. This makes people eat regardless if they are hungry or not.

3.   Fast-food, price, and advertising

Inspired by the movie *Super Size Me*

Most fast-foods are relatively inexpensive, available almost everywhere, and heavily advertised. Besides that, they are also deliciously made, and the average buyer who is not aware of disadvantages of such eating obviously gets influenced. Forty percent of the recent jump in US body weight is due to low price alone: $1.39 for a hamburger, $3.50 for a meal combo—who can beat that?

Of course, partially, it is everyone's responsibility to take personal action to evaluate what to eat, but unfortunately, not everyone is strong. Many people get easily influenced with advertising, great taste, smell, and low price. They know that fast-food is bad for them but consider it only until the next time they get hungry. The bombarding of TV and radio commercials and flyers continue doing their dirty jobs—fattening and killing millions of us. Those who are not educated about healthy ways of eating look at those commercials and decide this: "Look, it's on TV, it must be good. If it is allowed to be advertised—we can eat it!"

Vending machines are placed almost everywhere filled with similar low-quality junk—chocolate bars, candies, chips, and pop. What do our children eat when they get hungry? How can they learn otherwise if they see people snacking on the things that are on TV, radio, and on the flyers? They assume that it's OK.

Will this ever change? Will people ever be able to change a pocket candy for an orange or an apple? I believe that there is hope. When researchers dropped the price of more nutritious options by half and made them readily available in workplace vending machines and school cafeterias, adults and students quadrupled their purchases of fresh fruit and doubled their purchases on baby carrot sticks.

"It's hard enough for parents to guide their children's food choices, but it becomes virtually impossible when public schools are peddling junk food throughout the school day," said CSPI (Center for Science in the Public Interest) nutrition policy director Margo G. Wootan. "Many parents who send their kids off with lunch money in the morning have no clue that it can be so readily squandered on Coke, Doritos, and HoHos."

Despite the financial pressures on school systems that lead them to sell junk food in the first place, some schools are voluntarily setting higher nutrition standards for vending machine foods. As it happens, those school districts are doing well financially by doing good—they are not experiencing a drop-off in revenue by switching to healthier foods.

Enjoying an occasional calorie-rich treat doesn't make anyone obese or overweight, but because these foods are so heavily advertised, it makes overconsumption of these foods more likely. The government should reconsider allowance of advertisement of these products. While these sales help boosts the economy in one way, it takes billions of dollars away otherwise—making people sick, sluggish, and less agile. Healthy food restaurants should get promoted and supported by our system. All vending machine contents must be replaced with better choices.

4. Physical inactivity

In the last century, about 30 percent of people's energy was used on the physical labor and home duties. Today this is just 1 percent. The human muscle power has become unnecessary. Television, video games, and computer entertainment have replaced outdoor work and play as the major leisure time activity.

There will be more and more entertainment with Internet, television, and phones, and people will get more and more physically inactive.

What do we do?

Our life has now created the need for fitness and weight management, and if we want to live, feel and look better, we are left with no choice but to either go to the gym or participate in some kind of other physical activity.

I am afraid that with further technology development we will lose even that 1 percent of the physical labor at home or work. Scientists are presently thinking about robotic technologies and implementing it not only at our workplaces but also at home. Probably robots will be taking the dishes out from our dishwashers, washing our clothes, and cleaning our homes. What's left for us? Maybe we will learn how to type really, really fast or move our eyes quicker from TV to the computer monitor.

5.   Eating behaviors

What controls our eating behaviors? What happens when we get hungry?

Natural reactions of our body demand for food through gastric contractions of our stomach and digestive tract. This forces us to go and search for food. *Hunger* is triggered by the stomach hormone *ghrelin*, chemical and nervous signals in the brain, and other influencing factors such as weather, exercise, sex hormones, physical and mental illnesses, and others.

Many people assume that the amount of the food they eat depends on the sizes of their stomachs, and if they start controlling their portions, their stomach shrinks. But in reality, it is not the size of the stomach that changes as we change our eating habits, but the natural responses of the body's hunger. Our stomach can only shrink during prolonged starvations and usually remains the same size regardless of how much we eat. It slightly stretches when we *over*eat, but as soon as food is digested, it returns back to normal. Someone who decides to eat less may still feel hungry after the meals for a few days but eventually the body's hunger adapts quickly to changes in food intake. Later, large portions may even make that person feel uncomfortably full.

Hunger can be also triggered by the nutrient deficiencies in the blood. If something essential is missing in the blood, the body's hunger will force us to search for food.

When people go on restricted diets, food deprivation leads to hunger and stomach readaptation where at some point later hunger can return with "revenge" and can lead to overeating trying to make up for lost calories during deprivation. As the stomach capacity adapts to small meals, it can also quickly adapt back to larger ones.

Over the past few decades, the serving sizes in many fast-food restaurants have doubled. While this became good money-wise, it dramatically elevated the obesity problem.

Hunger is not the only signal that determines whether a person will eat. *Appetite* can also initiate the process of eating. The difference between hunger and appetite is that hunger is our natural life-or-death striving for survival while the appetite is rather emotional. A person can experience appetite without being hungry—smelling or seeing tasty foods can quickly stimulate one's appetite. Stress, on the other hand, can prevent a person from having an appetite, which eventually suppresses his hunger too.

Many other factors can trigger appetite:

- Seasonal foods and drinks. Many people like to eat or drink hot foods in cold weather or cold foods or drinks in hot weather
- Cultural or religious orientations
- Companionships
- Learned preferences (for example, having a dessert after each meal)
- Social interactions
- Stress
- Happiness
- Some forms of illnesses
- Flu
- Drugs
- Hormones and hormone imbalances
- Appetite stimulants or depressants
- What suppresses the hunger?

During each meal, at some point, the brain receives messages that enough food has been eaten. Those messages can come from different sources: stomach being full, enough of necessary nutrients, hormonal balance reached, emotional satisfaction, and others. After the brain detects those responses, it "commands" us to stop eating by suppressing our hunger. While the hunger and its unpleasant sensation is gone, we do other things in life—study, work, participate in physical and other activities, concentrate our attention on our feelings, emotional growth, etc. After a certain time, the digestive tract signals our brain for more food, and we start searching for food and eat again.

The amount of time between each meal depends on what we eat and how much. Researchers have found that foods high in fiber or water (or fiber with water) or even foods puffed with air suppress the appetite longer.

A meal providing protein may also quickly lend a feeling of fullness, and this explains the popularity of high-protein diets. Fat and protein combined together can trigger the release of a hormone produced by the intestine that slows stomach emptying and prolongs the feeling of fullness after each meal.

Source: Frances Sizer, Ellie Whitney "Nutrition Concepts and Contoversies" 2006. Some parts rephrased for easier reading and added with more information.

CHAPTER 18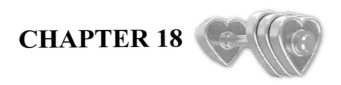

WHERE TO GET THAT ENERGY?

Most people I interview on their first visit to the gym complained on the lack of energy. "No energy to work, no energy to do home duties, no energy to exercise, no energy to even eat." It was bad enough to hear this from people who were in their late forties or fifties, but the worst of all was to hear such statements from youngsters and those who were not even twenty-five years old. How can you not have energy being so young? This is the age to be curious, spontaneous, and persuasive.

Many people think that the main reason for not having energy are their wrong eating habits or lack of exercise. While those things can be helpful, they are not the main reasons.

Our energy always starts in our minds. It is the state of our mind that creates our desires to do things. If we are not motivated, we will not do those things, no matter what we eat and how much we exercise.

Other people hope that supplements and boosting-energy solutions will help them to be energetic in life, while inside of their minds they are thinking down. The power of our mind is much stronger that any vitamins or energy drinks. Nothing will ever give you energy if you first don't try to find that energy inside of your thoughts. Only then supplements, food, and exercise can be helpful.

All the energy starts from our thinking. The body has no control over our mind, and only our thoughts possess the energy that we all are looking for.

Feeling down and concentrating on bad things always takes the energy away. Everyone of us sometimes gets caught on something bad throughout the day, and this can make us feel that we are losing our energy. But the willpower allows us not to get distracted by those things so we can keep our energy for doing things that we enjoy.

Of course, good-quality food, exercise, adequate rest, and fun are a big help to how energized we feel. But if our thoughts are refocused on the bad things, we will never be motivated to eat right, exercise, or feel at peace to rest.

CHAPTER 19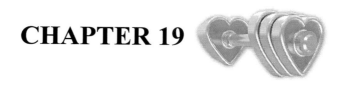

EXERCISE AND AGE

As much as 50 percent of the decline in physiological functions—weak muscles, stiff joints, low energy levels—are a result of inactivity and not the normal consequence of age. Most degenerative diseases associated with aging are the results of *not using the body*. If we exercise throughout our lives, many diseases may be prevented, and certain conditions may be reversed.

A report published in the *Circulation* journal of the American Heart Association concluded that middle-aged men were able to regain the cardiovascular levels that they had in their twenties. Even after thirty years of aging and living a relatively sedentary lifestyle, men were able to recover and maintain substantial fitness. The type of exercise was not as important as its *consistency*. After six months of regular exercise, the test subjects were able to reverse the aging process, boost their aerobic power by 15 percent, lower cholesterol, improve blood pressure, reduce heart attack risk, and enhance a feeling of well-being.

"Moderate amounts of exercise for one hour, four to five times a week can turn back the aging clock thirty years for middle-aged men," they stated.

It is not a surprise that after thirty-five it is harder to lose weight, gain muscles, or build strength. Your weight loss program can turn to an endless battle of starvation and exhausting workouts. You may also notice that whatever you were doing for a number of years is no longer effective: you are eating the same, exercising the same but still gaining weight. You may feel that you have reached a dead end plateau. How frustrating can this be?

What is the problem? Slow metabolism? Could be, but not only! The problem also lies in loss of hormones or a process—*menopause*. For women it begins anytime from midthirties to your late forties. For men it occurs around ages forty to fifty. Menopause starts slowly but progressively grows and can lead to serious health problems. Some of these problems are bone density loss, mood swings, loss of interest in sex, anger, and much more.

Does menopause affect men in the same way? Not necessarily. Men's menopause period is shorter than women's and has a little bit different effect on them: difficulties in gaining muscles, strength reduction, loss of interest in sex, growing potbelly, depression, and some others.

Hormones are produced by our body in the glands. If we take care of our body from a young age, the menopause period can be thrown away for much later years. Everything we do affects production of these hormones.

What exactly does our body need to fight menopause?

First of all, we need to learn how to manage stress in our life. In other words—build a positive attitude, self-esteem, confidence, and most importantly, control our emotions.

Second, we need to exercise. A properly designed fitness program can do 90 percent of work in that area. When we exercise, our body releases happy and other hormones. When we are happy, we do positive things, which make us even happier.

Third, we need to make some adjustments in eating habits. Certain foods promote hormone production while others do the opposite.

And *fourth*, we need to have quality sleep. Ninety percent of our hormones are "refilled" while we sleep. Lack of sleep not only exhausts hormones but can also lead to many other health problems.

A low level of estrogen in women is believed to be the main cause of unwanted symptoms like hot flashes, memory loss, or insomnia, but also the cause of more dangerous consequences like osteoporosis or even heart attacks.

For women it is very difficult to adjust this new stage in life. The first of many causes that set off early menopause symptoms is an *ovarian failure*. Women may either have ovaries that stop functioning well or do not produce enough hormones that are needed to ovulate.

There are three main choices when deciding on menopause treatments: synthetic hormones, bio-identical hormones, and natural herbs.

1. **Synthetic hormones/hormone replacement therapy**
   The hormones taken in HRT (hormone replacement therapy) are not molecularly the same as the hormones in your body. They don't balance your hormone level as much as they "turn off" the symptoms of menopause.

2. **Bio-identical hormones**
   These hormones are made in a lab and are molecularly the same as the hormones in your body. They are made from plants, and they focus on balancing your hormone levels.

3. **Natural herbs for menopause** (the best choice!)
   The menopause natural remedies (see table 3) contain phytohormones or plant hormones. These hormones are not the same as the hormones in our body, but they give the body hormonelike effects. Because herbs don't contain actual estrogen but phytoestrogen, they are also thought to help protect against cancer.

   Among other benefits, herbs can reduce hot flashes and night sweats and other symptoms of menopause.

Table 3. Best Natural Sources for Menopause

HERBS & VITAMINS	SYMPTOMS TREATED
Black Cohosh	Hot Flashes, Night Sweats, Vaginal Dryness, Depression, Cramps
Dong Quai	Night Sweats, Hot Flashes, Headaches, Vaginal Dryness, Digestive Problems
Feverfew	Migraines
Chasteberry	Hot Flashes, Irregular Periods, Depression, Tender Breasts
Licorice Root	Depression, Fatigue, Irregular Periods, Breast Tenderness, Yeast Infections, Digestive Issues
Alfalfa	Hot Flashes, Night Sweats, Digestive Problems
Vitamin D	PMS Symptoms, Osteoporosis
Calcium & Magnesium	Insomnia, Osteoporosis
Flaxseeds & Flaxseed Oil	Hot Flashes, Night Sweats, Vaginal Dryness, Digestive Issues

Source: Estrogen Source

CHAPTER 20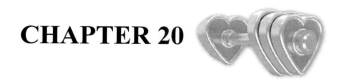

CANCER

In memory of one of my best high school students Iana Kalei

O nly in 2007 over 12 million new cancer cases and 7.6 million cancer deaths were estimated worldwide.

Every time I think about this number, I get disturbed when I compare it to the number of people living in my city, Toronto—one of the largest cities in the world. We have approximately 2.5 million living in the central area, so 7.6 million equals to 3 cities of Toronto.

Just think about it—20,000 people will die from cancer today or about 800 people within the next hour.

Just in United States alone, approximately 1.5 million new cancer cases and over half a million deaths from cancer were projected in 2009. The number of new cancer cases in Canada was expected to approach 171,000 in 2009, which represents approximately 470 Canadians diagnosed each day with some form of cancer. This represents an increase of 4,600 newly diagnosed cases and 1,500 deaths compared to 2008.

In *economically developed* countries, the three most commonly diagnosed cancers in men are prostate, lung, and colon cancer. Among women, they are breast, colon, and lung cancer.

Cancer doesn't feel sorry for anyone and doesn't discriminate if the person is rich or poor, nice or not, famous or unknown. Anyone can get it.

Even though we don't have the cure for cancer yet, everyone can do a lot to prevent this deadly disease by learning about it and passing this knowledge to others. Let's start from the beginning:

Normally, genes inside of each cell order it to grow, work, and reproduce. But sometimes these instructions get mixed up, causing the cells to form *lumps or tumors*, or spread through the bloodstream and lymphatic system to other parts of the body.

Tumors can be either *benign* (noncancerous) or *malignant* (cancerous).

Benign tumor cells stay in one place in the body and are usually not life threatening.

Malignant tumor cells are able to invade nearby tissues and spread to other parts of the body. Cancer cells that spread to other parts of the body are called *metastases*.

The first sign that a malignant tumor has spread (metastasized) is often swelling of the nearby lymph nodes, but cancer can metastasize to almost any part of the body. It is important to find malignant tumors as early as possible.

Cancers are named after the part of the body where they start. For example, cancer that starts in the bladder but spreads to the lung is called bladder cancer with lung metastases.

Carcinogen is a substance or agent that can cause cancer.

Cancer develops in four stages:

Stage 1: Exposure to a carcinogen

Stage 2: Entry of the carcinogen into a cell

Stage 3: Initiation—altering of the cellular genetic material by the carcinogen

Stage 4: Enhancement of cancer development by *promoters*, involving several more steps before the cell begins to multiply out of control; tumor formation

Stage 1 is the most important one because if we avoid the exposure to carcinogens, we will be able to control cancer. Most people can control that stage to a degree of their knowledge about carcinogens and also to the level of their self-awareness (many know that doing certain things can cause the cancer but still continue doing them).

Carcinogens can be found in multiple products that we use every day, including our food. Here are the most popular ones:

- *Formaldehyde.* This stuff is commonly used as a preservative in many household products, glue in particleboard, and in plywood furniture.
- *Paradichlorobenzene.* Found in toilet bowl cleaners and can cause harm to the central nervous system.
- *Perchloroethylene.* Commonly found in dry cleaning fluid, spot removers, and carpet cleaners.
- *Pesticides.* Used to control bugs and other vermin. They are loaded with carcinogens, including sodium 2, 4-dichlorophenoxyacetate. Overexposure has been associated with *lymphoma* and *leukemia.*
- *Tobacco smoke.* A well-known carcinogen that can harm you even if you don't smoke but are simply exposed to it.
- *City smog.* A well-known fact that the air we breathe has numerous carcinogens.

Many consumer products such as deodorants, soap bars, toothpaste, hair sprays, detergents, and makeup products contain carcinogens. While each product may only contain a small amount of cancer-causing agents, most of us use these products every day. Rolling a deodorant under the arms after a shower prevents odor, and antiperspirants effectively block sweat ducts. But at what price?

The list below consists of only some common consumer products that contain carcinogenic materials. These materials are usually hidden in the small prints of the product's bottles or packages.

Bath and beauty products

- *Dove Beauty Bar*: It's 99% water, but watch out for that other 1%. It includes *quaternium 15* and *formaldehyde*, known carcinogens, as well as irritants to the skin, eyes, and mucous membranes.
- *Johnson's Baby Shampoo and Magic Lotion*: Contains carcinogens *quaterium 15*, FD&C RED 40, which can cause dermatitis.
- *Crest Tarter Control Toothpaste*: This best selling toothpaste contains *saccharin* and *phenol fluoride*.
- *Talcum powder*: Talc, the main ingredient, is a carcinogen that increases the risk of ovarian cancer. Use corn starch instead.
- *Cover Girl Replenishing Natural Finish Make Up (foundation)*: This makeup includes *BHA, talc, titanium dioxide, triethanolamine*. These interact with nitrites to form nitrosamines and lanolin, which is often contaminated with *DDT* and other carcinogenic pesticides.
- *Organic Products:* 365 Organic Shower Gel, Alba Passion Fruit Body Wash, NutriBiotic Super Power Gel, JASON Pure Natural & Organic, Giovanni Organic Cosmetics, Kiss My Face, Nature's Gate Organics : 1,4-Dioxane.

  Look for the label "USDA Organic" when buying organic products made in USA or if this product made in other country look for the similar label.

Household cleaning products

- *Tide & Cheer Laundry Detergent*: Our favorite detergent contains *trisodium nitrilotriacetate*, a carcinogen.
- *Lysol Disinfectant*: While it makes the air sweet smelling, it contains the *dioxin*.

Food products

- *Oscar Meyer beef hot dogs*: Labeled ingredients in this American favorite include *nitrite*, which interacts with meat amines to form nitrosamines. Tests have also found other carcinogens such as *benzene hexachloride, dacthal, dieldrin, DDT, heptachlor, hexachlorobenzene*, and *lindane*. If you have to eat hot dogs, look for ones without nitrates in them.
- *Whole milk*: Certain containers contain *DDT, dieldrin, heptachlor, hexachlorobenzene, recombinant bovine growth hormone* and *Igf-1*. All of these increase the chances of getting breast, colon and prostate cancers. **Look for RBGH-free organic milk.**
- *Bottled Water*. A recent test has found the amount of a potential carcinogen known as *bromate* exceeded international standards in nearly 9 percent of bottled water products.

Seoul's environment ministry says seven out of 79 products tested contained up to point-0-2-2-5 milligrams per liter of bromate, surpassing the world's standard of point-0-1.

Bromate is a chemical that forms during the ozone sterilization processes used to kill microbes in drinking water.

The ministry says manufacturers of these products are switching to alternative sterilizing methods and were urged to voluntarily retrieve products already distributed.

The government is expected to adopt the international bromate standard for drinking water later this year.

- *McDonalds, Burger King, Kentucky Fried Chicken (KFC) and Friendly's Meals: PhIP*, a chemical that can increase a person's risk of developing cancer.

Pet products

- *Zodiac flea collars*: These dog collars include the labeled carcinogen *propoxur*. Try Trader Joe's herbal flea collars instead.

Other products

- *Carpets*: Some carpets are made or finished with petrolatum-based chemicals. These chemicals can "outgas" into the home. *Petrolatum* is believed to be a human carcinogen.
- *Some toys* made in China are reportedly being manufactured with a dangerous metal. An Associated Press investigation revealed high levels of *cadmium*, which is a known cancer-inducing agent. The AP tested 103 items—such as charm bracelets and pendants—bought in four states, including New York, late last year, and found 12 percent of them contained at least 10 percent cadmium. In one instance, levels were at 91 percent by weight. Testing also showed some toys easily shed the metal, raising additional concerns about exposure. Manufacturers turned to cadmium as an inexpensive alternative after calls increased for companies to abandon lead. But much like lead, research shows cadmium can hinder brain development in young children. The Centers for Disease Control's list of the 275 most hazardous substances in the environment ranks cadmium at number seven. A spokesman for the U.S. Consumer Product Safety Commission says the agency is opening an investigation and will take action as quickly as possible.

Source: www.encognitive.com

Of course, in today's world, it is nearly impossible to protect ourselves from all carcinogens, but minimizing the exposure is the key to reducing chances of getting cancer. For example, occasional use of your favorite shampoo will not kill you, but when you use it, try minimizing the time of it being on your body to seconds and prolong the time of being under the water trying to wash it off to minutes and not the other way around.

Some things that we do in life may not initialize cancer immediately but help to develop it over time. They are called cancer *promoters*. Among strongest cancer promoters are the following:

- High-fat diet
- Excessive alcohol intake
- Contaminated food intake
- High salt intake
- High sugar intake
- Low complex carbohydrate/fiber intake
- Low calcium intake
- Stress
- Sedentary lifestyle
- Smoking

These things work assisting carcinogens to initialize their actions. Nobody knows how much exactly is enough for the cell to get mixed up and start developing cancer, but if we put a substantial effort in protecting our own lives, we can significantly reduce the amounts of the exposure to carcinogens.

Things that we do to prevent cancer are called *antipromoters*. Antipromoters oppose cancer development. They are not only effective in cancer prevention but also work in treatment stages. Most powerful of them are the following:

- Vigorous exercise
- Balanced diet
- Positive attitude, mediation, and stress management
- Fresh air

Eliminating cancer promoters is strengthening the effect of antipromoters and vice versa. Become a label reader and do your own research. Don't immediately fall for the attractive commercials. There are many things they don't want you to know. Before you put something on the shelf in your household, read the small prints and research every ingredient of every product you buy.

CHAPTER 21

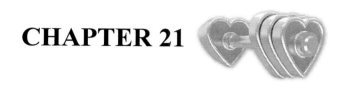

CANCER AND EXERCISE

An international team of cancer experts from Canada, United States, and Europe were brought together by Cancer Care Ontario, Canada to review scientific evidence regarding physical activity and variety of forms of cancer, including colon, breast, prostate, lung, testes, and endometrium or the uterus.

"Regular physical activity can reduce the risk of colon and breast cancer," a new Canadian study has found. The study's main recommendation—*adopt a moderate to vigorous regimen of physical activity to help prevent the often fatal disease.* Regular exercise is expected to become a key part of cancer prevention.

Cancer Care Ontario, which commissioned the study, immediately adopted the new measure, the first such public health recommendation regarding cancer prevention in Canada.

"We've had it for heart disease, and we've had it for diabetes," said Dr. Richard Schabas, Ontario's former chief medical officer of health. *"It is a well established part of the public psyche, but it has not been for cancer because the evidence has been slow in coming."*

"We've not had any public health recommendations from the field of cancer to link the benefits of physical activity to reduce your risk of getting cancer," added Dr. Schabas, head of preventive oncology for Cancer Care Ontario. *"So for Canada, this is a significant step forward in public policy around cancer prevention."*

"It is a good-news message for the public in terms of their own personal responsibility . . ." said Pat Kelly, a spokesperson with the Cancer Advocacy Coalition of Canada.

The report that found the evidence suggesting physical activity helps prevent colon cancer is very convincing and most likely a benefit for breast cancer as well. It also concluded that regular exercise may reduce the risk of getting prostate cancer.

Though more research is needed, Dr. Schabas said the success of exercising to prevent colon or breast cancer is primarily related to hormonal changes in the body caused by regular workouts. *"People should engage in at least 30-45 minutes of **moderate to vigorous** physical activity **most days**,"* he said. *"Moderate to vigorous workouts differ based on age."*

Source: *Toronto Star*

CHAPTER 22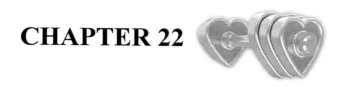

SMOKING AND EXERCISE

A cigarette contains about 4,000 chemicals, many of which are poisonous. Some of the worst ones are the following:

- *Nicotine.* A deadly poison
- *Arsenic.* Used in rat poison
- *Methane.* A component of rocket fuel
- *Ammonia.* Found in floor cleaners
- *Cadmium,* Used in batteries
- *Carbon monoxide.* Part of car exhaust
- *Formaldehyde.* Used to preserve body tissue
- *Butane.* Lighter fluid

Statistics still demonstrate how hard it is to give up smoking. If you smoke and think of quitting and start exercising regularly, then plan on starting exercising first. Quitting smoking is much harder commitment; exercising will help you along the way.

Smokers who take vigorous exercise while trying to kick the habit have more chance of success, a study has found.

Fear of gaining weight is one of the main reasons why women afraid to quit smoking, but research from US behavioral experts

201

found that exercise helped women stay smoke free. It found that the exercising women were twice as likely to stay off the cigarettes. 20% of the exercising women managed to remain cigarette free after the 12 weeks, compared with only one in 10 of the non-exercisers. The study did not use nicotine replacement patches.

Doctors should encourage smokers to exercise, as exercise is clearly proven to curb the cravings for cigarettes.

Source: BBC News

CHAPTER 23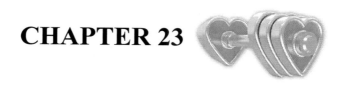

EXERCISE AND SEX DRIVE

S.H. *"I have gained approximately fifty pounds, mostly in my belly, and have no energy. My wife complains because I have no interest in sex. I tried to get Viagra, but my physician told me that I needed to control my weight first and get in shape."*

New research indicates that those who have sex three and more times per week look 10-12 years younger. Sex is an excellent workout, and if it's long enough, it can be compared to a good aerobics. During sex, your heart rate can reach the point of 180 beats per minute—approximately the same as world-class athletes have when they compete. The researchers also noticed that sex not only helped people to look younger. Most of those were also romantic, emotional, and happy in love. *"Regular exercise, well-balanced eating, moderate consumption of alcohol, sex, and positive emotions are the keys to a good health,"* researches stated.

Sex is one of the best preventative medicines of all.

Here are the different benefits of sex on the different health and psychological aspects of our lives:

Stress

A big health benefit of sex is lower blood pressure and overall stress reduction, according to researchers from Scotland who reported their findings in the journal *Biological Psychology*. They studied 24 women and 22 men who kept records of their sexual activity. Then researchers subjected them to stressful situations—such as speaking in public and doing verbal arithmetic—and noted their blood pressure response to stress. Those who had intercourse had better responses to stress than those who engaged in other sexual behaviors or abstained.

Another study published in the same journal found that frequent intercourse was associated with lower diastolic blood pressure in cohabiting participants. Yet other research found a link between partner hugs and lower blood pressure in women.

Immunity

Good sexual health may mean better physical health. Having sex once or twice a week has been linked with higher levels of an antibody called immunoglobulin A or IgA, which can protect you from getting colds and other infections. Scientists at Wilkes University in Wilkes-Barre, Pa., took samples of saliva, which contain IgA, from 112 college students who reported the frequency of sex they had. Those in the "frequent" group—once or twice a week—had higher levels of IgA than those in the other three groups—who reported being abstinent, having sex less than once a week, or having sex very often, three or more times weekly.

Cardiovascular Health

The researchers found that having sex twice or more a week reduced the risk of fatal heart attack by half for the men, compared with those who had sex less than once a month.

Cholesterol

Sex balances out the good to bad cholesterol ratio, as well as reduces the overall cholesterol count.

Pain

As the hormone oxytocin surges, endorphins increase, and pain declines. So if your headache, arthritis pain, or PMS symptoms seem to improve after sex, you can thank those higher oxytocin levels.

In a study published in the *Bulletin of Experimental Biology and Medicine,* 48 volunteers who inhaled oxytocin vapor and then had their fingers pricked lowered their pain threshold by more than half.

Prostate Cancer Risk

Frequent ejaculations, especially in men in their 20-s, may reduce the risk of prostate cancer later in life, Australian researchers reported in the *British Journal of Urology International.* When they followed men diagnosed with prostate cancer and those without, they found no association of prostate cancer with the number of sexual partners as the men reached their 30s, 40s, and 50s. But they found men who had five or more ejaculations weekly while in their 20s reduced their risk of getting prostate cancer later by a third.

Another study, reported in the *Journal of the American Medical Association,* found that frequent ejaculations, 21 or more a month, were linked to lower prostate cancer risk in older men, as well, compared with less frequent ejaculations of four to seven monthly.

Hormonal Balance

DHEA (a hormone produced by adrenal gland) is secreted during sex throughout the body. During orgasms or just before ejaculation, the level of DHEA in the bloodstream is five times its normal level. High levels of DHEA have been associated with longevity, enhanced libido, building muscle mass, and warding off depression.

Sex also improves other factors of our well-being:

Sleep

The oxytocin released during orgasm promotes sleep, according to research. Getting enough sleep has been linked with a host of other good things, such as maintaining a healthy weight and blood pressure.

Intimacy

Oxytocin, so-called *love hormone*, helps us bond and build trust. Researchers from the University of Pittsburgh and the University of North Carolina evaluated 59 premenopausal women before and after warm contact with their husbands and partners ending with hugs. They found that the more contact, the higher the oxytocin levels.

"Oxytocin allows us to feel the urge to nurture and to bond," Britton says.

Higher oxytocin has also been linked with a feeling of generosity. So if you're feeling suddenly more generous toward your partner than usual, credit the love hormone.

Self-Esteem

Boosting self-esteem was one of 237 reasons people have sex, collected by University of Texas researchers and published in the *Archives of Sexual Behavior.*

"One of the reasons people say they have sex is to feel good about themselves," "Great sex begins with self-esteem. If the sex is loving, connected, and what you want, it raises it."

Source: www.webmd.com/sex-relationships

Testosterone

Male sex drive is maintained by testosterone, a hormone produced primarily in the testes. The level of testosterone increases when men lose fat and gain muscles and vice versa.

What exactly does testosterone do to the body?

It elevates the nervous system activity level, enhancing *alertness*, *curiosity*, and *social interaction*. Loss of interest in sex could be a sign of low testosterone level in men. Researchers found that sexual dysfunction is more likely among those with poor physical health. Physically inactive people had negative experience with sexual relationships. "Your physical health affects your ability to perform sexually," they stated.

"Regular vigorous exercise, such as walking at least two miles or burning 300 calories a day, would lower the risk of impotence," concluded doctors at the New England Research Institute.

University of California also studied sedentary middle-age men: "One hour per day with three times per week of exercise would improve sexual function, more frequent sex and orgasm and greater satisfaction."

Sex is similar to cardiovascular activity. It requires endurance. Since cardiovascular exercise improves endurance, it also improves performance in sex. Sex will be longer, more frequent, and more satisfactory. Besides cardiovascular activities, weight training exercises focused on pelvis, buttocks, and upper leg muscles also can be very beneficial too. They increase blood flow necessary to maintain erection.

Regular exercise improves sex performance not only in men but also greatly in women. At the University of Texas, women between the ages 18 and 34 were studied in two groups—those who exercised for 20 minutes and the sedentary group. Both groups were proposed to watch an X-rated movie. After measuring the blood flow in women's genital tissue, it appeared that vaginal responses were 169 percent greater after exercising.

Exercise improves gland's functions in men for testosterone production, but the actual increase of testosterone level is happening during sleep or rest. This explains why men perform in sex better in the morning. Good night's sleep, well-balanced diet in combination with aerobic and weight-bearing exercises are crucial keys to improving one's sex drive.

CHAPTER 24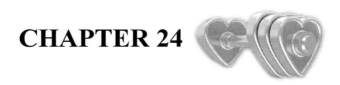

FAILURE OF MODERN MEDICINE

G.S. *I immigrated with my family to Canada about twenty years ago. What I've heard about Canadian medicine was that it was one of the most advanced medicines in the world and equipped with latest technologies. First couple of years living in Canada I felt very proud being protected by this medicine and felt secured about my family in case if anyone of us gets ill.*

I was very naïve and foolish. Terrible things happen, and it happened to me. While going through court procedures in order to get my landed papers, I've drawn myself into nervous breakdown, and this terribly affected my digestive system. One day, walking from English class, I started to experience shortage of breath and dizziness to the point that I had to stop and hold on to the tree. After a while, I somehow made it home and next morning called my family doctor. I explained to her my situation, and when she arrived, she asked me some questions. One of those questions was what I was doing last night. I told her that I went for my usual workout at the gym, and then went to the sauna . . .

As soon as she heard word sauna, *she exploded: "I always tell my patients, keep your bodies hydrated, drink a lot of water!" She did not give me anything and only recommended to drink more water.*

Next day while drinking more water all day I started to feel worse. I called my doctor again, and she came to my home for a second time. But this time I started asking her questions:

"Maybe it happens because I have a digestion problem?"
"Maybe!" she answered.
"Or a heart condition?"
"Maybe."
"Or low hemoglobin?"
"Maybe!"

After about ten more maybes I gave up. I realized that there is no help for me here. I thanked her for coming and said that I was feeling better.

Next morning I asked my friend to help me to go see another doctor. Holding me under my arm he took me into a local walk-in clinic. After about hour-and-a-half wait in line, a doctor took me in and started asking me the same questions I heard two days ago. After I answered them, he concluded, "I don't know what is wrong with you, but we need to do a full medical examination! You have to go to few hospitals for several tests . . . Altogether it will take about two weeks!" "OK," I thought to myself, "how am I going to manage that if I can hardly stand on my feet?"

Trying hard to put myself together I somehow made it through all those medical examinations. Pipes from all directions of my body, needles, electrodes, all sorts of drinking solutions nearly killed me. "Nothing is wrong with you!" concluded my new doctor after he saw my results and sent me back home. "This could be just some kind of stomach flu!" he said.

"The good news is that they didn't find anything, but the bad news is that I am still feeling awful!" I was thinking, and after I came home, I started to wait for my flu to be over.

Two more weeks later I had to call for an ambulance. My dizziness got so bad that I couldn't even go to the bathroom. My body was shaking most of the time, and I started to lose control. I lost thirty pounds and couldn't eat.

At the hospital, the nurse put me through new series of tests, and after receiving my results, the hospital doctor declared to me: "Nothing is wrong with you, darling. You can go home!" After I tried to explain to him my situation, he politely advised me to see my family physician and that was it.

Ambulance after ambulance from one hospital to another didn't bring any results. I lost forty-five pounds altogether and started to lose hope to recover.

*During the next **two years,** few more doctors looked at me but still didn't find anything. One of them tried to suggest antidepressants, but I refused. I realized that my life is going to an end and decided to spend the rest of it doing something that I loved. This was my exercise. I said to myself: "I'd rather die running than lying in my bed." Step by step somehow I made it to go outside. The whole world was spinning in my head, but I finally stepped on the grass. I looked around, took off my shoes, and "ran" expecting to collapse after a few meters. But amazingly, I didn't fall and actually in a couple of minutes started to feel that my moves were getting more stable.*

My run didn't last very long, but when I came home, some positive thoughts have crossed my mind. Day after day, minute by minute, I slowly "climbed up" to a ten-minute of continuous very, very slow jog. My weight started to go up, and the earth stopped spinning in my head. I was coming back to life.

Another six months later I pulled it through and decided to go to my last family doctor to share with him the story of my miraculous recovery.

Sadly, he did not believe me that the exercise was the actual cause of my recovery. Throughout our whole conversation he was sarcastically looking at me and in few minutes cut me off: "I am sorry, but I have another patient!"

....

Luba Grup, coauthor, *From early years, as long as I remember, I was always sick, constantly taking antibiotics, painkillers, and other drugs. Sinusitis infections, laryngitis, cysts, pneumonia, and many other illnesses were my best friends.*

That's how it lasted for many years including my life in marriage. But looking at me, nobody could ever tell or recognize how sick I was—I was a very slim girl and had a nice body. My naturally pale face was always covered with a lot of makeup.

Each of my three children was born healthy, but I had to fight for my life after each delivery. While some women try to lose weight after each baby, I was always trying to gain it, and besides all my previous health problems, I've got one more—lower back pain. I could not walk or stand for longer than five minutes, and most of my house duties I had to do sitting in a chair or stool. Having two babies and being alone in the house most of the time made my life extremely difficult. I was only twenty-two, but with all my physical problems, I felt like I was already eighty. Neither Extra Strength Tylenol nor any other painkillers help anymore. My family doctor's recommendations were prescribing more and more drugs. Each pill that I was taking eventually caused me new problems as side effects: nausea, diarrhea, dizziness, vomiting, etc.

I tried hard to get help from quite a few other doctors including emergency rooms at most local hospitals but was not successful. All doctors' advices always ended up with suggestions for more and more pills. I was even "convicted" by one doctor of having a mental disorder and was suggested to take antidepressants.

Hundreds of dollars spent on physiatrists and psychiatrists were a waste of time and money. I was running out of patience, and my life was slowly turning to hell for me. I knew that I had to do something different. Otherwise, I would just die.

My friend advised me to start exercising, but I did not take her suggestion seriously, and the assortment of my pills kept expanding.

Couple of years later I was diagnosed with brain tumor and was suggested for immediate surgery. Doctors told me that the end of that surgery was not a guaranteed success, and the consequences of it were unpredictable. They also advised that if I survive the surgery I may not be able to have any more children.

I really wanted to have another child. Risking my life, I postponed my surgery after a delivery.

They say that during pregnancy the mother's body is the strongest. I do believe that because during all pregnancy I was feeling much better. But as soon as I delivered the baby, all my health problems jumped right back on me bringing even more issues. New tumor in my nose, previous tumor in my brain, and as it appeared a little later, a new tumor in my uterus. Surgery after surgery, poisonous pills, needles, and IVs.

But this wasn't all. My marriage started to fall apart, and besides all my physical problems, I fell into a depression. Doctors were completely useless—pills, pills, and more pills, and now even stronger pills, antidepressants, and sleeping ones. My body weight went down to 102 lb. with my height of 5'7". When I was walking on the street I was afraid that the wind will drop me down on the ground. Somebody joked that I should consider carrying something heavy in my pockets.

I lasted another year like that. Life was a torture. Pain sometimes would reach such a degree that regular pills didn't help. I had to take something much more serious. I lost any interest to live. It felt like a dead end. There was no help from anyone including the doctors.

Another surgery! This time removing the tumor in my uterus. The conversation with my doctor who did that surgery ended up the same as with any of them before him—more prescription drugs and this time with injections of hormones and anabolic steroids.

This has reached my limit—I decided to give up on the help of all the doctors and save myself on my own. I completely ignored all the medical recommendations, threw away all my pills, and joined the gym. On my first fitness assessment, my trainer told me that I was underweight and all my muscles including my back were extremely weak.

I've decided to give up on buying anything new for myself including my clothes and signed up for personal training lessons. Slowly from 2 lb. dumbbells, one sit-up, and one halfway pushup, I started to feel better and better every day. I've also learned how to eat good food.

For the first time, it was very difficult. I have never exercised before, and doing this was new and strange for me. But I noticed the difference, and my friends noticed it too. I started to smile and look more alive even without my makeup. My weight started to go up. My strength and energy levels grew too. I even started to feel confident about myself, and my depression began to disappear. I gave up smoking.

I realized that life began to shape up for me all over again, and everything around me started to give me joy. I wanted to live and be happy.

And this all was done by me only and without any doctors. I feel so proud of my accomplishment, and I wanted to pass this alone to everyone.

•••

B.K. *In the middle of the night, my wife had a severe stomach pain, and at 3:00 a.m. I had to rush her to the hospital. After we arrived and registered at the front desk, we were forwarded to one of the hospital cubicles where a male nurse came and started asking my wife questions. One of his questions was how severe my wife's pain was. She answered that it was hurting her a lot. The nurse pulled out his syringe, filled it with medicine, and injected it in my wife's arm while asking more questions.*

"Are you allergic to Demerol?" was one of those questions.

214

My wife answered, "Yes."

But it was too late. The medicine was already injected, and it was the Demerol—full syringe. I panicked and asked what we should do. "Oh, don't worry about it. Just stay here, watch her and call me if there is anything wrong," said the nurse smiling at me and left.

Right after he left, my wife's eyes started to roll up. I ran to front desk to call for the doctor. "All doctors are busy with other patients. Someone will come as soon as he is free," the front desk girl coldly answered.

I ran back to my wife and noticed that her body skin started to turn blue. I checked her pulse, and it was less than 40 beats per minute. She was shaking and moaning how cold she was. I told about this at the front desk, and the new nurse came in. She put my wife IVs trying to flush out the Demerol and covered my wife with warm blankets.

After the new nurse left, my wife went unconscious. I tried to wake her up but was unsuccessful. Her pulse kept going down. With eyes full of tears I went down on my knees praying for God for help. This was my only option. I don't remember everything what I said, but I offered God everything including my life for my wife's recovery.

Praying and trying to warm up my wife's hands and feet, almost one hour later, I noticed how she moved. I checked her heartbeat. It was above 40. "Thank you, God!" I almost yelled out loud and kept rubbing her hands. Another half hour later, she opened her eyes.

"What happened?" she asked. I didn't tell her. "Why do you look so worried?"

"Nothing. I just want to take you home," I answered.

When the doctor came and I told him about what happened, instead of being empathetic, he turned the conversation another way.

Even after I told him that the nurse asked the question about the allergies after the injection of the medicine, he pretended that he

didn't understand me. "Your wife is OK now, and you can go home"
were his last words.

....

TV CHCH NEWS Report

(This is a transcribed article from the news report above.)

Sara Carlin was beautiful, she played hockey, loved her part-time job
and graduated as Ontario Schuler. As she prepared for university, she
felt overwhelmed and talked to her doctor about stress. He prescribed
the antidepressant drug Paxil.

"She told her sister," Sarah's mother says, "that it just makes you not
worry. It's good! She liked that because she did not have any more
anxiety about anything. "

Sara changed. She quit hockey, lost her job, started experimenting
with drugs and alcohol, and took a medical lee from her first semester
off Western. She went back to her doctor, and he doubled her dose of
Paxil. That was when she went really down the hill.

"It looked like she kind of been on the computer and taking off her
makeup," her mother described. "And then she just stopped. She still
had makeup on her face and went out of the room. My husband had
been wiring some lights. So there was electrical cable, pliers . . .
She just cut a piece and then . . . in an instant . . . decided to kill
herself."

After Sara's death, Sarah's mother and a reporter saw a Canada
warning against prescribing Paxil to teens because of an increased
risk of suicides. They also learned that it is dangerous to suddenly
stop taking Paxil, something Sara did days before her death when she
lost her pills. Then they discovered the drug had other side effects.

"She wrote in one note that she started to feel worthless," her mother
says. "But she did not understand what was going on. Those were the
side effects of Paxil. If she had known and we had known, we could

deal with that. You're confused, you're having nightmares, you can't sleep, and you don't know why these things are happening to you."

From the label

Until further information is available, PAXIL (paroxetine hydrochloride) should not be used in children and adolescents under 18 years of age (ie. pediatric patients), due to a possible increased risk of suicide-related adverse events in this patient population.

Terence Young (Drug Safety Canada):

> *"Patients die taking prescription drugs all the time. In fact, prescription drugs are the fourth leading death in Canada and United States."*

Terence Young found Drug Safety Canada after his daughter Vanessa had a fatal heart attack. The fifteen-year-old was taking Prepulcid for bloating, but shouldn't have been because she also had an eating disorder. He said, "The potential benefit of drugs have to exceed the potential risk. For example, ordinary anxiety that student gets from exams. Why would you give someone a drug that has a potential to kill him for ordinary anxiety?"

Reporter:

> *"So this is what I picked up from Shoppers Drug Mart. This is what they give out to patients who come in with new prescriptions of Paxil and side effects listed include diarrhea, unusual tiredness, nausea, and the list goes on. Nothing to do with suicide or potential risky behavior, anything like that. So obviously we can't rely on our pharmacist for information that we need. How much information should we expect from our doctors? How much information do our doctors even really have?"*

After the first part of this show aired many people contacted the CHCHNEWS telling similar stories with similar personal experiences with prescription drugs.

The Carlins want to be the last family to lose their daughter because they didn't know the side effects and dangers of her medication.

<u>Most adverse drug reactions are never reported to the Health Canada.</u> *This system is voluntary and has been set up forty years ago after the society finally realized that Thalidomide was deforming babies. Maryann Murray reported her daughter's death herself: "She was put on the drug and then the drug dosage was increased and then thirteen days later she had sudden cardiac arrest and was dead. She just died in her sleep.*

Twenty-two-year-old Martha was prescribed Lithium for bipolar disorder. And it killed her because of contraindication listed in her medical records.

Maryann Murray:

> *"This reaction between lithium and low potassium, certainly between lithium and cardiac conditions had been known for a long time. But if every previous case had been reported, we'd understand how great the risk was."*

Terence Young:

> ***"Family doctors are not getting proper warnings, and patients are in many cases getting absolutely no warnings. And that's the key problem."***

*An inquest into the death of Terence Young's fifteen-year-old daughter Vanessa fruitlessly recommended that patients get information leaflets with warnings in bold with every prescription. Young says that at least half of all the prescription drugs have serious side effects including deaths, but he says **doctors don't read all the drugs' literature** and that's something that pharmacist David Yu has noticed in his role at the Institute for Safe Medication Practices. He says **doctors aren't always aware of drug alerts**. **"They either don't get it, what's coming in,** or physicians are too busy sometimes. **They don't read every single thing coming in."***

*According to regional coroner and former clinician Dr. Jack Stanborough, **doctors hold back information to keep from scaring the patient**.*

"I found that people would actually be not complying with therapy. They are so afraid of the medication that I had negative outcome simply because they were in effect overeducated."

"Health Canada is looking at making it mandatory to report adverse drug reactions and it's developing a searchable database on drug information so you can inform yourself. Victim families think that coroner's inquest is the answer to raising awareness about these issues," Lisa Hepfner.

*In this province, the coroner's inquest office holds between fifty and eighty inquests every year, but vast majority are mandatory like construction site deaths. Inquests bring a lot of public attention to an issue, but the coroner's office won't call a discretionary inquest **unless top doctors all agree** that a jury can make recommendations to prevent similar deaths.*

When twenty-two-year-old Martha died from a heart attack, a coroner classified her death as natural even though the evidence blamed the prescription drug Lithium. "Young, seemingly healthy people don't just die in the night. We may not understand why they died, but there has to be a reason," says Martha's mom Maryann.

Regional coroner Jack Stanborough says death by appropriate medical treatment is classified as natural. "Of 2,800 deaths across my desk every year, a great number of them have drugs involved in the deaths either direct cause of death or a contributing factor."

Once or twice a month he reports a death to Health Canada as a possible adverse drug reaction. He says every unusual death is investigated, but the inquests are relatively rare.

Oakville MP Terence Young has been trying to help the Carlins to get inquest into their daughter's Sara's suicide to raise awareness about the links between antidepressants and teen suicide. Both they and the Murrays have been turned down by the coroner's office.

"The coroner's office is simply not doing their job. Their slogan is "We speak for the dead to protect the living," says Terence Young. "But no one is speaking for Sara Carlin."

Regional coroner Jack Stanborough says, "Probably 2 or 3 times a day I get a letter, an email or a phone call saying I would like an inquest into my loved ones death."

Lisa Hepfner reports, "Many deaths in Ontario have not been properly investigated. There is now a proposed amendment for an oversight body in the coroner's office. A minister in charge of community's safety can also order an inquest and he's been asked to do that for Sara Carlin. But he says that's premature."

In an interview with Community Safety Minister Rick Bartolucci Lisa said, "In a meantime it's been more than a year, and people could still be dying from the same cause."

Rick Bartolucci: "The reality is that they haven't exhausted all the avenues open to them. That's why I am requesting, I'm asking, I am encouraging them, and I will help them to arrange that meeting with the chief coroner."

Since CHCH News began this investigation, the chief coroner office has agreed to meet with the Carlins to discuss their concerns. We also heard from the makers of "Paxil" GlaxoSmith clients says Paxil or paroxetine has been safely used by tens of millions of patients for fifteen years and all precautions are on the drug label. But what they don't say is that the drug label is not the sticker on the pill bottle. It is extensive information patients have to go looking for if they want to know more about what they are taking."

"Tens of thousands Canadians die every year from first reactions of prescriptions drugs," recent study conducted and announced on November 3 of 2008 on CHCH News channel. "Safeguards put into effect more than forty years ago are no longer up to the job."

Here we are, fooled again, who have decided to entrust our health and our lives into hands of our doctors, who we think know everything about health, but who are actually studying diseases rather than health in their medical schools. Who, after all, don't read labels on the products they prescribe, and even if they read—don't tell us about their side effects.

Head hurts, Tylenol, leg hurts, Tylenol, stomach hurts, also Tylenol. That's the common procedure of today's doctors. It takes too much time and effort to diagnose why the head hurts or what caused that stomach pain. Why bother? The patient is looking for immediate relief, and the fastest way to do it—give him painkillers. Who cares what happens after and who cares if that painkiller has side effects? Just make the patient's pain go away and you will be a hero in his eyes. Whether Tylenol helped the cause of the pain, neither the doctor, nor the patient will ever know. But who cares about this now? Go, go, go. Next, next, next. More patients per day—more money. And when the patient leaves the doctor's office, the doctor will never find out if his patient has improved or if he developed some further complications, and the next time will come with more pain. What happens then? Stronger painkillers.

Modern medicine is not interested in making us healthy. By doing so they would be losing their profits. Relying that modern medicine will ever start thinking of preventing our diseases is useless. Modern medicine is only good to suck the money out of government's pockets, health insurance's, and ours. The rest of the times our medical attention is limited to mostly "greets and treats" at doctors' offices and then dangerous drug prescriptions.

What people need now is a government push on more detailed preventative health education starting from kindergarten. Every child needs to develop good habits and learn how our body works, how to heal small problems without pills, and how to prevent degenerative diseases. Small problems are usually body warnings about coming big problems. We should never treat symptoms unless we know the cause.

Our body has protective mechanisms. It can heal itself and regenerate its parts, but we have to provide a good environment for it, and that environment is *proper food, peace of mind, an adequate rest, and physical activity.* This all must come from childhood. Bad habits developed at a young age follow people throughout their lives and in many cases never get changed. Supported by television and media, these bad habits became our culture. We learn them from generation to generation and accept it as normal.

Until the government finally realizes that it is cheaper for the country and better for people to work toward preventions rather than treatments of all the diseases, our health problem will exist. By the statistics, only 15 percent of the populations are health enthusiasts. The rest need guidance how to do it. We need television, radio, and Internet to be involved globally. We need our leaders to set examples of a better lifestyle and speak out about it frequently.

Unfortunately, many of our doctors are not those who are passionate about their profession but are those who could afford to take this education or those who were forced by their parents to study medicine for financial benefits in the future. Beware!

CHAPTER 25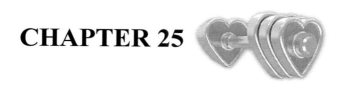

GYM BUSINESS—
CHICKEN FACTORY
(A Closer Look from the Inside)

W hen it comes to advertising, most gyms usually place pictures of young and good-looking people on their flyers and websites. Does everyone who wants to join the gym look like that? Sixty-five percent of people are now overweight, and this type of advertising can be very intimidating for those who are older and for those just looking to improve their health or getting into a little bit better shape. Looking at those flyers and websites, some people may assume: "Oh, no! Before I join the gym, I have to get in shape. See how those people look?" That is what I've heard from many people who have never been to a gym.

Even though the situation now has been changed somewhat and more of the "regular" population join gyms today, the mentality about gyms is still there—people feel intimidated by them.

We take it for granted. We (gym people) walk into a gym, any gym, and instantly we know what to do, how to do it, and where to go.

The reason, for people like us going to a gym (working in a gym) is second nature.

But let's think back to a time when it wasn't second nature. For me that was twenty-five years ago . . . before going to the gym regularly was part of my routine. In fact, I can remember very vividly my first experience: "I just don't want to look like a fool."

So I did the first thing that seemed to make sense . . . I lay down on a bench and began pushing some iron. The question is why did I do this? What would drive me to the bench when there were hundreds of other pieces of equipment to choose from? Let me go through the thought process (it was pretty short):

I had never been in a gym.
I knew I hated running on a treadmill.
I prefer to run outside.
All the other equipment were intimidating.

I had used barbells before, and I knew that I wouldn't look like a fool if I do it here too.

So let's not forget that most people don't feel comfortable in the gym. A lot of people are intimidated (one of the biggest reasons why people quit)! They have taken the first step, they joined your gym, now help them get the most out of it. Learn about them. Talk to them. Understand why they are there. Help them reach their goals!

But most gyms don't do any further steps. As soon as you join and did not purchase a package of personal training session—<u>you have been forgotten</u>.

Throughout my entire working career, I always witnessed the intimidation people feel when they come to the gym, especially when it comes to women. When a woman looks at the gym floor, she usually doesn't notice exercising machines there. For her this is a bunch of metal slam which, she thinks, she will never use. Handles here, handles there, seats, benches, pads, adjustments. "Forget it! This is something that men do!" She looks around, and I can see that in her mind she is searching for "What else can I do here besides these machines?"

Gym operators and managers assume that after joining, this woman will come to their gym, will stop at each machine and start reading the instructions written somewhere in the corner in fine print in language that is designed for only fitness pros. Hah! And if the other guy is exercising on that machine, puffing and sweating, she will just ignore him and continue reading those instructions!

Or maybe those owners and managers think, "Let's just get her banking information, and then it is up to her whether she exercises or not."

And no one will even notice her absence if she doesn't show up at that gym for the next few months. "Do your own research! Learn to survive! We've got your money!"

But when the year passes by and there is time to renew your membership, they will "kiss your behind" again to get your signature for another year. They will promise you mountains and will say that "this time they will take care of you" and "they will make sure that you will reach your fitness goals." Blah, blah, blah . . . As soon as your signature is down, everything stays the same.

Personal training might be a great idea for most beginners, but what if you cannot afford one? Sixty-five dollars to eighty-five dollars a session plus membership fees is affordable for only 10 to 15 percent of gym members. What about the rest of the 85 percent? How do they survive? Where do they learn how to use those machines?

Do gym owners know all that? Of course they do. They also know that young and agile populations keep memberships for longer. Those are self-driven, and all you need to do is sign them up. They don't need a special attention and education on the machines. Go, go, go! Sign up, sign up, sign up! More members—more profit.

Every year, in United States alone, 2 million of new members join gyms. But who are those people? Are they the ones among those

225

65 percent who are sick, obese, and overweight, or is it just people that are displayed on clubs' flyers—young, energized, and already physically active? Let's look at the fitness industry statistics.

By IHRSA (the International Health, Racquet & Sportsclub Association—the main fitness industry research source), the penetration of population belonging to fitness clubs in USA and Canada is approximately 15 percent. So 85 percent of people still don't consider exercise necessary. Or maybe they do, but don't exercise. Do gyms do anything about this problem? Are they trying to reach those people? Not really. Go, go, go! Sell, sell, sell! That's their strategy. Doesn't matter who joins, doesn't even matter if those who join actually exercise—as long as they pay their monthly dues.

Since 1984, the number of fitness clubs only in United States grew from 7,000 to 29,000, and the number of members joining those clubs grew from 15 million members to 41 million, but the sad statistics is that the number of overweight and obese people still more than doubled—from 30 percent in 1984 to 65 percent in 2006.

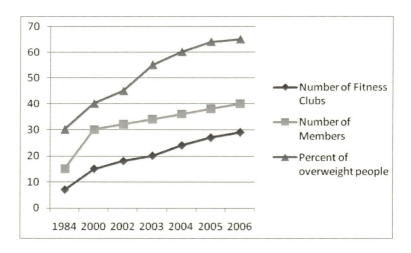

Gym business is doing well. But unfortunately, those who need exercise the most are still stuck at home watching their TVs or playing computer games. Neither the government nor the gyms create enough of awareness about necessity to exercise these days. It's "too hard" for them, and "too expensive"! Why bother about the obese when you can get those who are young and agile? Health education doesn't make profit, so why bother advertising it. It's so much easier to say, "We are open for everyone, and it's everyone's responsibility to take care of their health."

But what if those people don't know how to get that education? What if they can't read or write? What if they are immigrants, like most of the population in United States and Canada? Who is going to teach them how to exercise and eat right if not the gyms?

There is obviously not enough effort from the government and the fitness industry to change the statistics of our health today. The government is trying to find more money for more medical services instead of trying to prevent new diseases, and the fitness industry manufacturing members are like chickens at the farms where cheap meat is produced, caring only for productive ones. People joining? Good! Who is joining—it doesn't matter. As long as the cash is flowing in!

Most salespeople in gyms don't even have fitness backgrounds. Gyms hire people not based on passion for fitness or knowledge about health, but on ability to produce sales:

"What stops you from joining *today*?" or

"If I make your membership price affordable, would you be willing to commit *today*?" or

This is my favorite one—gym managers are forcing salespeople to learn this so-called question by heart—"We've talked about lot of things today, but one thing we didn't talk about is the initial investment. If it is affordable and within your budget, is there anything else stopping you to start attaining your goals *today*?"

And if this trick doesn't work on you to sell you the membership, get ready for the final push called in sales TO (turnover), where the so-called "supervisor" or a "manager" (usually just another colleague) steps in the sale process and tries to make you believe that you are the only one on this planet for "today's only" discount.

These sales pitches are used to sell cars, houses, time-shares, and now also to sell health.

When will gym owners snap out of this old-fashioned pressure-sale approach and start treating members like people and not like chickens? And when will they stop hiring people from McDonald's, Staples Business Depot, and Home Depot? It is hard to say because most gym owners and managers don't have fitness backgrounds themselves. Many of them don't even exercise or follow a healthy lifestyle. So why bother on studying fitness? They've decided to sell it by using an approach that worked on selling anything—by brainwashing and intimidating. Do they know how to crunch numbers? Oh, you better believe it. The only industry that can compare to fitness by its revenue is the movie industry—almost 15 billion dollars only in United States and 2 billion in Canada. Sounds impressive, huh? But while it is very good for the gym owners, it doesn't help the 85 percent of those who are in desperate need for health? Many of those who sign up cancel their memberships after a while or get lost without proper guidance. Who is going to give them that guidance? Salespeople? Remember, they get hired from McDonald's, Staple Business Depot, or Home Depot, and not trained to do fitness—twenty hours over club's sales manual and then—go, go, go, sell, sell, sell.

The main reason why gyms can't fix the obesity problem is because they don't care about obese and overweight population. Those people need special attention and very different approach. With the amount of members at most gyms, it is impossible to provide this special attention unless a new member purchases personal training sessions.

While the number of fitness clubs in the world is growing, obese, sick, and overweight population keeps growing too. A small fraction of the population keeps getting fitter while most are still in poor health. For the biggest part of it, the number of joining members is growing not because more people realize the need for exercise but simply because the population of earth is continuously growing. This is very easy to prove: the percentage of population who exercise regularly is still 15 percent and did not change for at least the past ten years. There is definitely not enough effort from the fitness industry and the government to reach the overweight and obese population.

Will gyms ever change their strategies? I highly doubt it. With competition growing in the fitness market, there will be less and less attention paid to each member because the competitive world dictates price reduction, and this automatically means the need for more members to maintain gym expenses. More members have never made any service better.

Unless some gyms decide to reinvest and start working toward the obese population, the situation will never change. Habits that obese people develop are extremely strong, and for them, a once-a-month flyer in their mail simply won't cut the deal. Obese people are looking for the emotional comfort, which most gyms today cannot provide.

I wrote all this not to discourage you from joining the gym. I love gyms. I just wanted you to know what to expect and be realistic when you join. Being a gym member has more advantages than disadvantages, but if you are hoping that a signed paper will automatically guarantee your success, think again. Expect to be forgotten as soon as you join and be treated just like another chicken head on the chicken farm. For most of the gyms, there is no such thing as customer service, so don't even expect it after you sign your agreement. I have seen too many people quitting gyms because of their overestimated expectations from those gyms, and I don't want you to be the one to quit for that reason. Gyms only offer you an open door, equipment, and other amenities within their hours of operation. The rest is on your own (unless you decide to sign up for an expensive personal training program).

*   *   *

Most people watch TV, and we need creative commercials, promoting healthy lifestyles, running throughout the day between every movie or TV show. Government, health insurances, big companies, and wealthy individuals who want to give back to their communities can invest in those commercials. People are busy, but if they are reminded not only to go shopping but also to go exercise, they will follow.

Those who invest in these commercials will benefit themselves because they will be reminded too, their families will be reminded, and most importantly, our children will learn the important message that "that's the way to live" and then will pass this message to further generations.

While gyms keep competing for 15 percent of the population, the rest of 85 is still floating in the air, getting overweight or sick or dying. There are lots of things that we can do together to prevent this from happening:

- Write to the government for a gym fees tax deduction
- Vote for more physical education in our schools and universities
- Make creative commercials on TV and radio
- Put fitness on billboards paid by the government
- Make advertisements in public transportation, etc.

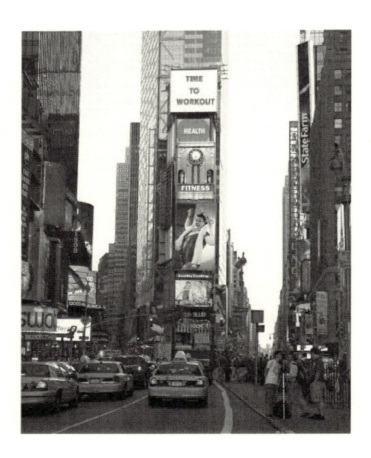

Until proper information overpowers all the commercial products that do no good to us, most people will still stay confused about the idea of how to stay healthy, live longer, and control the weight.

CHAPTER 26

IN THE GYM OR
AT HOME

I found out about fitness and bodybuilding at nineteen years old when I was serving the navy on the Russian submarine. Our ocean tours of duty were usually very short, and we spent a lot of time at bay. A couple of my friends and I rebuilt an old storage into a very primitive fitness room, where we had high bar for chin-ups, parallel bars for dips, incline bench, and some of the free weights.

They fed us really well in the navy, and within first three months of working out, we changed our bodies to the unrecognizable. From weak and flabby dudes, we turned ourselves into strong and rough boys who could perform over twenty-five chin-ups behind the head and could lift 200 lb. over the head ten times. Other guys sarcastically looked at us, how we usually, being half-naked, exercised, but eventually many of them joined us one by one, and when I left the navy, we together had planted a new tradition that was never recognized there before.

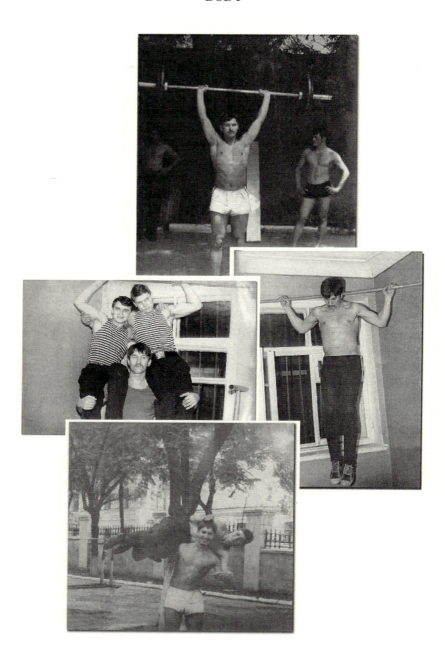

After I came back home from the navy, my father helped me to build some of the exercising machines, attachments to them, and I purchased some dumbbells and barbells so I could continue exercising.

For the first couple of months, everything was fine. But after a while, exercising alone started to seem boring. I tried to motivate myself with music, TV, posters of my favorite athletes, but none of it excited me.

One day I met my friend who was also a fitness enthusiast but who exercised at the local gym, and he invited me to try that gym.

When we came, I saw something that was very different from what we call a gym here: rusted dumbbells and barbells all over the floor, very primitive homemade machines, extremely low ceiling, and the worst of all—the smell. Inside my head, I named that gym Sweat Box. There were so many people there that we could hardly breathe, non-existing air-conditioning or any kind of ventilation, no windows, crumbled-down walls, broken ceilings and doors made you feel that you were in some kind of metal slam.

But there was something about that place. For some reason I performed better than ever that day. Maybe it reminded me about fun days in navy working out with my friends, but all my weights felt lighter even though I was using the same numbers as usual. I could not understand why this was happening to me but left for home with a very good feeling.

Next day I exercised at home and got very disappointed—I could not even get close to what I was lifting yesterday. I was very confused and decided to visit that gym again just to confirm that they had the same weight measures.

When I came, I was doing the same, and nothing felt any heavier.

Only later I discovered what was happening to me—I was motivated by the presence of other people. Doing the same under different circumstances makes you do it differently, so seeing other people exercising beside me made my muscles work harder without me even realizing it.

Eventually, regardless of all the inconveniences and discomfort at that gym, I still joined it and since then became a gym environment fan.

Before, in my navy days, I was always working out with my friends, and this is how I started, so this type of environment suited me best.

Many years passed, and now I am working out at a top-notch facility with huge swimming pools, very high ceilings, brand-new equipment, and great ventilation. But what attracts me the most here is still the same atmosphere that I experienced then—I love being surrounded by people, and they make me exercise harder.

Just a couple of decades ago gyms were mostly for fitness fanatics like me. Today more and more regular people realize the necessity of regular exercise, and among members we see those who just want to stay in good health and feel good. This makes me feel extraordinary happy about my profession. But what still worries me is that those who are obese—who need to exercise the most—still don't join gyms. Weight loss success stories on TV, radio, or in the mail about weight-challenged people are mostly about advertising some kind of suspicious so-called "magic" weight-loss programs. Many of those programs oppose gyms and put them down in order to get more business.

"Eat what you want and lose weight!"
"Twenty dollars plus the cost of food! Call now!" etc.

Everyone knows that those quick-fix programs don't last very long. Weight-challenged people don't need quick fixes. They've had enough of them. After every quick fix, they get back to where they were before. To change weight once and for all requires a lifestyle change.

I totally understand the intimidation of overweight people to join gyms. But I also wanted to encourage those who feel that way that the situation here is changing. Today's fitness market relies on regular population—those who are interested in improving health—and not on bodybuilders.

Overweight people are anxious that other people are going to judge them. But those days are over. Sixty-five percent of the population in most economically developed countries is now overweight, so for the

236

majority, one person is not very far from another in terms of his/her weight and look.

We see each other on the shopping malls and restaurants. These are the same people who go to gyms. So what is the difference where we meet?

Gyms don't care about you? Sure they don't! But your health is your health, and your life is your life, and only you can change it. Don't wait for someone to call you because most likely no one will. Take your life in your hands, and do whatever is necessary to make it better. And ignore what others might say or think because they won't—bodybuilders are too busy looking into the gyms' mirrors, and the rest—caring for their own problems and looks.

* * *

According to a survey done by IHRSA (the International Health, Racquet & Sportsclub Association), one given year, approximately 104 million Americans attempt to lose weight. The most popular weight loss strategies are outdoor exercise (48 million) and at-home exercise (47 million). Only a small fraction of those who did it at home achieved their weight loss goals. Those who exercised at health clubs to lose weight experienced much higher success rate.

When I was working as a personal trainer, I always tried to convince people not to waste money on the fitness equipment for home because of this statistics and also my past experience—I am a fitness fan and still could not do it at home. In my opinion, home is for relaxing. Throughout my twenty-seven years in fitness, I've seen very few people succeeding with their fitness plans at home, and home treadmills and other machines are usually being used for hanging clothes on them and not for exercising.

Exercising at home has few practical advantages. They are the following:

- Saving time travelling to the gym
- No time restriction—you can exercise anytime

- Privacy
- More hygiene

But exercising at home has also many disadvantages, and they are the following:

- Lack of motivation (big one!)
- Poor quality of equipment
- Poor variety of equipment
- Poor variety of activities and programs
- Lack of social environment (big one!)
- Lack of discipline (big one!)
- Relaxing atmosphere
- Distractions (children, friends, spouse, phone, etc.)
- Lack of information
- No guidance

Everyone is different, and some of you may "survive" exercising at home. I am not here to try reconvincing you but only to give a suggestion and share my own experience. But before you invest your money into your home equipment, make sure that you are aware of the above advantages and disadvantages. Exercising at home requires much more willpower and self-discipline, and it doesn't have any financial advantages—the money that you spend on your basic fitness equipment can cover your 5-6 year membership at a decent gym, where you can always find not only best equipment, but also lots of other things that you could never find at home. They are the classes, swimming pools, saunas, games, and most of all—motivation.

I have collected many stories and feedbacks from other people who have been members of different gyms. Here are the some of them:

F.K. *"What makes me keep coming to the club? The money I pay for my membership. I know that I paid—I have to go to get my monies worth. Sounds funny, but works for me, I stay fit."*

J.G. *"I like to alternate my program so I don't get bored. Plus, the quality of the machines, of course, is much better than you would buy for your home."*

238

A.P. *"I like to do yoga and Pilates classes. To hire a yoga or Pilates trainer, it would cost me a lot. To do it by myself—I am not always motivated. Here, everything is included in my membership, and I always get a good workout."*

K.L. *"Swimming is an excellent relaxation exercise for me. After my weight training, I like to go in the sauna and swim for 15—20 minutes. It makes me feel young again."*

R.H. and J.H. *"We both joined because we've got overweight and my husband stopped being interested in sex. He was always feeling too tired for it. We have only been coming to this gym for four months, and there are dramatic changes already. I can't complain anymore. Exercise keeps our sex life alive."*

M.D. *"I am fifty-eight. If I don't exercise, I start falling apart. My back hurts, I don't sleep well, and the weather affects every inch of my body. When I exercise, everything disappears. I feel young and energized. I tried to do it at home, but it's not the same. I need to feel that vibe."*

L.K. *"I am doing bodybuilding for twenty years. I am forty-one now. Many times I have to force myself to go workout. Not the workouts themselves make me come here but that feeling afterwards. Every time I finish my workout, I feel like I've dropped all my problems on the gym floor. I go home feeling a different person."*

CHAPTER 27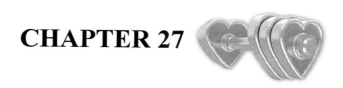

FIT AND FAT

Is it better to be slim or overweight? Even though the answer on that question might seem obvious, let's think about it first.

People often mistakenly associate slim people with fit ones. Appearance doesn't always describe one's fitness level, and neither does it describe a person's health. Being slim, of course, has certain advantages. It helps you to do the following:

1. Build confidence and pride in yourself
2. Change the way other people perceive you
3. Handle daily tasks and work with less effort
4. Participate in physical activities
5. Allow you to socialize and go out more.

But none of the above actually differentiates slim people from overweight when it comes to health.

A study published in the *International Journal of Obesity* involving more than 25,000 men tracked over a twenty-three-year period found that cardiorespiratory fitness was a better predictor of heart disease than weight. In other words, overweight men weren't necessarily at high risk for heart disease if they were fit. Unfit men were much more likely to die of heart disease than fit men—regardless of how much they weighed.

Fitness is a much more important factor in longevity than fatness. In fact, a 1999 study involving nearly 22,000 men lasted for an average of eight years concluded that being fit appeared to dramatically reduce the health risks of obesity that can lead to an early death. When it comes to living a long life, results indicated, *it is better to be fit and fat than thin and sedentary.*

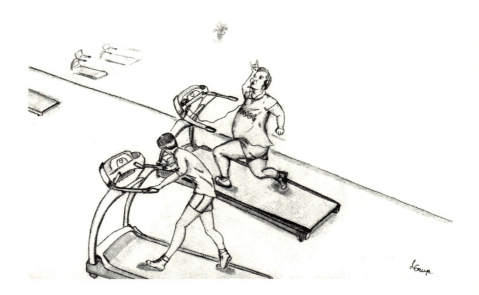

CHAPTER 28

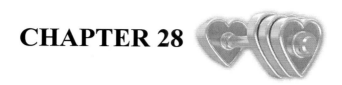

HOW DO I KNOW
IF I AM FIT?

L ook at the speedometer in your car. How many kilometers per hour can your car run? Most likely over 200. Will you ever drive with that speed? Probably not, unless you compete in car racing.

Why then do developers make those cars with such maximum speed?

Because cars need to have a reserve of power in case of emergency or extreme situations. Developers want to make sure that your car is not going to fall apart when it needs to perform hard, and that's what makes it reliable—if you decide to drive 150 kilometers per hour with reserve in your car of 260, your car will do it effortlessly.

The same rule works for our body. We need to have that reserve in our body so we don't fall apart in our emergency situations—when we are stressed out, need to catch a bus, climb long stairs, or do something intense.

As a car gets older, we fix it, tune it up, or repair its body so it looks good. Our body needs the same.

*   *   *

One of my friends is a car dealership manager. He used to sit all day at his desk and never exercised. Once we started talking about getting fit.

"I am fit!" he says. "Look at me! I am feeling fine! I am the top producer. I am running around this dealership all day!"

"OK," I said and asked him to show me some of his cars. First we looked at the Dodge Viper, the most expensive car in his dealership, and then at some cheaper models.

"All these cars look the same to me," I said, pretending that I don't understand anything about cars.

"Are you crazy!? You can't even compare Viper with any of these cars! It flies like a bullet. Those others will fall apart competing with Viper."

"But when they stand here beside each other, they look the same to me," I continued.

"You need to test the car before you say anything about it!"

"Well, it's just like our body, I guess—to say that you are fit, you need to test yourself too. Why don't we test you?"

"No problem," my friend answered, and we agreed to meet for his fitness test at the gym where I used to work.

Next morning, when my friend came, I put him on the treadmill and said, "I will set the speed on this treadmill assuming that you are fit for your age, OK? And you should be able to handle that speed with no problems—just like your Viper."

"Makes sense," my friend answered.

"Here it is," I said, speeding up the treadmill.

Someone suddenly called me to the front reception, and I had to ask my friend to stay alone for a couple of minutes. "Of course, no problem," answered my friend picking up the speed on his treadmill.

When I came back, my friend was sitting in the chair, and his treadmill was off.

"What happened?" I asked.

"Are you crazy? Did you want to kill me? I almost died running so fast."

"But you said that you were fit, and with this speed, you should be having no problem. I was only out for couple of minutes."

"Well . . . I guess I was not as fit as I thought . . ." said my friend, and the next day, he decided to join the gym.

*　　*　　*

What describes a person's fitness level? How do you know if you are fit?

Many people think that being fit is being able to run long distances or lift heavy weights in a gym.

But fitness is something quite different.

While fitness is based on results, these results are tightly connected with one's health. You could be trying to improve your strength, power, endurance, or anything else, but if it involves sacrificing your health, you are doing sports and not fitness. Fitness is almost everything what sport is but as long as you are not putting results ahead of your health. Physical results in fitness are based on norms in order to stay healthy, while in sports they are based on *only* maximum performance.

Fitness is also about body appearance, which is based on one's healthy body composition or, in simple words, how much of the *body fat* and how much of the *lean* tissue a body has. *Lean* is everything else except body fat—bones, muscles, organs, skin, etc.

Overall fitness is made up of five major components:

1. Cardiorespiratory endurance
2. Muscular strength
3. Muscular endurance
4. Body composition
5. Flexibility

Each of these components has its own norms. By performing specific tests, we determine how fit a person is on each of these components. There are few different ways to do that.

In this book I've included for you tests that do not require any fitness equipment. They are the following:

1. Resting heart rate
2. Blood pressure
3. Three-minute step (cardiovascular)
4. Push-ups (upper body strength)
5. Sit-ups (middle body strength)
6. Squats (lower body strength)
7. Plank (core stability)
8. Sit and reach (flexibility)
9. Body composition

After you perform all these tests you will be able to determine which feature or part of your body requires more attention.

1. Resting heart rate

This test is very simple, and it helps to establish the condition of your heart. It does not show exactly how your heart will perform under different resistance, but this test is still a good indicator of someone's fitness level. The slower your heart beats at rest, the fitter and healthier your heart is. With fewer beats per minute, your heart will spend more time at rest.

What's Needed?

- Timer

How to Perform

Find the pulse of your heart on your body. There are two most common places used to do that—your neck and your wrist.

On your wrist (see figure 4). Place the tips of your index, second, and third fingers on the palm side of your other wrist, below the base of the thumb.

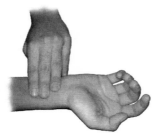

Figure 4. Wrist pulse

On your neck. (see figure 5). Place the tips of your index and second fingers on your lower neck, on either side of your windpipe.

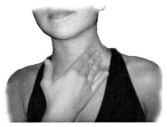

Figure 5. Neck pulse

Look at your timer or a watch and measure the number of your heartbeats per 10 seconds. Calculate beats per minute by multiplying that number by six:

Check your pulse: _____ × 6 = _____
                         (beats in 10 seconds)   *(your pulse)*

The best way to measure your resting heart rate is in the morning, while you are still in bed. You should be woken up by yourself (without alarm clock). If you use alarm clock or get off your bed and start walking around, your heart rate will go up, and your measurements will not be as accurate.

To get the most accurate number, measure your resting heart rate over at least three days and then average it out (because not every day you feel the same).

Refer to tables 4 (men) and 5 (women) for results.

Table 4. Resting Heart Rate Rating for Men, by Age

	18-25	26-35	36-45	46-55	56-65	65+
Athlete	49-55	49-54	50-56	50-57	51-56	50-55
Excellent	56-61	55-61	57-62	58-63	57-61	56-61
Good	62-65	62-65	63-66	64-67	62-67	62-65
Above Average	66-69	66-70	67-70	68-71	68-71	66-69
Average	70-73	71-74	71-75	72-76	72-75	70-73
Below Average	74-81	75-81	76-82	77-83	76-81	74-79
Poor	>82	>82	>83	>84	>82	>80

*Source: American Council on Exercise, Personal Trainer Manual

Table 5. Resting Heart Rate Rating for Women, by Age

	18-25	26-35	36-45	46-55	56-65	65+
Athlete	54-60	54-59	54-59	54-60	54-59	54-59
Excellent	61-65	60-64	60-64	61-65	60-64	60-64
Good	66-69	65-68	65-69	66-69	65-68	65-68
Above Average	70-73	69-72	70-73	70-73	69-73	69-72
Average	74-78	73-76	74-78	74-77	74-77	73-76
Below Average	79-84	77-82	79-84	78-83	78-83	77-84
Poor	>85	>83	>85	>84	>84	>84

*Source: American Council on Exercise, Personal Trainer Manual

Consult your physician if you are on any medication before measuring your resting heart rate because blood pressure pills, sleeping pills, antidepressants, and some others affect the heart rate.

Resting heart rate improves with aerobic activities such as walking, skiing, swimming, or sports games. The best results are achieved when those activities are performed for a minimum 20 minutes most days of the week.

2. *Blood pressure*

The pressure that blood exerts against the passing vessels is called blood pressure. Blood pressure is essential in maintaining blood flow and is defined by two pressures: *systolic* pressure and *diastolic* pressure. Both are measured in millimetres mercury (mm Hg).

Systolic is the pressure measured when the heart contracts. *Diastolic* pressure is the pressure measured when the heart is relaxed and filling.

Blood pressure readings are given as *systolic* pressure *over diastolic* pressure. A normative blood pressure reading is 120/80 mm Hg.

What's Needed?

* Blood pressure monitor

If you don't have blood pressure monitor, you can measure your blood pressure at any drug store. Even some grocery stores these days have blood-pressure-measuring stations.

How to Perform

* Don't eat or use caffeine, alcohol, or tobacco products 30 minutes before measuring your blood pressure.
* Empty your bladder before measuring your blood pressure.
* Rest for 3-5 minutes before measuring your blood pressure. Do not talk.

- Sit in a comfortable position. Do not cross your legs and ankles. Keep your back supported.
- Place your **left arm**, raised to the level of your heart, on a table or a desk, and sit still. Wrap the cuff smoothly and snugly around the upper part of your bare arm (see figure 6). The cuff should fit comfortably, but there should be enough room for you to slip one fingertip under the cuff. The bottom edge of the cuff should be **1 inch above the crease of your elbow**.

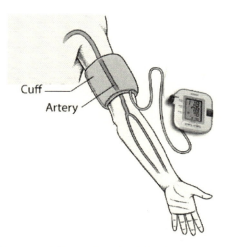

Figure 6. Measuring the blood pressure

3. *Three-minute step (cardiovascular)*

The **three-minute step** test measures your **aerobic (cardiovascular)** capacity. It determines *how quickly your heart rate recovers and returns back to normal* after exercise. The fitter you are, the quicker your heart rate returns to normal.

You will need to perform this exercise for 3 minutes nonstop and then calculate the total number of heartbeats for the next full minute, immediately after you finish the exercise.

What's Needed?

- A 12-inch-high step

- A metronome for accurate pacing. Pacing on the metronome has to be set at 96 bpm (beats per minute). If you don't have a metronome, you can get it off the Internet for free at www.MetronomeOnline.com
- Timer

How to Perform

1. Turn on the metronome.
2. Keeping a consistent pace based on the beats of the metronome, step on and off the bench for 3 minutes nonstop (figure 7). Check stepping rhythm throughout the test.
3. After completing 3 minutes immediately, sit on the 12-inch bench and begin counting your heart rate for one minute. You will notice how your heartbeat will be slowing down. Keep counting until the end of one minute. Refer to tables 6 (men) and 7 (women) for results.

   NOTE: This test is based on a 12-inch step, so use one as close to 12 inches as possible; otherwise, your results will not be accurate.

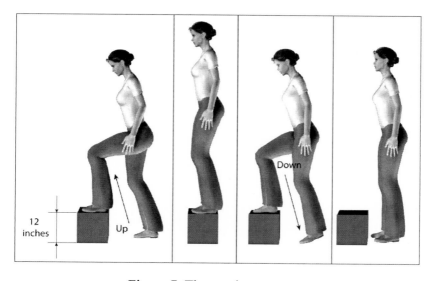

Figure 7. Three-minute step test

Table 6. Three Minute Step Rating for Men, by Age

	18-25	26-35	36-45	46-55	56-65	65+
Excellent	<79	<81	<83	<87	<86	<88
Good	79-89	81-89	83-96	87-97	86-97	88-96
Above Average	90-99	90-99	97-103	98-105	98-103	97-103
Average	100-105	100-107	104-112	106-116	104-112	104-113
Below Average	106-116	108-117	113-119	117-122	113-120	114-120
Poor	117-128	118-128	120-130	123-132	121-129	121-130
Very Poor	>128	>128	>130	>132	>129	>130

*Source: American Council on Exercise, Personal Trainer Manual

Table 7. Three Minute Step Rating for Women, by Age

	18-25	26-35	36-45	46-55	56-65	65+
Excellent	<85	<88	<90	<94	<95	<90
Good	85-98	88-99	90-102	94-104	95-104	90-102
Above Average	99-108	100-111	103-110	105-115	105-112	103-115
Average	109-117	112-119	111-118	116-120	113-118	116-122
Below Average	118-126	120-126	119-128	121-126	119-128	123-128
Poor	127-140	127-138	129-140	127-135	129-139	129-134
Very Poor	>140	>138	>140	>135	>139	>134

*Source: American Council on Exercise, Personal Trainer Manual

4.   *Push-ups (upper body strength)*

Push-up test is performed to define the strength of your triceps, frontal shoulders, and chest. The push-up position is different for men and women. Men use the standard position with only hands and toes in contact with the floor. Women use the modified bent-knee position. The rest of the procedure is the same as for men.

How to Perform (Men)

1. Assume the appropriate up position with your body rigid and hands about a shoulder-width apart (see figure 8, left).
2. Bend your arms and lower your body to about three inches from the floor. Make sure to remain your body rigid (see figure 8, right).
3. Strengthen your arms and return to primary position.
4. Score the total number of performed push-ups and refer to table 8 for results.

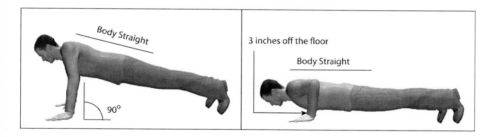

Figure 8. Push-up test for men

Table 8. Pushup Rating for Men, by Age

	17-19	20-29	30-39	40-49	50-59	60-65
Excellent	>51	>43	>37	>31	>28	>27
Good	35-50	30-42	25-36	21-30	18-27	17-26
Minimum	19-34	17-29	13-24	11-20	9-17	6-16
Below Minimum	4-18	4-16	2-12	1-10	0-8	0-5
Poor	<3	<3	<1	0	0	0

*Source: American Council on Exercise, Personal Trainer Manual

How to Perform (Women)

1. Assume the appropriate up position with your body rigid and knees on the floor, hands about a shoulder-width apart and arms perpendicular to the floor (see figure 9, left).
2. Bend your arms and lower your body to about three inches from the floor. Make sure to remain your body rigid (see figure 9, right).
3. Strengthen your arms and return to primary position.
4. Score the total number of performed push-ups and refer to table 9 for results.

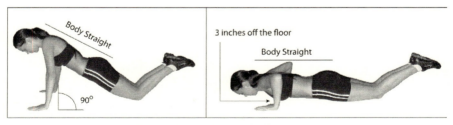

Figure 9. Push-up test for women

Table 9. Pushup Rating for Women, by Age

	17-19	20-29	30-39	40-49	50-59	60-65
Excellent	>32	>33	>34	>28	>23	>21
Good	21-31	23-32	22-33	18-27	15-22	13-20
Minimum	11-20	12-22	10-21	8-17	7-14	5-12
Below Minimum	0-10	1-11	0-9	0-7	0-6	0-4
Poor	0	0	0	0	0	0

*Source: American Council on Exercise, Personal Trainer Manual

5. Sit-ups (middle-body strength)

Sit-up test measures the strength and endurance of your abdominal muscles and also hip flexors. Abdominal muscle strength and endurance is important for holding your body and back support.

You will perform sit-ups *for one minute as quickly as possible* remaining in a proper position. The maximum number of sit-ups performed within one minute will determine the fitness level of your middle body.

What's Needed?

- Stopwatch or timer
- Exercise mat, cushioned carpet, or two-inch foam
- Spotter (someone who will hold your feet down to the floor)

How to Perform

1. Lie face up with your knees bent at right angle. Keep your feet flat on the floor, fingers next to your ears.
2. Have somebody hold your ankles firmly down to the floor or lock your ankles under the couch (see figure 10).

BODY

3. Squeeze your stomach and raise your body off the floor as quickly as possible. Touch the outer sides of your knees with your elbows still keeping your fingers next to your ears.
4. Return to the starting position rolling your back on the floor until your shoulders touch the floor. Keep your neck neutral throughout the motion.
5. Score the total number of performed sit-ups within a minute and refer to tables 10 (men) and 11 (women) for results.

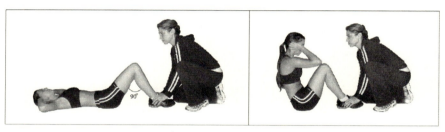

Figure 10. Sit-up test

Table 10. Sit-up Rating for Men, by Age

	18-25	26-35	36-45	46-55	56-65	65+
Excellent	>49	>45	>41	>35	>31	>28
Good	44-49	40-45	35-41	29-35	25-31	22-28
Above Average	39-43	35-39	30-34	25-28	21-24	19-21
Average	35-38	31-34	27-29	22-24	17-20	15-18
Below Average	31-34	29-30	23-26	18-21	13-16	11-14
Poor	25-30	22-28	17-22	13-17	9-12	7-10
Very Poor	<25	<22	<17	<13	<9	<7

*Source: American Council on Exercise, Personal Trainer Manual

Table 11. Sit-up Rating for Women, by Age

	18-25	26-35	36-45	46-55	56-65	65+
Excellent	>43	>39	>33	>27	>24	>23
Good	37-43	33-39	27-33	22-27	18-24	17-23
Above Average	33-36	29-32	23-26	18-21	13-17	14-16
Average	29-32	25-28	19-22	14-17	10-12	11-13
Below Average	25-28	21-24	15-18	10-13	7-9	5-10
Poor	18-24	13-20	7-14	5-9	3-6	2-4
Very Poor	<18	<13	<7	<5	<3	<2

*Source: American Council on Exercise, Personal Trainer Manual

6. Squats (lower body strength)

This test is to determine the strength of your lower body and your legs.

What's Needed?

- Chair or a bench

How to Perform

1. Place a chair behind you and stand close to it with your feet shoulder-width apart (see figure 11, left).
2. Squat down imitating sitting-down position and lightly touch the chair (see figure 11, right).
3. Stand back up.
4. Squat continuously without intervals.
5. Score the total number of performed squats until you are fatigued and refer to tables 12 (men) and 13 (women) for results.

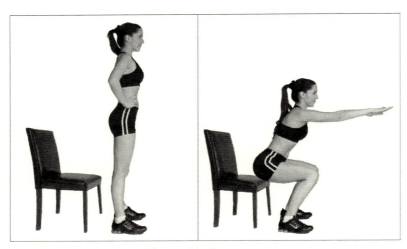

Figure 11. Squat test

Table 12. Squat Rating for Men, by Age

	18-25	26-35	36-45	46-55	56-65	65+
Excellent	>49	>45	>41	>35	>31	>28
Good	44-49	40-45	35-41	29-35	25-31	22-28
Above Average	39-43	35-39	30-34	25-38	21-24	19-21
Average	35-38	31-34	27-29	22-24	17-20	15-18
Below Average	31-34	29-30	23-26	18-21	13-16	11-14
Poor	25-30	22-28	17-22	13-17	9-12	7-10
Very Poor	<25	<22	<17	<9	<9	<7

*Source: American Council on Exercise, Personal Trainer Manual

Table 13. Squat Rating for Women, by Age

	18-25	26-35	36-45	46-55	56-65	65+
Excellent	>43	>39	>33	>27	>24	>23
Good	37-43	33-39	27-33	22-27	18-24	17-23
Above Average	33-36	29-32	23-26	18-21	13-17	14-16
Average	29-32	25-28	19-22	14-17	10-12	11-13
Below Average	25-28	21-24	15-18	10-13	7-9	5-10
Poor	18-24	13-20	7-14	5-9	3-6	2-4
Very Poor	<18	<20	<7	<5	<3	<2

*Source: American Council on Exercise, Personal Trainer Manual

7.   *Plank (core stability)*

The core muscles—the muscles in the abdomen, lower back, and pelvis. The strength and coordination of these muscles is very important for our daily life. They stabilize your spinal cord and provide firm base for practically every movement—help get out of bed, lift things, perform job duties, go places, have fun, and dance. Core muscles also provide assistance to perform other exercises.

How to Perform

1. Lie face down on the carpeted floor or exercise mat.
2. Place your elbows right underneath your shoulders arching your back, forearms parallel to each other.
3. Raise yourself up and form a straight bridge using your toes and forearms (see figure 12).
4. Maintain a straight line from your shoulders to your hips and knees. Keep your head aligned with your body.
5. Do not let your body sag down or raise your hips up. Remember to breathe.

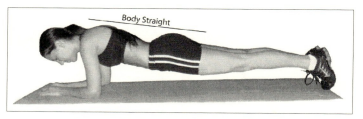

Figure 12. Core stability test (Plank)

Ratings

- **Strong**: Holding the position for longer than 60 seconds
- **Average**: Holding position for 30-60 seconds
- **Needs improvement**: Holding position for less than 30 seconds.

8. Sit and reach (flexibility)

What's Needed?

- Masking tape
- Yard ruler

How to Perform

1. Create a line on the floor using masking tape.
2. Lay down a yard ruler, allowing the line created by masking tape cross the 15-inch mark.
3. Tape the yard ruler firmly down to the floor on both ends.
4. Remove your shoes and sit down on the floor, placing your feet on the line, feet approximately 12 inches apart. Yard ruler has to be between your legs.
5. Keeping your knees fully straight, slowly lean forward with your arms straight and hands on top of each other, fingers aligned.
6. Slide your hands on the ruler and try to reach the farthest point.
7. Do three attempts, record the best result, and refer to tables 14 (men) and 15 (women) for results.

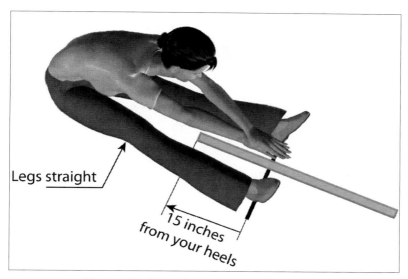

Figure 13. Sit and reach (Flexibility Test)

Table 14. Sit and Reach Rating for Men, by Age

	18-25	26-35	36-45	46-55	56-65	65+
Excellent	>20	>20	>19	>19	>17	>17
Good	18-20	18-19	17-19	16-17	14-17	13-16
Above Average	17-18	16-17	15-17	14-15	12-14	11-13
Average	15-16	15-16	13-15	12-13	10-12	9-11
Below Average	13-14	12-14	11-13	10-11	8-10	8-9
Poor	10-12	10-12	9-11	7-9	5-8	5-7
Very Poor	<10	<10	<8	<7	<5	<5

*Source: American Council on Exercise, Personal Trainer Manual

Table 15. Sit and Reach Rating for Women, by Age

	18-25	26-35	36-45	46-55	56-65	65+
Excellent	>24	>23	>22	>21	>20	>20
Good	21-23	20-22	19-21	18-20	18-19	18-19
Above Average	20-21	19-20	17-19	17-18	16-17	16-17
Average	18-19	18	16-17	15-16	15	14-15
Below Average	17-18	16-17	14-15	14-15	13-14	12-13
Poor	14-16	14-15	11-13	11-13	10-12	9-11
Very Poor	<13	<13	<10	<10	<9	<8

*Source: American Council on Exercise, Personal Trainer Manual

9.   Body composition

The *body composition* refers to the *proportion of body fat and fat-free mass (lean) in the body.*

Many people think that the less body fat they have, the better it is, but this is only true to a certain degree. Body fat is not our enemy as it may have been portrayed by the publicity, and we need to maintain a certain minimum of it in order to stay alive. Table 16 displays categories of different body fat percentages. Keep in mind that your lean mass (muscles, bones, organs, and skin) is always the difference between your total body mass (100 percent) and the percentage of your body fat. For example, if your body fat is 20 percent, your lean mass is 80 percent.

Table 16. Body Fat Percentage Categories

	Women (% Fat)	Men (% Fat)
Essential Fat	10-12%	2-4%
Athletes	13-20%	5-13%
Fitness	21-24%	14-17%
Overweight	25-31%	18-24%
Obese	32%+	25%

How do you measure your body fat?

There are few different methods, but I would like to stop your attention only on the most popular ones used today.

1. Bioelectrical impedance analysis

Handheld
Body Fat Analyzer

Body Fat Scale

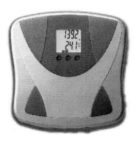

The bioelectrical impedance analysis (BIA) is the most popular, relatively inexpensive, convenient, but least accurate method. The main reason for inaccuracy is that during that process, the body fat doesn't get measured at all. BIA relies on measuring of the lean mass and then predicting the body fat percentage by subtracting it from the total mass (100 percent).

There is no one formula that accurately predicts body fat for the whole population. Differences in age, gender, ethnicity, body size, and fitness level all have a significant effect on the results. Another problem with BIA is that lean mass often varies—body position, the amount of water in your body, your food intake, skin temperature, and recent physical activity can all adversely affect the results, and as lean varies, so does the body fat prediction after the calculation.

2. Skinfold method

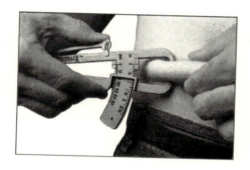

The skinfold method is based on pinching of the skin by *calipers* at several standardized points on the body to determine the fat layer thickness. These measurements are converted to an estimated body fat percentage by an equation. Some formulas require as few as three measurements, others as many as seven. The accuracy of these estimates is more dependent on a person's unique body fat distribution than on the number of sites measured.

The skinfold method is one of the most precise methods to determine your body fat but requires skills, and as such, they can be hard to perform for someone inexperienced.

3. Measurements method

This method is gender and height sensitive and is based on measuring of the body parts where fat concentrates the most: for men, abdomen, and for women, hips and waist. When women gain fat, they usually develop so-called "pear shape" where fat mostly settles around hips and waistline, but when men gain fat, their bodies widen mostly around their bellies creating an "apple shape." Some women as an exception to this rule might be born with an "apple shape," and some men, with "pear shape." Those need to use formulas of the opposite sex when trying to determine the body fat by this method.

Besides body parts with high fat concentration, this method relies on one more body measurement—neck—for both sexes.

This method is the most reliable for a reason that it depends on the body size changes in the areas with the highest fat concentration and is not affected by any lean fluctuations. This method is simple to perform and requires minimum skills.

What's Needed?

1. Measuring tape
2. Computer (Windows)

How to Perform

1. Refer to table 17 for appropriate measurements based on your gender, and write them down.
2. Refer to table 18 for body fat calculations.

Table 17. Measurements for Body Fat Calculations

Men	Women
Abdomen	**Waist**
Measure horizontally the *widest* circumference around the torso at the level of the navel (belly button). Exhale and keep the abdomen relaxed when measuring. The area should not be covered by clothing.	Measure horizontally the *narrowest* circumference around the torso at the level just below the bottom of the rib cage above navel (belly button). Exhale and keep the abdomen relaxed when measuring. The area should not be covered by clothing.
Neck	**Neck**
Measure horizontally, just below the Adam's apple. It may be necessary to angle the tape downward slightly in front to bypass the Adam's apple.	
	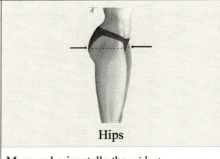 **Hips**
	Measure horizontally the *widest* circumference around the hips and buttocks. The area should not be covered by clothing.

Table 18. Body Fat Calculation on Computer (Windows)

1. Start > All Programs > Accessories > Calculator. 2. Click View > Scientific.

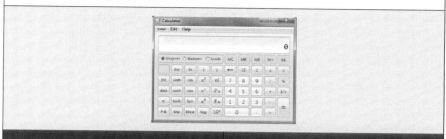

Men	Women
1. Type 86.01. 2. Click multiply "*". 3. Click "(". 4. Type your abdomen measurement in inches. 5. Click subtract "-". 6. Type your neck measurement in inches. 7. Click ")". 8. Click "log". 9. Click subtract "-". 10. Type 70.041. 11. Click multiply "*". 12. Type your height measurement in inches. 13. Click "log". 14. Click add "+". 15. Type 36.76. 16. Click the equals sign "=".	1. Type 163.204. 2. Click multiply "*". 3. Click "(". 4. Type your waist measurement in inches. 5. Click add "+". 6. Type your hip measurement in inches. 7. Click subtract "-". 8. Type your neck measurement in inches. 9. Click ")". 10. Click "log". 11. Click subtract "-". 12. Type 97.684. 13. Click multiply "*". 14. Type your height measurement in inches. 15. Click "log". 16. Click subtract "-". 17. Type 78.387. 18. Click the equals sign "=".

If calculating this way is too difficult for you, visit our website: www.gymbagbooks.com and use our online body fat calculator, or go to Downloads and download (for free) the Excel spreadsheet "Track Your Progress" where the formula is already installed and all you need to do is to insert your measurements.

CHAPTER 29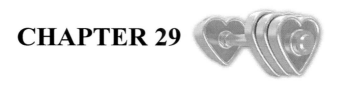

LOSING WEIGHT

Failure of Counting Calories Idea

Different bodies have different rates of burning the energy, and assuming that the same food will be burned with the same efficiency in two different bodies doesn't make any sense. There are so many factors that can modify the rate at which our body burns calories that narrowing down weight loss to just calorie count is losing yourself. Here are some of those factors:

- The caloric values of foods printed in books assume that foods containing those calories are burned completely. But in reality, our body burns some foods better than the others.
- Different people can burn the same foods with different efficiency. What works for some people may not work for others.
- Weight loss may be affected not only by the amount of calories at each meal but also greatly by their nutrient mix due to the fact that there are nutrients that help to burn body fat and there are others that promote fat gain. Striving for only reducing calories we, in the end, may be reducing the essential nutrients, and instead of losing weight, we will be losing health.

- The organically grown apple that is just taken from the tree will burn with different efficiency than the one that is grown using pesticides taken from the tree two weeks ago, transported, and repacked few times. But caloric books don't take that into consideration.
- The quality of foods affects their burning efficiency.

When creating a meal plan, we should first take into consideration the health benefits of each of our selection rather than count calories. We have very little control over the biochemical processes that take place after we swallow our food due to the individuality reason, but we can always improve our choices. With fad and junk foods, it is very easy to get the perfect number of calories per day, but what value does that food give you? Does it give you health, or does it slowly degenerate your cells year after year? When essential nutrients are missing, your body will not be functioning properly, leading to improper chemistry balance. How can we then expect that our body will burn fat, even if we exercise enough, and even if we eat proper amount of calories?

Fasting

Many people confuse what actually happens when we completely stop eating. In order to understand it better, we need to understand first how we store our energy.

Carbohydrates. Carbohydrates are broken down into sugars for absorption. Some of them are used to drive life, some for physical labor (if such exists), some gets stored in our body as glycogen, and the rest—as fat.

Glycogen is chains of glucose molecules put together for future use. Those who exercise regularly have bodies that build those chains better because they use them often. But those who don't exercise store extra carbohydrates as fat. Sugars can be very easily converted to fat but cannot be converted back to glucose.

Protein. After we eat protein-rich food, the protein needs to be first broken down into amino acids. Then our body uses amino acids to replace lost body protein or repair our muscle tissues. Not all amino acids are needed for that repair, and some of them get converted to glucose for energy. If that energy is not needed, protein converts to fat. After the protein is converted to fat, it cannot be converted back to proteins.

Fat. When we eat fatty foods, the fat breaks down to *glycerol* and *fatty acids*. The fatty acids then get used for various body functionalities, get broken down for energy, and if that energy is not needed—converted to body fat for future use. The glycerol is transported to the liver where it is reformulated into glucose and ultimately redirected for energy creation. The extra fat that we eat at each meal converts to body fat *in the most convenient way*. See figure 14.

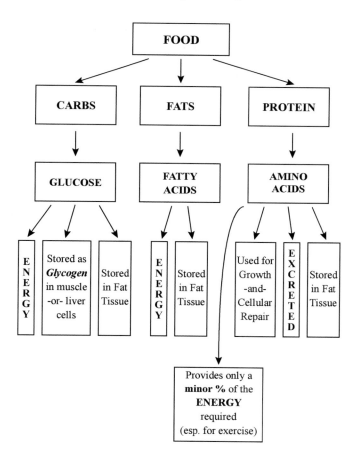

Figure 14. Food breakdown

Let's now reverse the energy flow and see what happens inside of our body when we are fasting.

If we don't supply food for one day or longer, our body gets into the body's storages and depletes them. "Oh, great!" you might say. "I will lose fat!" But unfortunately, our body does not choose to burn fat first because that process requires much more time and effort than to burn other quick sources of energy, such as glucose. To drive life, the body "doesn't have time" for long processes—the heart, brain, muscles, nervous system require immediate energy—and our organs cannot wait until the body will start burning fat.

Where does the body take glucose when we fast? First it depletes it from the liver. When those storages are emptied, the glucose is taken out of our muscles by breaking down the glycogen into glucose, and when those are gone too, the body starts breaking down our muscles to generate the required energy, basically *eating itself up*—skeletal muscle, the blood proteins, liver, digestive tract linings, heart muscle, and lung tissue—all vital tissues—are being burned as fuel.

Short-term fasting seems to benefit the body in some ways although there is no evidence that the body becomes internally "cleansed" as some believe. Fasting for a long time, however, *may harm the body*, when *ketosis* upsets the acid-base balance of the blood or when fasting promotes excessive mineral losses in the urine.

Ketosis is the second part of the process that takes place when our body's metabolism shifts from getting energy from carbohydrates to taking it from fat. When this takes place, this is the time that you lose the most fat. The name *ketosis* relates to the blocks of fat that are stored for release as energy, which are known as *ketones* or *ketone bodies*.

The main side effects of ketosis are bad breath and sluggish mobility—no energy. Bad breath is caused due to a change in the bacteria and enzymes throughout the digestive system, and slow movement because fat is much harder to use for energy production, making you low on energy.

Fasting remains alive only until their stores of fat are gone almost completely or until half their lean tissue is gone, whichever comes first.

Wise people in many cultures have practiced fasting as a periodic discipline. Fasting could be your great tool to test the willpower, but if you want to lose weight, fasting is not the best way because of the lean tissue degrading and nutrients' depravation. During fasting and even sometime after, the body also slows down its metabolism trying to conserve the energy.

Source: (Frances Sizer, 2006), p. 330. Rephrased for easier reading and added with additional information.
Please put full name of the source

Dieting

Many diets are created for people with specific medical problems, but a large number of people attempt to apply the weight loss characteristics to those diets. For example, a Dr. Bernstein diet is primarily for those with diabetes and issues with insulin resistance. Pritikin's high-complex carbohydrate, low-fat diet helps to reverse many degenerative changes that appear due to American diet.

High-Protein, High-Fat Diets

High-fat, low-carbohydrate diets include Atkins, Stillman, Zone, Protein Power, Sugar Busters, Drinking Man's, and some other diets. The psychology that supports the idea of these diets is that from the ancient times man has always been a hunter and has always eaten a diet high in protein and fat (which could be debatable).

When it comes to losing weight, these diets work because fats are digested slower, and they suppress appetite longer than carbohydrates. Fats also produce ketones, which reduce hunger even more. But the biggest disadvantage of these diets is that due to ketosis, they can lead to ketone-induced kidney damage. Also, too much protein produces an excess of ammonia, a toxic product after the protein breakdown. Ammonia can damage the kidney, liver, and even the brain. Our body has the ability at some point to turn ammonia into less harmful urea. But urea is also a toxin that in excess can cause gouty arthritis.

High-protein diets may develop allergies since proteins are potential allergens, which in return can create digestive and absorptive problems, nutrient deficiencies, and immune system damage.

High-protein diets de-emphasize high-carbohydrate, high-fiber plant foods. These foods help lower cholesterol. Consuming too much protein and fat raises cholesterol levels and increases cardiovascular risk.

High-protein diets don't provide some essential vitamins, minerals, fiber, and other nutritional elements.

High-Complex Carbohydrate, Low-Fat Diets

The Pritikin, Dean Ornish, and Paavo Airola diets are the most popular of the many high-complex carbohydrate (80 percent), low fat (10 percent or less) diets.

Pritikin and Ornish diets work for people who overate themselves fat and are sick of typical American diet rich in protein, white flour, sugars, and hard fats. These diets help to reverse many degenerative changes that appear due to American diet—rheumatoid arthritis, hypertension, diabetes, and cardiovascular disease.

But after a person becomes healthy, high-carbohydrate, low-fat diets may become dangerous because of low content of essential fats. Some vitamins are fat soluble and can be only absorbed with the help of fats. Those are vitamins A, D, E, and K. When total fat intake is below the body requirements, absorption of these vitamins may become problematic leading to health issues. For example, diets with less than 5 percent fats are correlated with cancer in Philippines, most likely due to low absorption of vitamins A and E, which protect against cancer-causing free radicals.

Pritikin and Ornish diets are very low in omega-3 and pay no attention at all to this crucial component of any balanced diet.

Pritikin initially developed his diet for himself. He was obese and clogged his arteries in his forties. He managed to clean them, and this fact was proven after he died in his sixties when the autopsy on his body was done. But Pritikin died of suicide after battling leukemia.

High-complex carbohydrate, low-fat diets may be a good first step to a healthier life but in a long run can still develop some health problems or even death due to a low volume of essential fats that are so important to our health.

Source: Udo Erasmus, 1999, *Fats That Heal, Fats That Kill*

Dr. Bernstein and Low-Carbohydrate Diets

Dr. Bernstein diet promotes that everyone should strive for normal blood glucose (around 85 mg, prediabetes is 100 mg, and diabetes is 126). The idea of this diet is very simple—you eat what you want but within very clear guidelines: very low carbohydrates and doing it forever.

Dr. Bernstein has been on his own diet since 1969. Only motivated people will be able to stay on it because of its restrictions. Diabetes can be a great motivator for it, but weight loss and health might not be.

The biggest disadvantage of this diet is that due to its restrictions it can be very difficult to continually get enough of all the vitamins, minerals, and nutrients needed for optimal health. While supplements can take care of vitamins and minerals, getting a range of other nutrients is difficult on any low-carbohydrate diet.

This diet also gets very boring for those who like to cook and prefer the creativity with their meals.

Any diet too low in carbohydrates eventually brings the same effects as fasting. When the glucose from food carbohydrates and body storages runs out, the body starts breaking down fat and protein for energy and creates ketone bodies to feed the brain. While breaking down the fat may sound good for those who are trying to lose some pounds, breaking down the muscle tissues is never a good idea.

Low-carbohydrate or low-carbohydrate, high-protein diets have been heavily promoted for weight loss, and they take many credits for their initial success. But this success quickly fades away after the dieter returns to normal eating—the body, deprived in carbohydrates gains all the weight back, and often with some extra. The enormous effort in trying to lose weight and sudden disappointment leads people to quit trying and give up on the hope to ever improve their body permanently.

Scientific Report on Dieting

Many popular diet books have hooked millions of overweight, meat-loving readers with this tempting advice: eat unlimited calories of protein and fat, and you will lose weight provided that you avoid the carbohydrates. Scientific evidence is mixed on whether a high-protein, low-carbohydrate diet produces leanness especially when it comes to maintaining it.

Research indicates that among 28,000 participants tested *within laboratory* where energy intake was held constant, those who consumed a high-protein diet had a higher BMI values than those who consumed a more balanced diet, and no difference was observed in weight loss between both groups. But the picture changed for people who lived *outside the laboratory* if they had a free choice on how much to consume. Obese people choosing from a high-protein, low-carbohydrate diet lost more weight during the first six months than those on low-fat, adequate carbohydrate diet. During the next six months, weight loss was achieved in both groups, and the gap between groups was narrowed to the minimum. The average weight losses for high-protein, low-carbohydrate diet was only significantly higher only during the first three months of dieting. How do scientists explain this greater initial loss? First, when glycogen stores are lost, as in low-carbohydrate diets, substantial water loss followed. Second part of explanation is that people on low-carbohydrate diets generally consume fewer calories due to the suppressed appetite caused by protein and fat.

At twelve months, when both groups were off their diets, the low-carbohydrate group regained weight more rapidly, while the low-fat group remained more stable.

*When weight loss occurs on high-protein, low-carbohydrate diet, it is because people **lose water** and **eat less due to suppressed appetite by protein and fat**, and not because of some kind of magic or "super secret" of this diet.*

Dangers and Risks of Dieting

Diet books recommend replacing carbohydrate-rich foods with those rich in protein. Do the authors of these books really present an evidence of long-lasting experience of those who fixed their health problems by such diets, or are these diets only a representation of a quick-fix solution with no permanent results?

Based on the healthy eating index, a measure of how well the diet meets dietary recommendation, saturated fats from animal sources are implicated in worsening a woman's risk of breast cancer. High-protein, high-fat diets also clearly raise the risk for heart and artery disease, osteoporosis, kidney stones, kidney disease, and many cancers.

Diets low in carbohydrates produce chronic ketosis, which further leads to health problems and vitamin and mineral deficiencies.

Complex carbohydrates increase our levels of serotonin (happy hormone), so when we eat them, we feel better. When our serotonin levels are higher, we are happier. It's that simple.

Fad diet authors often promote and profit from supplements and meal replacers. They claim that those supplements and meal replacers provide all the elements missing from the diet. Such assumption does not have any scientific proof, and many of those superficially created products don't even have their own controlling industry. They mostly belong to enthusiasts and business people. The production of most of the supplements is still not controlled by FDA.

Facts from many latest studies confirm that consumption of more whole grains, fruits, vegetables, and low-fat milk products collates with lean body and good health.

Eliminating or greatly reducing intakes of whole grains, vegetables, milk, and fruits is baseless. By doing so, we will be eliminating many nutrients, fibers, and other necessary body elements with proven health benefits.

Lies and Truths of Fad Diets

Lie: You'll lose weight fast without counting calories or exercising because the diet or product alters metabolism.

Truth: No known trick of metabolism produces significant weight loss without proper eating or exercise.

Lie: On this diet, you can eat all you want and still lose weight.

Truth: Unless the diet is composed entirely of celery or lettuce, basic laws of governing energy disapprove this claim. Energy consumed must be used to fuel the body or is stored as fat.

Lie: You'll never regain the weight even after you've stopped using the diet product.

Truth: Maintenance of a new lower weight requires lifelong changes in proper eating and exercise.

Lie: Eat all the fat, sugar, or other foods you want and lose pounds every day because this product blocks absorption of energy nutrients.

Truth: Losing 2 lb. of body fat (7,000 calories) per week through malabsorption would require passing about 1,000 calories of undigested fat or carbohydrate out of the digestive tract each day, an unlikely outcome and losing 2 lb. a day in this manner is physically impossible.

Lie: This product is 100 percent successful in producing weight loss.

Truth: The causes of obesity are multiple, and even prescription medications and stomach-shrinking surgeries are not 100 percent effective.

Lie: You'll lose weight just by wearing the product or rubbing it on your skin.

Truth: No over-the-counter patch, cream, wrap, ring, bracelet, other jewelry, shoe inserts, or other gimmick is known to cause loss of weight or fat.

Lie: Reset your genetic code to be thin.

Truth: You inherited your genes, and no diet can alter them.

Lie: Stress hormones make you fat.

Truth: Supplements sold to block stress hormones and produces weight loss do neither.

Lie: High-protein diets are so popular because they are the best way to lose weight.

Truth: See previous chapter.

Lie: High-protein diets energize the brain.

Truth: The brain depends on carbohydrates for energy.

Sources: Federal Trade Commission, Deception in Weight-Loss Advertising Workshops: Seizing Opportunities and Building Partnerships to Stop Weight-Loss Fraud, a Federal Trade Commission Staff Report, December 2003, available at www. ftc.gov; Food and Drug Administration, Counting Calories: Report of the Working Group on Obesity, March 12, 2004, available at www.cfsan.fda.gov/~dms/owg-rpt. html; S. Barrett, Impossible Weight-Loss Claims: Summary of a Federal Trade Commission Report, December 16, 2003, available at www.quackwatch.org.
Taken: Nutrition Concepts and Controversies., Frances Sizer, Ellie Whitney

CHAPTER 30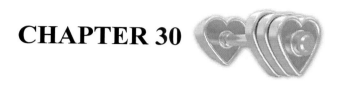

GETTING STARTED

D on't expect to lose weight overnight. Our body is not a water tank that you can just open the plug and when you are done—just pour it out. It will take some time.

Setting Goals

Set realistic goals and be persistent—this is the most important in any goal. Regardless how little your steps may be, they are your steps, and they will move you forward.

Research clarifies the gap between high expectations and reasonable goals. At the beginning of each year on a weight-loss program, *obese* women named four potential weights to achieve:

- Dream weight—110 lb.-145 lb.
- Happy weight—approximately 160 lb.
- Acceptable weight—approximately 170 lb.
- Disappointed weight—approximately 185 lb.

By the end of the year, most women had lost an average of 35 lb., or 16 percent of their starting weight, which was more than reasonable. But the women still felt discouraged because of their unrealistic expectations at the beginning. Despite experiencing remarkable physical, social, and psychological benefits, they still were dissatisfied because they have not even met their "disappointed" weight.

Most rapid weight loss programs do not consider health benefits along the way, while modest weight loss programs, even when the person is still overweight, lead to improvements in control over many health problems such as diabetes, blood pressure, and other issues. They also improve body functionality, efficiency, and boost self-esteem.

The best way to set goals is to write them down. The evidence confirms that if we keep our goals inside of our minds and don't write them down, we are not always firm on them. When everything is "mixed" in our mind, living throughout each day, we often forget about our goals.

What is first in losing weight?

For the overweight person, first reasonable goal is to prevent further gain. As this is accomplished, a following goal might be to reduce body weight by about 5 to 10 percent over a year's time. If you reach your goals sooner, you can set your new goals, but 10 percent per year is reasonable. For example, if your weight is 230 pounds, losing 5-10 percent will be equal to 12-23 pounds per year.

The most difficult part in the weight loss is not the weight loss itself, but the weight maintenance. Millions of people lose weight every year but only a small fraction of them maintain it.

Keeping Records

Keeping records is crucial. Recording your food intake and exercises will help you see where you are at and where you are going and also will identify what to improve.

Track all your progress! Surest way to do it is to do the following:

- Have a calendar on your fridge door (this is the place where you go often). The calendar has to be big enough to notice it. Your main daily goals have to be highlighted in red.

- Have a journal.
- Put reminders on your door, computer, and your phone—at home and at work.
- Program your TV or computer to shut down when it is time to go exercise, eat or cook your food.

Acting Upon Knowledge

"Knowledge is power" they say. I have seen quite few big posters displaying this slogan.

But the knowledge is only power if we're getting use of that knowledge. Otherwise it becomes useless baggage of information. Many people read and study all their lives but still never get successful. So how does that knowledge make them powerful?

Only power is power! The ability to act upon your knowledge. First time I realized about this was when I was twenty-two years old and was starting to work as a physical education teacher while studying in university. This was the best way to learn my profession because while I was learning all the theories at the university I was immediately practicing them at work. I still remember most what I've learned because I was learning with small steps—little bit of knowledge and then a little bit of practice.

When you practice what you learn, you find the best possible ways to use your knowledge.

Always act upon your knowledge. There is a big difference between knowing what to do and doing what you know. Don't wait until you learn everything because there is no such a thing. There will always be more and more information every day. And while you are acting upon your knowledge, you keep getting more knowledge.

Staying Firm

"Why did you quit the first time?" I asked those who were joining gym again after quitting.

"Life gets in the way," I've heard from many of them.

"And what about this time? What if life gets in the way again?"

"This time I am serious!" most people would say.

"On the scale from 1 to 10, where would you put yourself how serious you are this time?"

"Between 8 to 10!"

You know what happens after they go home? For many—life gets in the way. And all those nice words that they told me quickly dissolve in their every day's routines.

Many people, who join gyms, come mentally unprepared. They don't make it firm enough for themselves that joining the gym was what they really wanted.

"I will try for few months, see what happens," or "I don't want to commit to a year, I want to have an option to cancel my membership at anytime." These are not firm words, and there is no commitment in them.

I tracked people who didn't want to commit to a year membership and noticed that these were the ones who usually quit in a few months. Such a thing happened to them not because their "life got in the way" but simply because they never made it firm enough for themselves.

When you know what you want, you don't doubt it, and what you want is just as clear as the nose on your face. But when you doubt it, you work toward it with halfway strength. Halfway efforts bring halfway results, and halfway results bring halfway satisfaction, and then, guess what? You give up because no one likes halfway satisfaction.

When we make it clear, we work with maximum effort. Maximum effort always brings maximum results, and then we are happy.

In order to succeed, from now on, you simply cannot allow yourself to do the following:

- Say you are too tired
- Postpone your workout without a valid reason
- Wait for inspiration
- Plan to get rigid tomorrow or next Monday
- Give up because you skipped some workouts
- Give up because you are not getting results fast enough
- Tell yourself that you are too old or too young to start
- Blame others or your family for lack of free time
- Say your job is too demanding to allow you to get better with your workouts
- Tell yourself that you are never going to change your body or improve your health

CHAPTER 31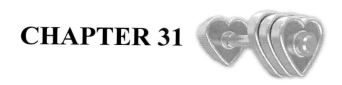

NUTRITION

Planning Your Meals

Contrary to the claims of those who promote fad diets, *no particular food plan is magical*. You are the one who will have to live with this plan, and you should design it yourself because we all grow up in different cultures and are accustomed to eat different types of foods. Your meal plans should be designed around your culture and not around the opinions of faddists. This will make the process of adjusting to a new way of eating much easier.

Trust Mother Nature

We, humans, always claim that we know better than Mother Nature. We decide that our fruits need to be blended to juices, grains to flour, and our food needs to be heated and processed before we eat it. We invented sandwiches, donuts, crackers, cookies, candies, cakes . . . you name it. Then we decided that this is not enough and started inventing meal replacements—powders, shakes, smoothies, protein and energy bars, and even pills that are supposed to be feeding us just as good as natural products.

But how can we claim that we know better than Mother Nature if we can't even cure cancer, prevent heart attacks, or stop diabetes? How can we even take any credit for food inventions and say that this is all good if most of those foods are practically killing us? Was Mother Nature wrong inventing an apple? Why then do we destroy it—remove its skin, blend it, and drink instead of chewing it?

Because we think we know better.

We are now having a new trend called organic food. Hah?! Finally we are getting back to where we started—allowing our chickens to run, growing fruits without pesticides, and even making beauty products and soaps as hundred years ago. We like the word *natural* on the labels of the products we buy. This word would not even need to be there if we always trusted Mother Nature.

We've opened up the stores that we call health stores. Does this mean that all other stores are nonhealthy ones? Looks like it. Most of the foods that are sold in traditional supermarkets, convenient stores, gas stations, cafés, sports bars, gyms, and fast-food restaurants are human inventions—blended, processed, refined, heated, sweetened, salted, and wrongfully mixed.

30.1 Carbohydrates

Unfair Anticarbohydrate Propaganda

"My personal trainer told me that I had to cut down on my carbohydrates and get my energy source mostly from protein. He said that this is the best way to lose weight and recommended not to eat fruits too. It seems working—I am losing weight, but I read that too much protein could damage your liver. I really want to know the truth, so I don't end up in the hospital after such diet."

For the past decade, carbohydrates took unfair blame for the people's fatness. Without going into research, everybody started to cut down on carbohydrates. Did we get any slimmer? We only got fatter and now even sicker.

What are carbohydrates? How much is enough? What kind of carbohydrates should we eat and what kind to avoid? We need to know these answers before we judge if carbohydrates are good or bad for us.

Carbohydrates are the *ideal* nutrients to meet your body's energy needs, feed your brain and nervous system. They also help keep your digestive system in good condition, and *within calorie limits, help you to stay lean.*

Carbohydrates are substances from food that provides us with energy—*glucose*. Glucose is used in our body to drive our life. Carbohydrate-rich foods are the ones that come from mostly plants; milk is the only animal-derived food that contains significant amounts of carbohydrates.

The sun provides energy for plants through sunlight and a process within a plant called *photosynthesis. Chlorophyll*, the green pigment in a plant is responsible for capturing that energy from the sun.

Carbon dioxide (CO_2) that we breathe out from our lungs and that is produced by our cars gets absorbed into the plant leaves and then with water from soil, forms the most common of the sugars—the single sugar **glucose**. Scientists tried to reproduce glucose by the same chemical reactions, but could not do it due to some secrets that are known only by Mother Nature. Only plants can make this happen.

In books, the glucose molecule is displayed as a ring of 6 atoms (simplified symbol) or as a ring of 5 carbons, 1 oxygen plus a carbon "flag" (see figure 15).

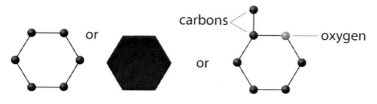

Simplified Symbols

Figure 15. Glucose molecule structure

Within the plant, the *light energy becomes chemical energy,* forming the six-atom glucose molecule. Glucose provides energy for plant's roots, stem, flowers, and fruits of the plant. But not all energy is being used, and some of it remains available for humans and animals.

Carbohydrates can be in two forms: *simple carbohydrates* and *complex carbohydrates.*

Simple carbohydrates are sugars. These kinds of carbohydrates can be easily digested in our body. They are in table sugar, soft drinks, cakes, cookies, pies, candies, ice cream, jam and jellies, and many other desserts. Refined, empty calorie carbohydrates are likely to cause us to gain fat. They also cause us to overeat because they don't have fiber—one of the ingredients that "turns off" hunger. By the time we feel full with these concentrated-calories, fiber-poor foods, we've eaten more calories than we need, and the excess turns to fat. This also applies to all juices. For example, it takes up to twelve oranges to make one glass of orange juice.

Complex carbohydrates are the ones that takes longer to digest. They are mostly in seeds or leaves of a plant. Complex carbohydrate contains *starch and fiber*. The best sources of complex carbohydrates are brown rice, legumes, whole grains, wheat bran, barley, oats, oat bran, rye, vegetables, fruits, and others.

Even though fruits and some vegetables contain sugars, they are categorized as complex carbohydrates because of the value of fiber in them. Fiber slows down the absorption of these sugars and has other health benefits. Juices, especially nonpulp ones, don't have many advantages over any other sugary drinks in terms of sugar due to nonexisting fiber.

Simple carbohydrates are called simple because they have fewer molecules (see figure 16). Complex carbohydrates have many molecules connected in chains (see figure 17).

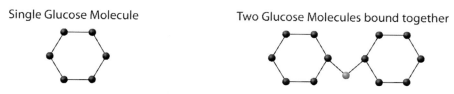

Figure 16. Simple carbohydrates

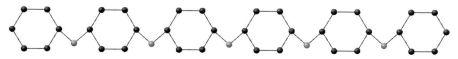

Figure 17. Complex carbohydrates chains

The longer the glucose chains, the more time our body needs to break it down.

The energy in our body burns with a certain speed depending on how physically active we are at a given moment. When a marathon runner drinks something sweet, his body will burn the simple carbohydrate in his drink fast because his body is working fast too. But if the person who sits on the couch drinks the same drink, he will only use some of the simple carbohydrates for energy, and the rest will be converted to fat. His body is working slowly, and he would be better off having complex carbohydrates that digest slowly as well. Whether we eat simple carbohydrates or complex, our body can only absorb as much as it needs to drive our life at any given moment. The excess of it will be stored as fat.

Glycogen

Glycogen is a chain of glucose molecules. About two-thirds of these chains are stored in our muscles. The other one-third accumulates in our liver. Why do we need it, and what is the importance of this storage?

First of all, it is great that the excess of carbohydrates that we eat is not collected as fat. And the second advantage is that we have immediate energy available for our physical and mental activities when we run out of available glucose from food. Our body can tear these chains apart and send glucose to blood for energy.

The muscle cell starts breaking down glycogen into glucose only when the glucose level in the blood begins to drop. If there is food in the stomach, the body will take glucose first from there. Then, if it's not enough, or if breaking down of food takes longer than the body requires, muscles will deplete its glycogen into glucose.

Nonfit people do not store very much of glycogen in their muscles simply for the reason that they don't need it. Their muscles move rarely, and immediate energy required is also rare. Why would their muscles "bother" to develop a new feature that will never be used when it can store the excess of carbohydrates in more a "convenient way"—as fat?

Fit people, on the other hand, constantly and regularly use a lot of glucose for physical activity, and their bodies get rebuilt to better glucose collecting and burning machines. The accumulation of glycogen is a natural response of our body to protect itself and prepare for the next physical activity.

Those who exercise regularly have a significant advantage over nonexercisers in terms of what type and how much of carbohydrates they can "afford" to eat. They can turn excess of carbohydrates into *glycogen* within their muscle tissue instead of fat in their fat depots, and the fitter the person, the better he stores carbohydrates as glycogen and not as fat. All people can store glycogen, but the percentage is higher for those who exercise regularly.

Fiber

There are two types of fiber: soluble and insoluble.

- **Soluble fiber** can dissolve in water and can also help to lower blood fats and maintain blood sugar. Primary sources are *beans*, *fruits*, and *oat products*.

- **Insoluble fiber** cannot dissolve in water, so it passes directly through the digestive system. It's found in *whole-grain products* and *vegetables*.

Fiber comes *only from carbohydrates* and has tremendous benefits to our health. Insoluble fiber is a hard structure of a plant that supports the leaves, stems, roots, and seeds. It is a chain of sugars but not digestible by the human body.

Fiber is not available in animal proteins or fats, and without adequate amount of fiber, our body degenerates developing many illnesses including heart diseases and cancer.

If there were no fiber, there wouldn't be complex carbohydrates. Without fiber, starch would stick together or digest just as simple sugar. Highly processed carbohydrates are broken down into too little pieces. They have very little fiber. A good example is white flour, which is made from whole grains by instant mechanical process. The less grains are ground, the better the quality of the flour. Whole-wheat flour is less processed and accordingly has more fiber.

Besides fiber and starch, carbohydrates have other important nutrients such as vitamins and minerals. By refining the carbohydrate, these nutrients are lost in the process and cannot be recovered. Some processed foods have labels: Vitamins and Minerals Added. Those vitamins and minerals are not always added in a proper combination, as it would naturally be in original carbohydrate. This makes the digestion of that carbohydrate problematic.

During digestion, fiber from complex carbohydrates has the ability to absorb fat from food that we eat. Then the absorbed fat never reaches the bloodstream. It passes through the digestion tract together with fiber, making our diet less fattening even though we eat fat. In many countries in Europe, food is rich in fat, but because it is also rich in fiber, this makes the whole diet much healthier.

To understand better what fiber does to the fat inside of our body, spill a little bit oil on your kitchen countertop and then cover it with a regular paper towel. You will notice how oil will immediately get sucked into that paper towel. Paper towel is also made out of fiber—very similar to the one we eat. So if you eat fatty food, combine it with salad, and you will reduce the amount of it digested.

Starch

Starch is a plant's storage form of glucose. As a plant matures, it stores the energy in its seeds for the next generations. If there was no starch, glucose would be washed away by the rains because glucose is water soluble.

Glycemic Index of Carbohydrates

All carbohydrates have *glycemic index*—a value that describes how fast the carbohydrate can provide its glucose into the bloodstream. Those carbohydrates that deliver glucose faster have higher glycemic index, and those that are slower have lower index.

All carbohydrates are divided into three glycemic index categories depending on the speed of releasing of the glucose.

Pure glucose itself is given a value of 100. All other carbohydrates are described relative to glucose. For example, if a carbohydrate is releasing its sugar slower than pure glucose by 30 percent, then this carbohydrate will receive index 70 (100 [glucose] - 30 = 70)

If we eat too much of carbohydrates with high glycemic index, two things can happen:

1. We can develop diabetes.
2. We can gain fat.

What makes a carbohydrate release sugar fast? There are two things:

- High level of sugar in it, and
- How refined carbohydrate is (physically broken down). A good example of highly refined carbohydrate is a white bread.

Glycemic Index Range

low—55 or less
medium—56-69
high—70 or more

Glycemic Load of Carbohydrates

Even if we choose to eat carbohydrates with low glycemic index but we eat too much, we can still gain fat or develop diabetes. The glycemic load of carbohydrates gives us more understanding about carbohydrates.

To understand glycemic load better, imagine a gun. If we say that a gun is loaded with 7 bullets, we can also say that 1 serving of a particular carbohydrate is loaded with 7 units.

A high glycemic index food consumed in small quantities would give the same effect as larger quantities of a low glycemic index food. For example, white rice has high glycemic index, so eating 50 g of white rice at one sitting would give a particular glucose curve in the blood, while 25 g would give the same curve but half the height. Since the peak height is probably the most important parameter for diabetes control, multiplying the amount of carbohydrates in a food serving by the glycemic index gives an idea of how much effect an actual portion of food has on blood sugar level.

Glycemic Load Range

low—10 or less
medium—11-19
high—20 or more

Food manufacturers are creating new food products in a faster rate than glycemic index testing can be performed on them. Each year, tens of thousands of new packaged-food items are added to grocery shelves, but only a few hundred foods are tested for glycemic index.

Because of this, it's doubtful that we'll ever reach a point in time where glycemic index is known for all foods. The most productive glycemic index testing laboratory is based in Australia, so a larger portion of the currently tested foods are of Australian origin.

Just to give you an idea about some of the most popular foods tested for glycemic index and glycemic load, I've created tables below from which you can learn how to make better selections when creating your meal plan. If you don't find your favorite foods in those tables, there are multiple websites on Internet displaying that information, and you can search there by the product you are looking for. One of the most detailed one is www.mendosa.com. This website has great variety of tested foods for glycemic index and glycemic load.

When using my tables, remember that foods in them are rated by glycemic index. Keep an eye on the glycemic load when choosing foods for your meal plan because some of the foods with low glycemic index may have high glycemic load. Those are color-coordinated for your attention.

Today, the use of the glycemic index for reducing weight remains uncertain even though there are some great results achieved by many people. Everybody is different, and the effect of glycemic index depends on many factors: body type, body size and weight, metabolic rate, etc. The food's glycemic effect may also vary depending on how the food is prepared, its ripeness, and which other foods accompany it in the same meal. Meanwhile, dietary guidelines still suggest choosing foods ranking low on the glycemic index and glycemic load for weight and blood sugar level control.

Table 19. Fruits & Vegetables by Glycemic Index & Glycemic Load

	FRUITS (per 120g)	GI	GL		VEGETABLES (per 80g)	GI	GL
LOW	Cherries	22	3	LOW	Spinach	6	1
	Grapefruit	25	3		Broccoli	6	1
	Prunes	29	20		Cabbage	6	1
	Apples	38	4		Asparagus	8	1
	Plums	39	3		Lettuce	10	1
	Peaches	42	4		Mushrooms	10	1
	Strawberries	43	1		Onions	10	1
	Oranges	43	4		Red Peppers	10	4
	Pears	43	5		Green beans	28	1
	Grapes	46	8		Tomato, ripe	38	4
	Kiwi fruit	52	7		Carrots	49	3
	Mango	55	8		Green peas	48	4
MEDIUM	Grapes black	59	11		Yam	51	7
	Cantaloupe	65	4	MEDIUM	Sweet corn	60	11
	Pineapple	66	6		Sweet potato	61	9
HIGH	Kiwi	67	7		Potato, boiled	63	6
	Figs	67	32		Beets	64	5
	Bananas	71	16	HIGH	Potato, baked	73	14
	Raisins	72	56		Pumpkin	75	3
	Watermelon	80	5		Parsnips	97	12

GI = Glycemic Index, GL = Glycemic Load

Table 20. Snacks & Cereals by Glycemic Index & Glycemic Load

	SNACKS (per 50g)	GI	GL		CEREALS (per 30g)	GI	GL
LOW	Peanuts	15	1	LOW	All-Bran	38	9
LOW	Chocolate Milk	54	14	LOW	Special K	54	11
LOW	Popcorn	55	15	LOW	Frosties	55	15
MEDIUM	Power Bars	56	18	LOW	Bran Buds	58	7
MEDIUM	Croissant	67	15	LOW	Bran Chex	58	11
MEDIUM	Oatmeal Cookie	58	18	LOW	Life	66	16
MEDIUM	Muffin, carrot	62	18	LOW	Nutrigrain	66	10
MEDIUM	Raisins	64	23	LOW	Muesli	66	16
MEDIUM	Snickers Bar	68	19	LOW	Puffed Wheat	67	13
MEDIUM	Rye Crackers	68	22	LOW	Grapenuts	67	13
HIGH	Mars Bar	70	23	LOW	Shredded Wheat	72	13
HIGH	Water Crackers	71	22	LOW	Raisin Bran	73	12
HIGH	Soda Crackers	72	24	MEDIUM	Bran Flakes	74	13
HIGH	Corn Chips	73	18	MEDIUM	Cheerios	74	15
HIGH	Doughnut	76	18	MEDIUM	Corn Bran	75	15
HIGH	Vanilla Wafers	77	28	MEDIUM	Rice Krispies	82	21
HIGH	Rice Cakes	80	34	MEDIUM	Corn Chex	83	21
HIGH	Jelly Beans	80	37	HIGH	Cornflakes	83	21
HIGH	Puff Crispbread	81	30	HIGH	Crispix	87	22
HIGH	Pretzels	83	27	HIGH	Rice Chex	89	23

GI = Glycemic Index, GL = Glycemic Load

Table 21. Beverages & Juices by Glycemic Index & Glycemic Load

BEVERAGES & JUICES (per 250g)	GI	GL
Smoothie	33	14
Tomato Juice	38	4
Apple juice	40	12
Carrot juice	43	10
Pineapple juice	46	16
Grapefruit juice	48	11
Orange Juice	50	13
Pepsi	58	15
Cranberry Cocktail	68	24
Coca Cola	63	16
Poweraid	65	13
Fanta	68	23
Sports Plus	74	13
Gatorade	89	13
GatorLode	100	51

LOW (Smoothie–Orange Juice), MEDIUM (Pepsi–Fanta), HIGH (Sports Plus–GatorLode)

GI = Glycemic Index, GL = Glycemic Load

Most legumes and dairy products are low in glycemic index unless they are sugar added, such as ice cream.

Insulin Dependency on the Fat Storage

After we eat sugary foods, the pancreas, a large organ lying near the stomach, secretes into the bloodstream a hormone called *insulin*, whose job is to lower the blood sugar level. While insulin is lowering the sugar level, few things are happening:

- Insulin commands the body to *stop breaking down glucose and the body fat* because it "wants" to use up the excess of just-eaten sugar.
- Body starts *"packing up"* just-eaten *sugar into glycogen* trying to store it wherever possible including converting it to body fat.
- Insulin commands to put *breaking down of proteins on hold,* making muscle-building process difficult.
- If the spike of sugar level in the blood is too high, pancreas may produce too much insulin leading to lowering the blood sugar level below the normal. Then we start feeling run-down, and our body starts craving for sugar again. Eventually, the body may get "confused" about the normality of the sugar level in the blood.

30.2 Fats

Seventy percent of people die from three main causes involving fatty degeneration: cardiovascular disease (approx. 44 percent), cancer (approx. 22 percent), and diabetes (approx. 2 percent). Most of these deaths are due to ignorance and misconceptions about fats. Simplistic half-truths advertised on TV, radio, some magazines and newspapers have created a lot of confusion. While some TV programs and food channels claim to promote healthy ways of eating or cooking, they still utilize fats incorrectly.

Most doctors, who are supposed to give us advice on how to prevent the degenerative diseases, unfortunately also have very limited understanding about healthy and unhealthy fats.

Many fad diet books advice to reduce the fat content in your diet without taking into consideration that some fats are absolutely required for health, some help to reduce body fat, and some clean our heart arteries. In order to lose body fat but still stay healthy, it is absolutely essential to understand the difference between good and bad fats. Fats play an enormous role in keeping our body in "good working condition."

A Closer Look at Fats

Our cell membranes are made of fat, and when we eat right fats, our body uses those fats to protect and regenerate those membranes. Some fats are used for energy, brain work, and hormonal balance.

Understanding about fats can only come from understanding their molecule structures. Without this fundamental knowledge, we will always be lost in the opinions of others. Let's take a closer look on a fat molecule to identify good and bad fats:

The fat molecule, whether it is solid fat like butter or liquid like vegetable oil, is made up of one molecule of *glycerol* and three molecules of *fatty acid*. The most common name for fats used in books is *triglycerides*. It might sound complicated to you, but this name explains itself: if you break it down into two words, *tri* and *glycerides,* you will remember it faster: *tri* is three molecules of *fatty acids,* and *glyceride* is one *glycerol* molecule holding those fatty acids together.

To understand the fat molecule structure better, I am offering here a step-by-step diagram-to-diagram lesson, the simplicity of which I have tested on my kids and people who don't know about chemistry at all. If you pay a little attention to what you read further, I can almost guarantee that in 15-20 minutes you will know everything you need to know to differentiate good and bad fats.

Let's get started.

Step 1

Take a look at figure 18. This is the fat molecule in the most simplified way—no atoms or connection between those atoms shown—just blocks. This can be compared to looking at the house that you intend to buy from the outside.

You can see here how 1 molecule of glycerol is holding 3 fatty acids together.

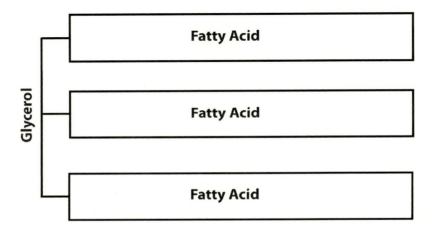

Figure 18. Fat molecule structure (Simplified view)

Step 2

Let's open up each block of the fat molecule just to get a basic idea about how atoms are connected there. Compare to the house that you intend to buy again. This will be as going inside the house and browsing quickly around without going into details.

You may notice from figure 19 how the glycerol molecule has a straight shape with 3 atoms connected together and fatty acids have zigzag forms and how they are different in length. Each fatty acid within a single fat molecule can be different in length and its structure.

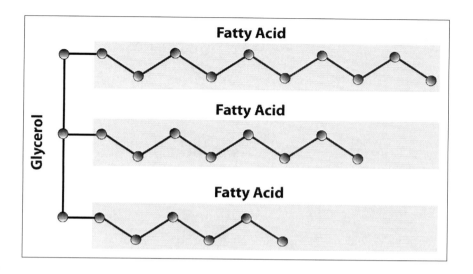

Figure 19. Fat molecule atoms connection

Step 3

For better understanding, cross-refer figures 18 and 19 with the next one, figure 20, which for simplicity displays all 3 fatty acids with their same length and structure.

Comparing to the house you intend to buy, this step is going into details of each room, and the rooms on figure 20 are the blocks shown in light gray color. What do we see there? The same straight glycerol molecule with more details in it and the same fatty acids zigzags but also with more details in them.

Let's find out those details.

Every fat molecule consists of carbon atoms (C), hydrogen atoms (H), and oxygen atoms (O). Those atoms are color- and size-coordinated. Carbons are *larger* **black** balls. Hydrogens are *smaller* **gray** balls connected to carbons, and oxygen atoms are *larger* **gray** balls also connected to carbons.

Fat Molecules (Triglycerides)

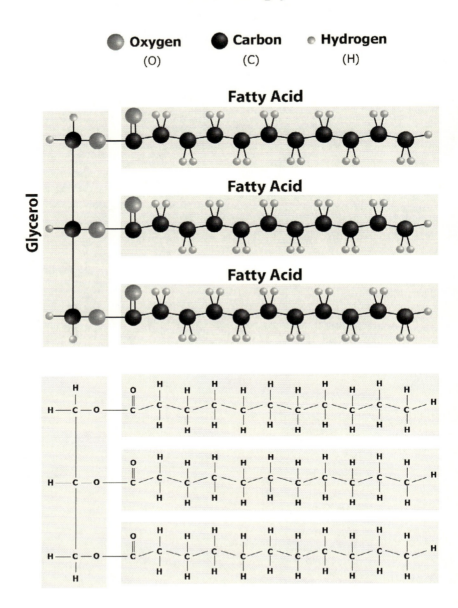

Figure 20. Fat molecule structure (Detailed view and formula)

The carbon connection with their hydrogen varies from fatty acid to fatty acid, but the fatty acid's structure plays a major role in recognizing good and bad fats, and this is what we are going to learn further.

Saturated and Unsaturated Fats

In terms of molecule structure, saturation refers to whether or not all the carbons in a fatty acid are holding their hydrogen atoms. If every available bond from the carbons is holding hydrogen, the chain forms a *saturated* fatty acid (see figure 21, "Saturated"). Notice how every carbon is holding at least two hydrogen atoms.

Saturated fats occur naturally in many foods—plants and animal sources, including meat and dairy products. Examples of the most saturated are beef fat, lamb, pork, poultry fat and skin, beef fat (tallow), lard and cream, butter, cheese, and other dairy products made from milk.

Sometimes in a fat molecule, carbon can lose one hydrogen atom and then reconnect differently forming so-called *double bonds*. Those fatty acids are called *unsaturated*.

Unsaturated fats that have one double bond are called *monounsaturated* (mono means one), and those that have two and more double bond are called *polyunsaturated* (see figure 21, "Monounsaturated" and "Polyunsaturated"). Unsaturated molecules bend when forming double bonds. Saturated fatty acids stay straight.

Good examples of unsaturated fats are most nuts, olive oil, flaxseed oil, and hemp oil, avocados, and some fish, such as salmon.

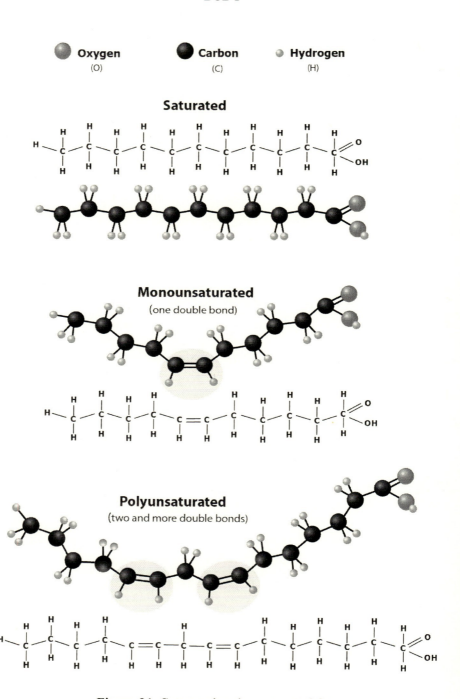

Figure 21. Saturated and unsaturated fats

Plants can modify saturated fatty acids, and they can "insert" one or more double bonds into their chains, changing those chains into unsaturated. They are doing that to support their life, recreating fat formulas depending what type of fat is more needed for them. Plants can insert double bonds between any two carbons in a carbon chain, as close as 3 and 6 carbons from *methyl end* (methyl end is where fatty acid connects to glycerol molecule, figure 21, left). This ability enables plants to produce two "families" of fatty acids very well known as omega-3 (3-d carbon is to create first double bond) and omega-6 (6th carbon to create first double bond). These two fatty acids are called *essential fatty acids*. They both are vital to human health and must be provided with food. Our body cannot produce them or modify from any saturated fats (as plants do).

Essential Fatty Acids (EFAs)

The key components of healing **(good)** fats are the *essential fatty acids*. They are *linoleic acid omega-6* (shortly abbreviated as **LA** or **18:2w6)**, and *alpha-linolenic acid omega-3* (abbreviated as **LNA** or **18:3w3**).

LA (omega-6)
18:2w6 abbreviation means 18 carbons in the chain, 2 double bonds, and the first double bond starts at carbon number 6 from the methyl end (left).

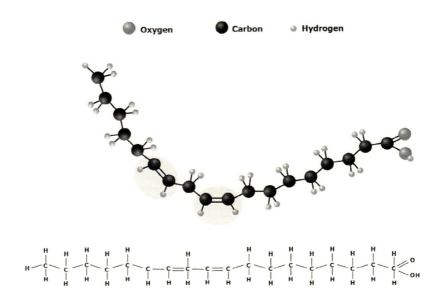

Figure 22. Linoleic Acid (Omega 6)

Some of the richest sources of omega-6 (LA) are the following:

- Safflower oil—the richest natural source
- Sunflower oil
- Corn oil
- Sesame oil
- Hemp oil (best balance of omega-6:omega-3)
- Pumpkin oil
- Soybean oil
- Walnut oil
- Wheat germ oil
- Evening primrose oil

LNA (omega-3)
18:3w3 means 18 carbons, 3 double bonds, the first of which is number 3 from methyl end.

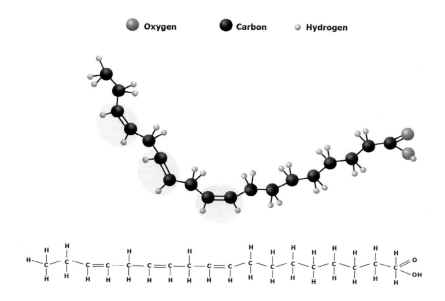

Figure 23. Alpha-Linoleic Acid (Omega 3)

Some of the richest sources of omega-3 (LNA) are the following:

- Flax—the richest natural source
- Salmon
- Soybean
- Chia
- Hemp
- Walnut
- Wheat germ
- Kukui (candlenut)
- Rice bran
- Pumpkin

Both of these unsaturated fatty acids are polyunsaturated because they both have two or more double bonds.

Importance and Functions of EFAs

Essential fatty acids in plants mostly come from their seeds. If you take a seed in your hands, you may notice how most of these seeds have a hard shell. That shell is designed by Mother Nature to protect the oil in the seed from light, heat, and air, and seeds were meant to be consumed by humans and animals in that original form. But because we are so "inventive," we eat them in a completely different form now. We destroy those seeds, exposing oils taken out of them to all possible processes including heat, light, and air.

If those fatty acids are consumed not in their original form, their molecule formula does not match with molecule formulas of our body, making the healing and regenerating process impossible. Fatty acids with unrecognized formulas eventually get stored as body fat instead of constructive use. Then not only do we get fat but also sick because we are lacking the important ingredients to support our life.

Light, the greatest enemy of EFAs, produces free radicals in oils and speeds up 1,000 times oxidation of oil with oxygen from air.

Oxygen breaks down oil even when the oil is not exposed to light. In plants, all the seeds are firmly sealed into their shells. If some seeds open up, they get rapidly oxidized and rancid.

Heat, used to *deodorize, hydrogenate*, and *fry* also destroys EFAs by twisting their molecules.

Essential fatty acids are involved with producing life energy in our body from food and then moving that energy throughout our system. EFAs regulate growth, vitality, and mental state. Many people these days complain about the low energy level even when they eat a sufficient amount of calories per day. This is partially due to our food "modernization" and lack of EFAs in that food.

Essential fatty acids are responsible for the most vital processes in our body functionality:

Cells

EFAs are part of each and every cell membrane in our body. They help to hold proteins within the cell membrane by the electrostatic forces of their double bonds. They also move substances in and out, helping cells stay alive and maintain their stability.

Hemoglobin production

EFAs help to produce red blood pigment from simpler substances. They are also involved in a process of delivery of oxygen to our tissues.

Energy production

EFAs hook up oxygen, electron transport, and energy in the process of oxidation, a process that helps to "burn" the food to produce the energy.

Oxygen transfer

EFAs transfer the oxygen from air into our lungs. Oxygen then gets carried by our blood to all our cells. Burning body fat requires oxygen too, and EFAs help that process in many ways.

Recovery from fatigue

Both EFAs substantially shorten the time for muscles to recover from fatigues after exercise. They convert the lactic acid (soreness experienced after intensive workouts) into water and carbon dioxide. This is especially important for athletes or those who exercise intensively.

Brain development

During the first year, around 50 percent of an infant's daily calories come from fat. Mother Nature knows how important fat is for babies. Fats are major components of the human brain cell membrane.

Fat burn

At the levels above 12 to 15 percent of total calories, in some cases, EFAs show the increase of the rate of metabolic reactions in our body and burn more fat into carbon dioxide, water, and energy resulting in weight loss and energy production.

How do we know that we are lacking EFAs? Our body is designed to let us know when EFAs are missing by various symptoms:

LA (Omega-6) Deficiency Symptoms

- Eczemalike skin eruptions
- Loss of hair
- Liver degeneration
- Kidney degeneration
- Behavioral disturbances
- Excessive water loss through the skin
- Failure of wound healings
- Sterility in males
- Miscarriage in females
- Arthritislike conditions
- Heart and circulatory problems
- Growth retardation

LNA (Omega-3) Deficiency Symptoms

- Growth retardation
- Weakness
- Impairment of vision and learning ability
- Motor incoordination
- Tingling sensations in arms and legs
- Behavior changes
- High blood pressure
- Edema
- Dry skin
- Mental deterioration
- High triglycerides

Deficiency symptoms if caught on time can be cured just by adding EFAs back to the diet.

Essential fatty acids are called essential because they govern every life process in our body. Life without them is impossible, and we, as humans were designed to receive them through our food. But for the past 50-70 years, we destroyed most of the products that contained

EFAs. We grind grains to produce cereal and breads. We developed mass production of many products that required heating, toasting, and roasting, which completely killed the EFAs, and we also invented fast-foods, some of which contain no EFAs at all.

Source: Udo Erasmus, *Fats That Heal, Fats That Kill*

EFAs Balance

How much of each essential fatty acid is enough, and in what combination should it be to provide the best benefit to our health?

Due to food modernization, our current consumption of omega-6 has doubled from 1940. Excess of intake of omega-6 can cause increased water retention, raised blood pressure, and raised blood clotting. By comparison, our intake of omega-3 fatty acids has shrunk to one-sixth.

Because omega-6 and omega-3 "compete" with each other, the proper ratio between them is extremely important.

The omega-6:omega-3 ratio in our brain is 1:1; in the fat tissue is 5:1; other tissues, about 4:1. Studies suggest that the evolutionary human diet rich in animals, seafood, plants, and fruits may have provided a ratio between 1:1 and 4:1.

As estimates of the World Health Organization suggest, approximately 6 percent of total calories should come from the source from omega-6 and 2 percent from omega-3. This makes the ratio between omega-6:omega-3, 3:1.

What does it mean in terms of grams and calories? For an average person who consumes 2,000 calories per day, the amounts of calculations will follow:

Calories

omega-6: 2,000 × 6% = 120 calories per day
omega-3: 2,000 × 2% = 40 calories per day

Grams

1 gram of fat equals to 9 calories. So the calculations will be as follows:

omega-6: 120 calories / 9 =13.3 grams (1 tablespoon or 6 gel capsules)

omega-3: 40 calories / 9 = 4.4 grams (less than 1 teaspoon or 2 gel capsules)

The Standard American Diet provides an omega-6: omega-3 ratio of between 10:1 and 30:1 instead of suggested 3:1 ratio. People who eat a Western diet rarely have omega-6 deficiencies because omega-6 is found in most vegetable oils and even processed foods. Omega-3 is most important nutritionally to the people who eat the Standard American Diet (SAD). Americans are more likely to get too much of omega-6 than too little.

Tips

1. Some people may assume "If I buy a proper supplement blend of omega-6 and omega-3, which is 3:1, from a health store, I will solve the problem.

    But let's think about it first. If your present diet, for example, is a Standard American Diet with ratio of omega-6:omega-3 10:1, adding a ratio 3:1 is not going to make your total ratio 3:1. It will be 13:2.

    To get the proper ratio, you need to take into consideration the *total number of calories* per day and not just the ratio of your supplements—you need not only to increase the consumption of omega-3 but also to reduce the consumption of the omega-6.

2. Someone with good mathematics skills may decide to add only omega-3 to the diet to make the ratio mathematically also 3:1, even though in reality it is 18:6. But while mathematically this is correct, adding more fat calories to the diet is not healthy. The ratio 18:6 is not the same as 3:1. Calculations should be

based *not* on proportional coincidence of numbers but on the total amount of calories consumed per day. To get the 3:1 ratio between omega-6 and omega-3, not always omega-3 should be added to the diet but often the consumption of omega-6 should be reduced.

In order to be effective, the essential fatty acids need the "support" of vitamins C, B_3 and B_6, and magnesium, and zinc. Without these important components, EFAs' digestion and outcome of the EFAs is also impossible.

Essential Fatty Acids and Hunger

Because essential fatty acids are essential, the body survival mechanism works the way that it will always keep you hungry until you finally get enough of essential fatty acids. You may be eating enough of carbohydrates, protein, and other fats, but until you provide a bare minimum of essential fatty acids, your body will not give up "asking" for more food.

To help yourself balance your omega-6:omega-3 ratio, please refer to table 22 that compares the contents of saturated, monounsaturated, and polyunsaturated fatty acids in various fats and oils.

Table 22. Comparison of Dietary Fats

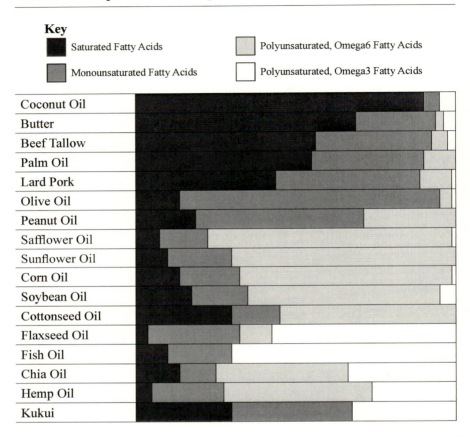

Saturated Fats

Misconception that saturated fats are somehow bad for you lately went beyond any logic. Saturated fats are blamed for everything—fatness, heart problems, cancer, and even diabetes. Should we also blame wine for alcoholism and food for overeating?

If we are talking about overconsumption, that's a different story. But overconsumption of the essential fatty acids can damage our health just as fast as the overconsumption of saturated fats.

Saturated fats are like essential fatty acids; they can build our cell membrane, and they are also an excellent source of energy. But

NUTRITION

unfortunately, in many magazines and newspapers, saturated fats are represented as our enemy or dietary monsters hiding in our food just to cause problems.

Mother Nature knows best, and we should always trust it. Take a look at table 20 again and notice how all natural products have saturated fats—even olive oil, and even flaxseed oil—they all have saturated fats.

Although we don't normally consider saturated fat as an essential nutrient, it is just as vital to good health as the essential fatty acids. We need saturated fat for proper digestive function, growth, and a host of other processes.

Saturated fats portraying bad is a profit-generating propaganda to sell other products. Fad diet books or weight loss programs may tell you to avoid saturated fats in order to make a sale of their own products. Those who sell essential fatty acid capsules or vegetable oils may also try to bend you over into this idea.

Before the twentieth century, mostly saturated fats were used by humans, and we didn't have vegetable oils then. Did we get better with our heart diseases, cancer, and other health issues by replacing saturated fats with vegetable oils? Statistics says the opposite.

A 2004 article in the *American Journal of Clinical Nutrition* raised the possibility that the supposed causal relationship between saturated fats and heart disease may actually be a statistical bias. The authors take the example of the "Finnish mental hospital study" in which saturated fat intakes were monitored more closely than were total fat intakes, therefore ignoring the possibility that simply a larger fat intake may lead to a higher risk of coronary diseases. It also suggests that other parameters were overlooked, such as carbohydrate intakes.

A 2010 meta-analysis in the American Journal of Clinical Nutrition looked at twenty-one unique studies containing over 350,000 people. They found no association between saturated fat and an increased risk for coronary heart disease, stroke, or cardiovascular disease.

A study of 297 Portuguese males with acute myocardial infarction (heart attack) found that "total fat intake, *lauric acid*, *palmitic acid* (two common saturated fats), and *oleic acid* (a monoinsaturated fat) were inversely associated with heart attacks and concluded that *low intake* of total fat and lauric acid from dairy products *was related to acute heart attack*". The authors suggest that "recommendations on fatty acid intake should aim for **both an upper and lower limits**".

Blaming saturated fat for our diseases does not fit the facts and is inconsistent with the historical record. *The Lancet* (medical journal) reported a study of 2,000 men who went on a low saturated fat diet to see how that would affect cardiovascular health. The study found that those participants didn't experience any reduction in heart attack death risk over a two-year period.

Of course you can find the researches proving that overconsumption of saturated fats lead to heart problems and other diseases. But again, they are talking about *over*consumptions.

Life is about balance. Overconsumption of saturated fats was proven to be bad, but this doesn't mean that we should be avoiding them. Whether we overconsume with carbohydrates or with saturated fats—it doesn't matter—overconsumption is an overconsumption.

Dietary Recommendations for Saturated Fats

A 2004 statement released by the Centers for Disease Control and Prevention (CDC) determined that "Americans need to continue working to reduce saturated fat intake." Additionally, reviews by the American Heart Association led the association to recommend **reducing** (please mention, not avoiding) saturated fat intake to less than 7 percent of total calories according to its 2006 recommendations. This concurs with similar conclusions made by the World Health Organization (WHO) and the US Department of Health and Human Services, both of which determined that reduction in saturated fat consumption would positively affect health and reduce the prevalence of heart disease.

Cholesterol

Cholesterol is another victim of today's commercialized halfway truth information. The anticholesterol propaganda is a big business for doctors and drug companies. It is also a powerful marketing gimmick for vegetable oil and margarine manufacturers and those who advertise their products to be "cholesterol free."

Cholesterol plays both a vital and detrimental role in our health, but most people, being misinformed, consider cholesterol only as an ugly beast hiding in our body with a purpose to kill.

What is cholesterol? Cholesterol is the hard fatty and waxy substance that melts at 149°C. The most important function of cholesterol is to provide protective coating to our arteries and its surrounding walls. Cholesterol also regulates our cell membranes' fluidity. Nature has equipped each cell with the ability to generate its own cholesterol. Just think about it—why would Mother Nature do that if the cholesterol was bad? When a membrane of a cell gets too loose, the cholesterol gets added to it to stiffen the membrane, and when a membrane gets too hard, the cholesterol gets removed from it.

Another important function of cholesterol is to make steroid hormones. *Estrogen, progesterone* (female hormones), and *testosterone* (male hormone) are the productions of this functionality. *Estrogen* has an important role on skin tension, making of bones stronger, and protection against arteriosclerosis.

Progesterone was named after its only known action of that time, "pro" meaning support of, and "gestation" meaning pregnancy. It is now also known as involved in the female menstrual cycle and embryogenesis.

Testosterone is the principal male sex hormone and an anabolic steroid. It plays a key role in the development of male reproductive tissues such as the testes and prostate as well as promoting secondary sexual characteristics such as increased muscle and bone mass and hair growth. In addition, testosterone is essential for health and well-being as well as preventing osteoporosis.

Cholesterol is the best source of getting energy, libido, fertility, and vitality. It also aids in digestion and boosts mental performance. In digestion, cholesterol plays an important role synthesizing bile acids. When those acids are secreted into intestine by the liver, they are used to mix fat with water-soluble enzymes to digest the fat and fat-soluble vitamins. Vitamin D is also made in our body by the functionality of cholesterol.

Cholesterol regulates water balance in our body through our kidneys, increasing sodium retention and also regulating cortisone balance, which promotes the synthesis of glucose to prepare our body for stress and to suppress the inflammation. In medicine, large doses of cortisone are used to suppress the inflammatory reactions.

Why then in spite of all these good things, cholesterol is still being portrayed as our enemy? First of all, because cholesterol has been always misunderstood, and second, those who want to sell their own products or services represent cholesterol only from his bad side.

Good and Bad Cholesterols

Almost everyone at least once heard about *good* and *bad* cholesterol, and we are always being warned and programmed to control the cholesterol we eat.

But the majority of cholesterol in our bloodstream comes from the manufacturing in our liver and not from food as it is usually presented by the media and the doctors. Many people still think that dietary cholesterol is a major factor in elevated blood cholesterol, which is not true.

The Faculty of Health and Medical Sciences, University of Surrey, Guildford, Surrey, UK, has conducted the study to determine whether the *increased dietary cholesterol* intakes *increase the LDL*, so-called bad cholesterol:

Methods used. Two groups of free-living volunteers on an **energy-restricted diet** were studied for 12 weeks: one group was instructed to consume two eggs a day, and the other, to exclude eggs.

Results. Energy intake fell by 25 and 29 percent in the egg-fed and non-egg-fed groups, resulting in a moderate weight loss of 3.4 kg and 4.4 kg, respectively. The daily intake of dietary cholesterol increased significantly in the egg-fed group from 278 to 582 mg after 6 weeks. The concentration of LDL cholesterol *decreased* in the non-egg-fed groups after 6 weeks and in the *egg-fed and non-egg-fed at 12 weeks relative to baseline.*

Conclusions. An increased intake of dietary cholesterol from two eggs a day *does not increase total plasma or LDL* cholesterol *when accompanied by moderate weight loss.* These findings suggest that *cholesterol-rich foods should not be excluded from dietary advice* to lose weight on account of an unfavorable influence on plasma LDL cholesterol.

Elevated levels of LDL (low density lipoprotein) cholesterol are usually associated with an increased risk of coronary heart disease. LDL deposits cholesterol on the artery walls, causing the formation of a hard, thick substance called cholesterol plaque. Over time, cholesterol plaque causes thickening of the artery walls and narrowing of the arteries, a process called *atherosclerosis.*

HDL on the other hand is always trying to compensate for our flaws—it "works hard" to shuttle cholesterol away from tissues, arteries, *delivering it back to our liver.* That is why HDL is called the "good cholesterol."

Why is HDL taking cholesterol back to your liver? Why does your liver make sure that you have plenty of cholesterol? And why not take it right to your kidneys or your intestines to get rid of it?

Let's think about that.

From your liver, the cholesterol gets put back into other particles or taken to tissues and cells that need it. *Your body is trying to make and conserve the cholesterol for the precise reason that it is so important, indeed vital, for health.*

Why then, about two-thirds of the North Americans, European, and affluent populations worldwide still suffer from cholesterol deposits?

For the last fifty years, there are few different theories developed about the causes of cardiovascular problems due to cholesterol:

1. **Free radicals**
Free radicals are created by environmental pollution, cigarette smoking, and poisons like cleaners or herbicides. This theory suggests that arterial walls are first damaged by the free radicals in our bloodstream and that cholesterol deposits are part of the mechanism that attempts to repair that damage.

   The deficiency of minerals and vitamins allows free radicals to be present.

2. **Antioxidants**
This theory revolves around too low levels of antioxidants in our blood that causes arterial damage and thickening.

3. **Overconsumption of refined foods**
Nutrient-poor sugars and processed foods may cause our body to manufacture more cholesterol, which in the long run causes clogged arteries.

4. **Vitamin C deficiency**
This theory was proposed by the team of Dr. Rath and Pauling—the winners of two Nobel prizes for Chemistry and Peace. It is based on idea that vitamin C is required for the synthesis of the "glue" that surrounds our cells, and it makes them unified and consistent and keeps our tissues from falling apart.

   Vitamin C is the strongest antioxidant. It prevents free radicals from damaging our cells and tissues. It helps to utilize proteins, make our arteries, bones, teeth, cartilage, and other tissues stronger. Tissue strength is particularly important in our arteries since they are constantly under pressure. The Standard American Diet is deficient in vitamin C and leads to develop a weakness of the connective tissues in our arteries.

Narrowed arteries to our heart produce chest pain and may result in a *heart attack*. If an artery to our brain is blocked, a *stroke* occurs. Depending on the size and location of the blocked artery, the stroke may be minimal or fatal. If a clot blocks an artery in our lungs, *pulmonary embolism* occurs. A blocked artery in our leg results in impaired circulation that can lead to *gangrene*. *Blindness* and *deafness* can occur when arteries supplying sense organs are blocked. Atherosclerotic deposits may also lead to high *blood pressure*, resulting in heavier load on our heart and kidneys.

Source: Udo Erasmus, *Fats That Heal, Fats That Kill*

Other Causes of Raised Cholesterol

The vitality of cholesterol in our body is so important that our body has created a system to generate cholesterol without the necessity for us in obtaining it from food. Because cholesterol is the stress precursor of stress hormones, our body generates more cholesterol when we are under stress. Our body can manufacture cholesterol out of sugars, proteins, and fats, especially when all these foods are consumed in excess. The more excess is consumed, the more pressure there is on our body to start producing cholesterol.

The excess of cholesterol from food may create "no need" for the body's cholesterol production. This makes our regulating body system "lazy" because our body always compensates for cholesterol intake by reducing the amount synthesized. If the consumption of dietary cholesterol is continuously high, the body system to produce its own cholesterol may appear to be too slow-paced which can affect our health.

Dietary cholesterol is available only in foods from animal sources. Plant foods are cholesterol free. The average North American adult consumes about 800 mg of cholesterol daily. About 45 percent comes from eggs, 35 percent from meat, and 20 percent from dairy products. Only about half of the cholesterol consumed is getting absorbed and used by their body. The rest passes through unused.

The American Heart Association recommends limiting cholesterol intake to less than 300 mg per day. Table 23 represents some of the popular foods by their cholesterol level, and it will help you to control your intake.

Table 23. Foods by Cholesterol

	FOODS	SERVING SIZE	CHOLESTEROL (mg)
LOW	Low-Fat Milk	1 Cup	10
	Cheddar Cheese	1 oz.	30
	Whole Milk	1 Cup	33
	Lean Ground Beef	3.5 oz.	78
	Pork Tenderloin	3.5 oz.	79
	Chicken (skinless)	3.5 oz.	85
	Pork Chop	3.5 oz.	85
	Salmon	100g	87
	Duck Meat	100g	89
	Crab	100g	89
	Lard	100g	94
	Beef Chuck	100g	105
	Pork Shoulder	100g	114
	Pork Ribs	100g	121
	Hamburger large single patty	226 g	122
	Sardines	100g	142
MEDIUM	Cheeseburger, double patty	1 each	141
	Shrimp	100g	173
	Pork Liver Sausage	100g	180
	Veal	100g	184
	Butter	100g	218
	Turkey Giblets	100g	289
HIGH	Beef Liver	3.5 oz.	389
	Chicken Giblets	100g	442
	Eggs fried (2 large)	100 g	480
	Chicken Liver	100g	561

Do not get confused by completely avoiding foods from the bottom of the table because moderate amounts of those foods may be very beneficial to your health.

Liver and cod liver are nutrient-packed superfoods that can help boost your energy, libido, muscle growth, brain power, and general health. They are abundant sources of nutrients that are difficult to obtain elsewhere. Liver contains an unidentified "antifatigue factor" that was found to greatly boost endurance. It is extremely rich in energy-related nutrients that have not been sufficiently researched.

Eggs, especially ones that are produced by free-run chickens have high levels of omega-3 fatty acids.

Milk and cheese from grass-fed cows may also be also good sources of omega-3.

Antioxidants

Antioxidants are the group of vitamins and compounds that helps fight free radicals and even some aspects of aging as well. They are vitamin C, vitamin E (mostly coming from nuts, seeds, vegetable oil, and wheat germ), beta-carotene (principally from carrots, tomatoes, and squash), the mineral selenium (mostly from fish, shellfish, red meat, grains, eggs, chicken, garlic, and liver), and a variety of other compounds found in fruits and vegetables.

Fiber and Cholesterol

Dietary *fiber* has the ability to remove cholesterol from the body. If the fiber is absent, up to 94 percent of the cholesterol is reabsorbed.

Physical Activity and Cholesterol

Physical activity considerably helps in lowering LDL and elevating HDL cholesterol, fighting the developing coronary artery disease. Even moderately intense physical activity such as brisk walking is beneficial when done regularly.

Garlic and Cholesterol

In people with high cholesterol, garlic's lowering effects extend to a range of anywhere between 10 to 20 percent. A growing number of studies have shown positively that garlic can lower cholesterol.

Anticholesterol Pills

Lowering cholesterol with pills doesn't solve the problems of cholesterol levels, and the main cause of cholesterol buildup is not the cholesterol itself but *bad diet, physical inactivity, stress, nutrient deficiencies*, and *some other problems*. Treating cholesterol levels with pills is placing patches on infected wounds, and, statistically, increase death rate from suicide and cancer.

Using the conventional medical thinking that is being used for cholesterol would lead one to believe that doctors should reduce the risk of Alzheimer's disease by taking out everybody's brain.

Removing cholesterol will do nothing to improve the underlying problems, the real roots of chronic disease.

Some of the so-called experts recommend that a person's cholesterol should be as low as possible, and in order to sell their products and services, they also say that it cannot be achieved by diet, exercise, or any known lifestyle modification. Therefore, they prescribe cholesterol-lowering pills adding to the $26 billion in sales of drugs each year.

Major scientific organizations have chastised medical journals for allowing the pharmaceutical industry to publish misleading results and half-truths in a convenient way to generate more profits. Their studies usually show only one-way results with a purpose to sell more drugs.

Lowering cholesterol levels with pills have been shown to worsen patients with congestive heart failure, a life-threatening condition where the heart becomes too weak to effectively pump blood. For those who still have healthy hearts, the side effects of cholesterol-lowering drugs may not show immediately. This is why doctors feel so comfortable prescribing them. If that person dies in the process, the doctor always covered with an explanation to his death—"high cholesterol level history." And no one can ever prove that that person actually died of the cholesterol-lowering drug.

Cholesterol-lowering drugs have been shown to cause nerve damage and to greatly impair memory. The way they work—they inhibit a vital enzyme that manufactures cholesterol in the liver. The same enzyme is used to manufacture coenzyme Q10, which is a biochemical needed to transfer energy from food to our cells to be used for the work of staying alive and healthy.

Most cardiologists insist that lowering cholesterol is reducing the risk of heart attacks, but very few of them can actually say that lowering cholesterol with pills actually leads to a reduction in the risk of death. It has never been conclusively shown that lowering cholesterol with drugs saves lives. In fact, several large studies have shown that it is actually correlated with an increased risk of death and also risk of cancer.

Bottom line

Cholesterol is **a vital component in our body** and is **not an evil** as it is presented to us by the media and many doctors. In fact it is one of our best friends. We would not be here without it. **The actual evil is overeating, wrong food, stress, and physical inactivity**.

Trans-Fatty Acids

When it was discovered that overeating saturated fats increases the risk for coronary heart disease, the food industry turned to *partial hydrogenation*. This process lowered the content of saturated fat in vegetable shortening and margarine, but, oops! dramatically increased the amount of a certain kind of fat—*trans* fat. While suppliers praised processed vegetable oils as healthy unsaturated and cholesterol-free substitutes for animal fats, there is now strong evidence that introducing trans-fatty acids into our diets *does much more harm* than consumption of saturated fats.

327

The Harvard School of Public Health has issued a warning against intake of trans fats:

> Trans-fats are even worse for cholesterol levels than saturated fats because they raise bad LDL and lower good HDL. While you should limit your intake of saturated fats, it is important to *eliminate* trans-fats from your diet.

Vegetable oils have molecule structure with kinks—double bonds. These double bonds give oil ability to stay liquid at room temperature. Traditionally, vegetable oils are cheaper, but as liquids, they are not a suitable alternative, and this is why in the early twentieth century *hydrogenation* was invented.

Since the first time hydrogenated oils were introduced, we keep producing these products, even though we know they kill us because fat and oil industry is a big business. Only in the USA, market oils and fats constitute about 5 billion dollars or about 25 percent of the world market. The vegetable oil sale alone is about 1.3 billion dollars.

There is nothing good to be said about trans fats, and you don't need a single milligram of it. Trans fats cause about 50,000 premature deaths each year only in United States alone—with the restaurant industry accounting for roughly one-third of them. Cookies, crackers, chips, hamburgers, cakes, french fries, processed nuts, and many others have trans fats.

Prolonged consumption of trans fats leads not only to atherosclerosis, inflammatory joint diseases but also development of birth defects.

Just a century ago we were comfortable using animal fats like butter and lard for baking and other cooking processes, and we were much healthier then. Deep-fry oils and baking fats that are high in saturated fats, like palm oil, tallow or lard, can withstand extreme heat (of 180-200°C) and are *resistant to oxidation*, while many vegetable oils when heated up turn to trans fats. A 2001 parallel review of a twenty-year dietary fat studies in the United Kingdom, the United States of America, and Spain concluded that polyunsaturated oils like soya, canola, sunflower, and corn *degrade easily to toxic compounds and trans fats* when heated up.

Scientists asked global health authorities *not to recommend* consuming large amounts of polyunsaturated fats *without considering a protection of these fatty acids against heat—and oxidative-degradation.*

Not many people understand that polyunsaturated fats displayed on the food labels can actually be trans fats or other chemical compounds produced by heating of the oil. When people hear recommendations to consume more of polyunsaturated fats instead of saturated, they usually go by those labels, but not all labels display trans fats, even though it is required by the Food and Drug Administration since January 1, 2006. When people eat food at food courts and restaurants the situation is even worse—food is often cooked with vegetable oils (because they are cheaper), which immediately converts to trans fats.

Identifying *trans* fats helps to make heart-healthy food choices, which helps reduce risk of cardiovascular diseases. Let's look at molecule structure of fats again to understand better what happens when unsaturated fats turn into trans fats.

Take a look at the figure 24. Double bonds in unsaturated fats can come in two forms—*cis* (good fats) and *trans* (bad fats). In *cis*-compounds, two hydrogen atoms that form double bond are on the same side (*cis* means same side). In *trans*-compounds, two hydrogen atoms are on opposite sides of the double bond. Saturated fats don't have double bonds.

The shape of *trans*-fatty acids is in between that of *cis* fatty acids, which are bent, and that of *saturated* fatty acids, which are straight. The straighter the molecule, the easier it can become solid. Thus, *cis*-unsaturated fatty acids *are liquid at room temperature*, whereas *trans* fats are solid at room temperature (they melt at 44°C).

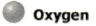

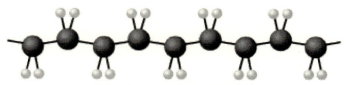

saturated - no double bonds

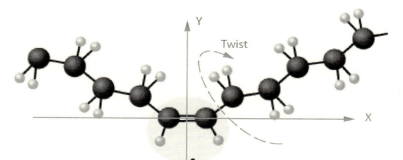

**unsaturated - *cis* compound
(both hydrogen atoms on same side)**

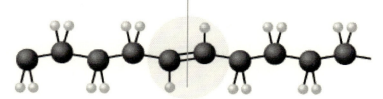

**unsaturated - *trans* compound
(hydrogen atoms on opposite sides)**

Figure 24. Cis-compounds (good fats)
to Trans- compounds (bad fats) conversion

When some oils get heated up, one side of the *cis* configuration turns around in the middle of the double bond forming a *trans*-configuration.

A very slight change—the rotation within the molecule where hydrogens appear on their opposite sides—makes a drastic change in properties of the fat molecule. It turns that molecule into unnatural configuration. That configuration can cause many serious problems inside of our body. *Cis*-molecules are similar to the ones in our body. *Trans*-molecules are biologically different and act differently.

Within a single fatty acid, there can be few different configurations formed. Some of the double bonds can be twisted *trans*-way while others remain *cis* (see figure 25).

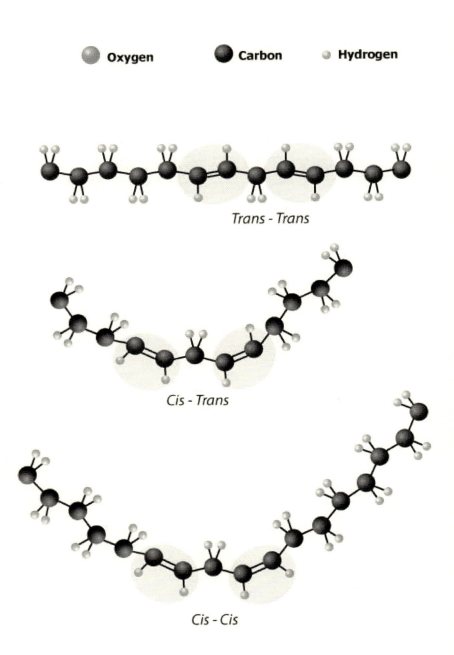

Figure 25. Cis-Trans fatty acids variations

The number of the *trans*-compounds formed in the oil depends on the damage done to that oil. Why molecules choose to turn when heated, nobody knows. I choose to believe that it just hurts them. Fresh oils are alive substances, just like us, and once we put them under extreme temperatures, they twist and turn just like we would twist and turn if someone put the fire on us.

Cis and *trans*-compounds are different molecules, with different physical and chemical properties. Once *cis* configuration is turned into *trans*-configuration, few things happen:

Melting point. *Trans*-configurations are packed differently, and that changes their melting points. They become solid at room temperature. This makes them hard for our body to deal with because the melting point of *trans*-configurations is approximately 44°C, while the temperature of our body is around 37°C. This makes *trans fats* sticky inside of our body that leads to the following problems:

    b.   Heart overload

Our heart's normal fuel is fatty acids. When *trans* fats are present, our body's enzymes try to break them down to produce some energy for our heart. But because *trans*-configurations are unnatural, our body gets confused and breaks them down slower than other fats. This lowers the ability of the heart to perform. In situations of increased activity, stress, or crisis, lowered heart performance could have fatal consequences.

    c.   Clots

Unnaturally sticky molecules create clots in small blood vessels causing strokes, heart attacks, or circulatory problems in many organs, such as lungs, extremities, and even sense organs.

Holes in cell membranes. Trans-fatty acids destroy protective barriers around cells, which are vital for our cells to stay alive and healthy. Trans-fatty acids also create holes in those cells through which some harmful molecules get in. As a result, allergic reactions may be developed and the immune function may be impaired.

Energy. Trans-fatty acids are substances that don't exist in the nature; thus, they are not familiar to our body structure and our energy flow. When our body receives molecules that are wrong in shape, size, or properties, body energy flow gets thrown off the normal pattern.

Source: Udo Erasmus, Fats That Heal, Fats That Heal. Rephrased and added for easier reading.

Food Sources of Trans-Fatty Acids

Animals and plants naturally do not produce trans-fatty acids. Milk and beef contain some of trans-fatty acids, produced by bacteria that help cows digest foods in their digestive systems. However, most of the trans fats in our current diet originate *from **_processed vegetable fats_*** (see figure 26).

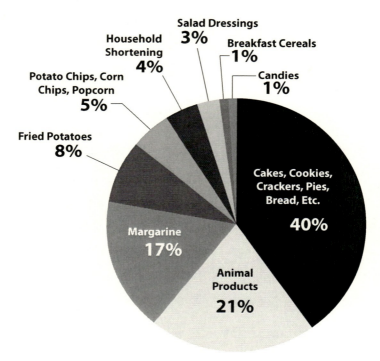

Figure 26. Foods containing trans-fatty acids

According to the US Food and Drug Administration, adult Americans consume on average about 5.8 g of trans fats or 2.6 percent of calories, per day, while the medical research shows that daily intake of about 5 g of trans fat is associated with a 25 percent increase in the risk of heart disease. One large cup of hot chocolate, for example, contains up to 4 g of trans fats, a large portion of onion chips or french fries up to 10 g, some sandwiches and pies—up to 8. Many precooked and frozen products sold in grocery stores have vast amounts of trans fats.

The American Heart Association's Nutrition Committee strongly advises the following guideline for healthy Americans over age two:

Limit trans fat intake to less than 1 percent of total daily calories or less than 2 g per day.

The food industry is constantly changing, and it is very hard to list all products that contain trans fats, but many food manufacturers have been working to reduce the amount of trans-fatty acids in popular products by exploring new technologies and/or using soybean oil with improved fatty acid profiles for enhanced stability. As a result, a variety of cookies, crackers, potato chips, energy bars, popcorn, and other snack foods now contain zero grams of trans fats. Many companies in order to stay in business had to readjust their products' quality due to today's demand. But still there are plenty of other products, restaurants, and cooking approaches that can damage your health.

In order to minimize the consumption of trans fats in our diet, the three easy measures can be taken:

1. **Avoid restaurants.** Some restaurants claim that they have changed their ways of preparing the food and they now use better oils for deep-frying. But those oils are still highly processed, eventually still containing trans fats. There is no way for you to know if there are no trans fats in your meal at any restaurant, even though their nutritional guides may say so.

Trans fats in restaurants are unavoidable.
2. **Read labels.** Before you put anything on your shopping list, make sure that this product is safe for you and free of trans fats. Be especially careful with precooked and frozen products. Read labels.

3. **Avoid frying.** Frying and deep-frying produces trans-fatty acids.

Frying and Deep-Frying

Fried foods smell good and taste delicious, and for many people, they seem harmless. "How can it be bad if it tastes so good?" But after we eat fried food, besides the trans-fatty acids, our body has to fight many other toxic substances. It may not harm you immediately but over five, ten, twenty years of continuously consuming fried foods, your cells may accumulate the damage and you may develop some degenerative diseases.

If the frying temperature is too high, many nutrients including vitamins and minerals are destroyed. Proteins turn into substances promoting cancer, and starches, sugars, and fats go through massive molecule damage turning into smoke by destruction of fatty acid and glycerol.

Frying and deep-frying is not recommended, and in order to stay healthy, we should try avoiding this process. There is no such a thing as safe frying unless it is done on water. Temperatures destroy most of the vegetable oils, especially when it comes to essential fatty acids—omega-6 and omega-3. Many people are still confused by using these oils for frying assuming that if that oil is good for salad, it will "behave" just as good on the frying pan. But it isn't so. Essential fatty acids when heated up turn into "ugly monsters" producing much more toxic elements than saturated fats.

If you need to fry at all, the best sources after water are the following:

- *Coconut*
- *Palm*

- *Palm kernel*
- *Cocoa butter*
- *Butter*

These fats are destroyed minimally during frying, thus leading to less damage to our health. But because they are saturated, they should be used in small amounts.

Fried butter and tropical fats, used in moderation, create fewer health problems than other frying fats. Margarines and shortenings should not be used for frying at all because they contain too many altered molecules to begin with, and frying only makes them worse.

Olive, sunflower, and *safflower* oils are acceptable for frying but only on low temperatures.

Traditional Chinese cooks first put water when they fry, and only then add oil. Water brings the temperature down to 100°C, a nondestructive temperature for many frying oils. In European gourmet cooking, vegetables are placed in the frying pan before oil is added to protect those oils from overheat and oxidation.

Avoiding frying will help you to prevent cancer, heart problems, and many other degenerative diseases. There are many other alternative ways of preparing food and making it delicious.

Conclusion: The American Heart Association's Nutrition Committee strongly advises these fat guidelines for healthy Americans over age two:

- Limit total fat intake to less than 25-35 percent of your total calories each day.
- Limit saturated fat intake to less than 7 percent of total daily calories.
- Limit trans fat intake to less than 1 percent of total daily calories.
- The remaining fat should come from sources of monounsaturated and polyunsaturated fats such as nuts, seeds, fish, and freshly made vegetable oils.

- Limit cholesterol intake to less than 300 mg per day, for most people. If you have coronary heart disease or your LDL cholesterol level is 100 mg/dL or greater, limit your cholesterol intake to less than 200 mg a day.

Table 24 below represents some of the popular foods by their fat content, but as per the cholesterol table from before, do not get confused by avoiding foods from the bottom of this table, such as for example, nuts. Even though they are very high in fat, those are good fats, and moderate amounts of them are very beneficial to our health.

Table 24. Foods by Fat Content

	FOODS	SERVING SIZE	CAL	FAT (%)	SAT (%)	MONO (%)	POLY (%)
LOW	Tuna	3 oz	99	6	2	1	3
	Shrimps, boiled	3 oz	90	14	3	2	6
	Chicken breast	½ breast	142	20	6	7	4
	Beef, top sirloin	3 oz	158	30	11	13	1
	Soy milk, Vanilla	1 cup	100	32	5	7	19
	Oysters, raw	1 cup	169	33	10	4	13
	Liver, chicken	1 cup	234	35	11	8	11
MEDIUM	Yogurt, whole milk	1 cup	170	42	26	10	2
	Turkey leg, roasted	546 g	1136	43	13	12	12
	Lamb, loin	3 oz	172	44	17	18	4
	Goat milk	1 cup	140	45	26	11	2
	Drumstick, roasted	1	112	46	13	18	10
	French fries	1 small	271	48	11	28	8.3
	Ham, regular	3 oz	139	48	16	24	5
	Salmon, cooked	3 oz	175	54	11	20	20
	Tofu	¼ block	117	55	8	12	31
	Chicken wings	1 wing	159	60	16	25	14
	Egg	1 large	78	62	18	23	8
	Swiss cheese	3 oz	324	66	42	18	3
	Cashews	1oz	156	72	13	37	13
	Pumpkin seeds	2 Tbs.	114	72	15	24	35
	Pistachios, roasted	1 oz	161	72	9	39	22
	Cheddar cheese	3oz	342	74	47	21	2
HIGH	Sausage , pork	1 unit	92	75	25	32	10
	Peanuts, roasted	1 oz	166	76	11	38	24
	Peanut butter	2 Tbs.	188	77	16	37	22
	Pork spareribs	4 oz	310	78	26	32	6
	Almonds	30 nuts	160	79	6	48	19
	Cream, half & half	3 Tbs.	60	80	50	23	5
	Avocado	1 med.	322	82	12	55	10
	Walnuts	¼ cup	196	89	8	12	65
	Cream Cheese	3 oz	297	90	56	25	4
	Salad dressings	1 Tbs.	60-75	91-100	14	20	40
	Butter, 1 stick	113 g	810	100	64	27	4

Best and Worst Oils

Why are some oils so expensive? At a health store, you can spend over $30 per liter; when at a supermarket, some oils cost less than $5 per 4 L jar.

Cheap oils are made differently. They are highly processed while those sold at health food stores are freshly made. This is where the price difference is: it takes much more product to produce good oil. Manufacturers of low-quality oils know that people these days don't have time to do their own researches. How many people really know what the "cold pressed" oil means? If the label on the bottle says "cold pressed," should we automatically trust it and consider that oil as good? Not exactly. There are many tricks manufacturers use to take your attention away.

Hundred years ago "cold pressed" oils were made on manually operated presses. It took a lot of time and produce to squeeze very little oil.

We don't use manual presses today, but the best oils are made on similar machines using similar technologies. That's why those oils are so expensive.

"Cold pressed" today means nothing. It is usually subject to different regulations, depending on the part of the world where the oil is made. In the United States, oil labeling is not regulated, so "cold pressed oil" *may not be actually cold pressed oil at all*.

Pressing cold seeds, nuts, or vegetables does not produce a lot of oil. Heat increases the yield of oil. In some countries in Europe, "cold pressed" means 27°C, but here in North America, it can mean a lot of things. Some manufacturers preheat the seeds for an hour and deodorize them before pressing. After the seeds are fully pressed, they may go for another round of preheating and deodorization, and this time they may even add some water to increase the oil yield. Grinding seeds, nuts, or vegetables to a very refined paste produces even more oil. Paste also goes through *malaxation* process—mixing for about forty minutes. Sometimes this paste gets heated up too. But when the oils are actually pressed, the press itself is not heated, so the manufacturer can say that his oil was "cold pressed." Can anyone argue that? It is cold pressed, isn't it? But is this the oil you are looking for?

Most of the oils that are sold in supermarkets are very low in quality and *should never be consumed by humans*. Extra-virgin olive oil is probably the only one that deserves attention there.

Most of the freshly made oils except for extra-virgin olive oil require refrigeration. They are very fragile and can get very quickly rancid at room temperature.

The best oils today are made by hydraulic press, the ancient method to produce any oil at that time. They are very lightly preheated to safe temperatures. The only two materials that will yield enough oil without heating them are the sesame seeds and olives. Therefore sesame oil and olive oil from hydraulic press are the only oils that could be truly called "cold pressed."

Best Quality Oils

Olive Oil
When you take a bottle of olive oil in your hands, read very carefully what the label says.

"Cold pressed" refers only to the processes of olives being pressed under a cold hydraulic press. It does not refer to anything else. The olives may have been heated prior the pressing or turned to a paste or even bleached.

The word *virgin* describes that this oil is of its best quality. It means that olives were pressed first time, in their freshest state, and without any heat.

The "extra-virgin cold pressed" or "extra virgin 100 percent pure first cold pressed" are the closest possible to their natural state. If you see the Organic label on your bottle, it is even better because organic merchants will not condole misleading labeling.

Other Oils

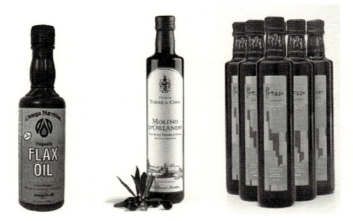

Other unrefined truly cold pressed seeds and nut oils are also fresh expeller-pressed, but they are pressed at very low temperatures (30°-33°C/86°-92°F for EFA oils, 30°-43°C/86°-110°F for culinary oils). This process is done without any exposure to damaging light, oxygen, and reactive metals. Because these seeds and nuts are harder than olives, they require a low heat to soften them up, but low temperatures do not damage the oil in any way. After oils are extracted, they are immediately placed in special containers to protect from light and refrigerated to protect from rancidness. At home they must be refrigerated.

Medium Quality Oils

These oils are made on the press with rotating worm shaft, applying temperatures between 200 and 250 degrees. Obviously these oils cannot be considered as "cold pressed" but sometimes are still labeled this way. Organic merchants will not "play this game," and on their bottles, these types of oils are labeled as "expeller pressed."

Even though these types of oils are "not perfectly made," they still may not be considered as refined because some seeds and nuts can withstand higher temperatures, and the oils out of those seeds may be considered as healthy. An example is coconut oil.

Low Quality Oils

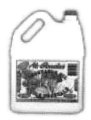 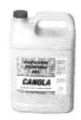 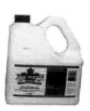 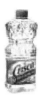

"Consuming partially hydrogenated and processed oils is like inhaling cigarette smoke. They will kill you—slowly, over time, but as surely as you breathe. And in the meantime, they will make you fat!"

Source of this quote: TreeLight, www.treelight.com

The process of refining vegetable oil damages the fats and makes them very unstable and prone to going rancid quite easily. Rancid oils in any form are particularly bad for your health because they introduce cancer-causing free radicals into your body, without the benefit of including an antioxidant like vitamin E.

Here is how low quality oils are made: a nasty process

Step 1. Crushing and Heating

All the seeds without any reselection of good and bad get crushed to a paste and then get heated up to a temperature of 180 degrees.

Step 2. Pressing of Seeds

The seeds are put through a high-volume press, which uses high heat and friction to press the oil from the seed pulp.

Step 3. Bathing in Oil and Pulp in Hexane

Hexane is produced by the refining of crude petroleum oil. Chronic intoxication from hexane has been observed in recreational solvent

343

abusers and in workers in the shoe manufacturing, furniture restoration, and automobile construction industries where hexane is used as glue. The initial symptoms are tingling and cramps in the arms and legs, followed by general muscular weakness. In severe cases, atrophy of the skeletal muscles is observed, along with a loss of coordination and problems of vision.

In this step, the seed pulp and oil are put through a hexane solvent bath and steamed again to squeeze out more oil.

Step 4. Final Squeeze

Now the seed/oil mixture is put through a centrifuge, and phosphate is added to begin the separation of the oil and seed residue.

Step 5. Water Degumming

In this process, water is added to the oil, and a large part of water soluble and even a small proportion of the non-water-soluble phosphatides (natural components of cell membranes) are removed.

Step 6. Neutralization

Any free fatty acids, phospholipids, pigments, and waxes in the extracted oil promote fat oxidation and lead to undesirable colors and odors in the final products. These substances are removed by treating the oil with caustic soda (sodium hydroxide) or soda ash (sodium carbonate). All this settles down to the bottom and then gets drawn off. This is why refined oils are lighter in color, thinner, and more prone to oxidation.

Step 7. Bleaching

The major purpose of bleaching is the removal of off-colored materials in the oil. The heated oil is treated with various bleaching agents such as fuller's earth, activated carbon, or activated clays. Bleaching promotes fat oxidation since some natural antioxidants and nutrients are removed along with the impurities.

Step 8. Deodorization

Pressurizing steam at extremely high temperatures **(500 degrees or more)** is used to remove volatile compounds that could cause off odors and tastes in the final product. A light solution of citric acid is often added during this step to inactivate any metals such as iron or copper present in the final product.

Canola Oil—Canadian Poison or Remedy?

The name *canola* was born in Canada from two words, *Canada* and *oil*, and there is no such seed, nut, or a vegetable in the nature that is called canola. This product is developed from rapeseed, which was originally used as a lubricant, fuel, soap, and synthetic rubber base, as well as an illuminant for slick color pages in magazines. If taken internally, original rapeseed is poisonous to humans due to high content of *erucic acid* and *glucosinolates*. *Erucic acid* is used in polyesters, plastics, and nylons.

Some researchers indicate that the substances in the rapeseed can cause red blood cells to clump together.

Rapeseeds were widely used in animal feeds in England and Europe between 1986 and 1991 and caused animals to go blind and mad (mad cow disease).

How did we end up eating rapeseeds?

The "invention" of canola oil as a food is credited to Baldur Stefanson at the University of Manitoba, who took original rapeseed and bred it with some other seeds that were low in the erucic acid and glucosinolates. Originally this product was called LEAR—low erucic acid rape and only later renamed to canola oil.

By the source of Young Again and many others, the Canadian government paid the FDA (Food and Drug Administration) a sum of 50 million dollars to have canola oil placed on the list of generally recognized as safe foods (GRAS).

And here you go, the new industry was created, and the former lubricant came to our tables and kitchens. An instant top seller, canola oil is now on the tip of everyone's tongue.

Well . . . if we could eat hydrogenated oils for so many years, why not rapeseed? Soon, probably, we'll be eating motor oil disposed from our cars, and it will be called "motorola." Oh, I am sorry, this name is already taken by an electronics company. But what is the difference anyway—industries lately are getting mixed up "a little."

"The high praise for Canola is propaganda put forth by the Canadian government because canola, a hybridized rape plant, is one of that nation's chief export products," states the report by Tom Valentine and Maryland-based Mary Enig, PhD. *"Consumers search out various products with Canola oil in them because they believe this is somehow much healthier than other oils. All food grade Canola, including the varieties sold in health food stores, are deodorized from its natural stink with 300 degree F. high temperature refining. You cannot cook a vegetable oil at that temperature and have behind anything much edible. Health food store operators parrot the hype without checking any facts."*

Research at the University of Florida-Gainesville states that as much as 4.6 percent of all the fatty acids in canola are "trans" isomers, due to the refining process.

In 1996, the Japanese announced a study where a special canola oil diet had actually killed laboratory animals. As a reaction to this study, Canadian scientists verified this fact using piglets where piglets were dying because they were depleted of vitamin E. Canadians reported that other vegetable oils did not appear to cause the same problem. The idea of something depleting vitamin E rapidly is an alarming development because vitamin E is absolutely essential to human health.

On January 26, 1998, Omega Nutrition, one of the major producers of organic, cold-pressed oils for the health food store market, published a press release. The release stated, *"If you are cooking with Canola oil of any quantity, you might as well be using margarine."*

Rapeseed is lubricated oil used by small industry. It has never been meant for human consumption. It is derived from the mustard family and is considered a toxic and poisonous weed, which when processed, becomes rancid very quickly. It has been shown to cause lung cancer. (Wall Street Journal, 6/7/1995)

Rape seed is very inexpensive to grow, and this is probably the main reason why government stands behind it—good profit. Some typical and possible side effects include loss of vision, disruption of the central nervous system, respiratory illnesses, anemia, constipation, increased incidence of heart disease and cancer, low birth weights in infants and irritability. Generally Rapeseed has a cumulative effect, taking almost 10 years before symptoms begin to manifest. Canola is a Trans-Fatty Acid, which has shown to have a direct link to cancer.

Studies of Canola oil done on rats indicate many problems. Rats developed fatty degeneration of heart, kidney, adrenals and thyroid gland. When the Canola oil was withdrawn from their diet, the deposits dissolved, but scar tissue remained on the organs.

Reading all these researches, I was just wondering why there were no studies done on humans before the Food and Drug Administration placed canola oil on the GRAS list? Oh, I get it!—50 million dollars had speeded up that process.

"Strange new diseases involving the nervous system may be caused by Canola oil which dissolves the **myelin sheath** *off the nerves throughout the body,"* studies report.

Myelin is an insulating layer that forms around nerves, including those in the brain and spinal cord. It is made up of protein and fatty substances. The purpose of the myelin sheath is to allow rapid and efficient transmission of impulses along the nerve cells. If the myelin is damaged, the impulses slow down. This can cause diseases like multiple sclerosis.

"The nervous system, once the insulation is stripped, can be compared to your home with bare wires inside the walls—a

dangerous situation. In the body, symptoms may be many and varied:

1. *Tremors, shaking, palsy due to malfunction of nerve impulse transmissions*
2. *Uncoordinated walking, writing and other automatic physical movements*
3. *Slurred speech*
4. *Excessive salivation*
5. *Deterioration of memory and thinking processes*
6. *Blurred vision*
7. *Fuzzy or low audio levels*
8. *Difficulty urinating/incontinence*
9. *Environmental sensitivity/allergic to smells, food, clothing, electrical equipment*
10. *Breathing problems/short of breath*
11. *Nervousness or nervous breakdown*
12. *Numbness and tingling in extremities*
13. *Heart problems/arrhythmia"*

Of course, those who sell canola will always support and promote the researches "proving" that canola is somehow good for our health. Canola today has already "penetrated" in hundreds of products that are sold in our supermarkets—breads, cookies, candies, pizzas, and hundreds more. It's cheap, and why wouldn't companies making those products buy it?

In my opinion, until there is enough research done on humans with canola, we should refrain from using it. Clean up your fridge and kitchen from all the products containing canola in them. *Read labels.* If you eat out, choose restaurants that don't use canola (ask). Why should you use such a controversial and suspicious product when there are much better alternatives available from hundreds of years ago—fats that have been used for generations.

Meanwhile fast-food restaurants are so proud implementing their new so called "healthy" technologies using canola oils for their deep-frying. Who knows, maybe those fast-food restaurant people know better about human's health than the PhD professors.

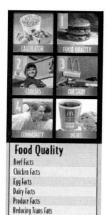

Reducing Trans Fats (TFAs) Facts
See What We're Made Of ™

McDonald's® Canada has been working with government and industry experts to decrease and, where possible, eliminate trans fats (TFAs) from our menu items. This approach has been North American in scope.

In 2007, Health Canada adopted the recommendations of the Trans Fat Task Force, limiting the trans fat content of vegetable oils and soft, spreadable margarines to 2% of the total fat content and the trans fat content for all other foods to 5% of the total fat content.

Food Quality
Beef Facts
Chicken Facts
Egg Facts
Dairy Facts
Produce Facts
Reducing Trans Fats

Reducing TFAs
In early 2008, we successfully completed our transition to a trans fat free Canola Oil Blend cooking oil in all McDonald's Canada restaurants. Our customers continue to enjoy the same great taste of McDonald's.

We're proud that all of our fried menu items meet Health Canada's voluntary trans fat limits -- including our world famous French fries, hash browns, all chicken choices, and Filet-O-Fish®. As part of this process, we also successfully reduced saturated fats.

McDonald's Canada has also successfully reduced trans fats in our baked goods.

Sources: www.aspartame.ca, www.controlincognito.com, www.dldewey.com, http://urbanlegends.about.com/library/blcanola.htm, http://www.buzzle.com, http://www.realmacaw.com, and many others.

30.3 Proteins

Protein in Greek means "of primary importance." Proteins are somewhat much more complicated than many people think. Books and books can be written about what types of proteins there are and what are their molecule structures. The whole human body is made out of protein—*organs, muscles, ligaments, tendons, hair, nails, skin,* and *blood*; our *enzymes* and *hormones* are protein too, and there are other ten to fifty thousand kinds of protein that make up many vital functions. We use protein to create new cells throughout the body and also to repair existing cells.

To sustain life, we need a daily consumption of protein; our body cannot store proteins the way it stores glucose and fat.

Proteins are build up of amino acids—chemical units or "building blocks." When we eat protein-rich food, our body breaks proteins down into those blocks and then rebuilds new proteins for the body's different purposes. Each individual type of protein is composed of a specific group of amino acids in a specific chemical arrangement. Each protein type is tailored to a specific need, and proteins are not interchangeable.

Not all building blocks would fit into all the functions and structures. Certain amino acids are necessary for brain functions and some enable vitamins and minerals to do their "jobs" properly. This is why balanced eating is so important—the lack of some components can lead to deficiency of others. For example, the low level of amino acid *tyrosine* may lead to iron deficiency, low level of *methionine* and *taurine* has been linked to allergies and autoimmune disorders, etc.

The Essential and Nonessential Amino Acids

Just like *essential fatty acids*, essential **amino acids** cannot be synthesized by our body, and they have to be provided with food. There are eight essential amino acids:

1. *Tryptophan*. Necessary for the synthesis of neurotransmitter serotonin (happy hormone). It helps relieve migraine and depression.
2. *Tyrosine*. A precursor of dopamine, norepinephrine, and adrenaline. It enhances positive mood. It is also an antioxidant.
3. *Valine*. Essential for muscle development. Side effects of high levels of valine in the body include hallucinations.
4. *Isoleucine*. Necessary for the synthesis of hemoglobin, a major constituent of red blood cells.
5. *Leucine*. Beneficial for skin, bone, and tissue wound healing. It promotes growth hormone synthesis.
6. *Lysine*. Component of muscle protein and is needed in the synthesis of enzymes and hormones. It is also a precursor for L-carathine, which is essential for a healthy nervous system function.

7. ***Methionine.*** An antioxidant. It helps in the breakdown of fats (!) and aids in reducing muscle degeneration. It is also good for a healthy skin and nail.
8. ***Phenylalanine.*** Beneficial for healthy nervous system. It boosts memory and learning. It may be useful against depression and suppressing appetite.[10]

Best sources of the essential amino acids are *eggs, fish, meat, fowl,* and *dairy products.* These products fall into the category of protein called a *complete protein,* meaning that they contain all eight essential amino acids. Plant proteins may not contain all the essential amino acids in the necessary proportions, and they fall in another category—*incomplete protein.* A protein that is low in one or more amino acids is also called a *limiting protein.*

Protein quality is usually defined according to the amino acid pattern of *egg protein, which is regarded as the ideal.* Many plant proteins are low in one of the essential amino acids. For instance, grains tend to be short of lysine, while pulses are short of methionine.

But this doesn't mean that those who are vegetarians are always lacking the essential amino acids. Vegetarians achieve the perfect combination by *combining* plant proteins, such as, for example, a grain with a pulse. Soya is a high-quality protein on its own, which can be regarded as equal to meat protein. The limiting amino acid tends to be different in different proteins. This means when two different foods are combined, the amino acids in one protein can compensate for the one lacking in the other. This is known as *protein complementing.* Here are some tasty and healthy complete protein combinations:

- Beans on toast
- Corn and beans
- Hummus and pita bread
- Nut butter on whole-grain bread
- Pasta with beans
- Rice and beans, peas, or lentils
- Split pea soup with whole grain or seeded crackers or bread

- Tortillas with refried beans
- Veggie burgers on bread

Source: the Veggie Table

Our body is continuously breaking down protein to amino acids, but the types of proteins get build up from those amino acids only when the need arises. If we eat too much of protein when amino acids are not needed, our body turns them into fat. This process is irreversible, and our body cannot turn fat back to protein.

It is crucial to have all the necessary amino acids come together. Even if one amino acid is missing, the body cannot continue proper protein synthesis. This can lead to various physical problems and body dysfunctions.

Sometimes body dysfunctions themselves can lead to improper protein synthesis: infections, trauma, stress, age, or just impaired absorption can often interfere with the body's ability to build or break down proteins properly.

Some of the effects of a diet deficient in essential amino acids include the following:

- Reduced energy levels
- Slow metabolism
- Sleeping disorders
- Chronic fatigue
- Digestive problems
- Hair loss and skin ailments
- Nervous reactions
- Emotional upset
- Stress and general poor health

Other possibly life-threatening symptoms of essential amino acids deficiency include obesity, malnutrition, and buildup of wastes in the bloodstream. All these effects can be extremely detrimental to an individual's well-being, so a balanced intake of amino acids becomes extremely important.

The *nonessential* amino acids are the following:

1. *Alanine.* Removes toxic substances released from the breakdown of muscle protein during intensive exercise. Side effects of excessive alanine level in the body is associated with chronic fatigue.
2. *Cysteine.* Component of protein type abundant in nails, skin, and hair. It acts as antioxidant (free radical scavenger) and has a synergetic effect when taken with other antioxidants such as vitamin E and selenium.
3. *Cystine.* The same as cysteine, it aids in removal of toxins and formation of skin.
4. *Glutamine.* Promotes healthy brain function. It is also necessary for the synthesis of RNA and DNA molecules.
5. *Glutathione.* An antioxidant and has antiaging effect. It is useful in removal of toxins.
6. *Glycine.* A component of skin and is beneficial for wound healing. It acts as neurotransmitter. The side effect of high level glycine in the body is that it may cause fatigue.
7. *Histidine.* Important for the synthesis of red and white blood cells. It is a precursor for histamine, which is good for sexual arousal. It also improves blood flow. Side effects of high dosage of histidine include stress and anxiety.
8. *Serine.* A constituent of brain proteins and aids in the synthesis of immune system proteins. It is also good for muscle growth. Read more.
9. *Taurine.* Necessary for proper brain function and synthesis of amino acids. It is important in the assimilation of mineral nutrients such as magnesium, calcium, and potassium.
10. *Threonine.* Balances protein level in the body. It promotes immune system. It is also beneficial for the synthesis of tooth enamel and collagen. Read more.
11. *Asparagine.* It helps promote equilibrium in the central nervous system—aids in balancing state of emotion.
12. *Aspartic acid.* Enhances stamina, aids in the removal of toxins and ammonia from the body, and beneficial in the synthesis of proteins involved in the immune system. Read more.
13. *Proline.* It plays a role in intracellular signaling.[10]

The nonessential amino acids are called nonessential not because they are less needed in our body, but only because our body can synthesize them. When we eat other foods like fats, carbohydrates, and other amino acids, our body has the ability to produce nonessential acids out of those foods. Some nonessential amino acids get synthesized even without food.

Defining the Quality of Protein-Rich Foods

Fat Content in Proteins

Best sources of protein are animal sources, but they all contain saturated fats. Overconsumption of saturated fats can lead to developing a cardiovascular disease, and we have to be always careful when selecting animal proteins. For example, the amount of protein in 100 g of tuna and 100 g of pork is the same—27 g, but the amount of fat is very different—4 g, and 20 g respectively. Consuming 100 g of tuna instead of 100 g of pork will reduce the fat content in the diet by five times providing the same quality. Proteins are poorly digested when combined with fat because fat slows down the digestion. Most vegetables help proteins to digest better by adding vitamins and also removing extra fat by their fiber.

Table 25 will help you to get an idea how to get the best source of protein without overloading your diet with fat.

Table 25. Complete Proteins by Fat Content (per 100g)

	FOODS (100g)	PROTEIN (g)	FAT (g)
LOW	Milk, skimmed	4	0.4
	Lobster, meat only	27	1.3
	Cod fish, fillet, baked	22	1.4
	Milk, 2%	4	2
	Chicken breast skinless, fillets	27	3
	Trout, steamed	17	3.3
	Cottage cheese	14	4
	Tuna fish, grilled	27	4
	Milk, whole	4	4
	Steak, fillet, grilled	30	6
	Chicken legs, skinless	27	6
	Salmon fish, grilled	20	8
	Rabbit	27	8
	Pheasant, roast	30	9
MEDIUM	Eggs, 2 large	12	10
	Roast, beef	26	11
	Veal, fillets, roasted	30	12
	Cheese, low fat	30	14
	Pigeon, roasted	13	14
	Pork Chops	29	16
	Lamb	25	17
HIGH	Beef sausage	15	19
	Cheese, feta	16	20
	Chicken wings	22	20
	Pork Sausage	13	24
	Goose, roasted	30	25
	Parmesan cheese	23	31
	Duck, roasted	20	30
	Cheeses, cheddar	25	30
	Bacon	28	45
	Cream cheese	3	46

Cholesterol Content in Proteins

Some proteins may be low in fat but still high in cholesterol. For example, eggs are the best source of protein, have the most balanced proportion of amino acids, reasonably low in fat, but are very high in cholesterol—two eggs contain a full daily recommended allowance for cholesterol.

For more details about the cholesterol content of some of the most popular foods and to help yourself control the cholesterol content in your diet, please refer to table 23 page 324.

Incomplete Proteins by Carbohydrate Content (Attention, Vegetarians!)

Most animal proteins don't have carbohydrates in them, but for people who are trying to avoid consuming meats and for vegetarians, it is a good idea to overlook the carbohydrate content in their proteins. Since vegetarians are also using nuts in their diets, the fat content in nuts should also be a concern.

Table 26. Incomplete Proteins Rich in Carbohydrates

FOODS	Protein (g)	Carbohydrates (g)
Brown Rice	3	23
Noodles	5	25
White Rice	3	27
Whole Wheat Macaroni	6	27
Fried Rice	6	29
Whole Grain Brown Rice	4	30
Spaghetti	6	31
Whole Wheat Bread	13	41
Naan Bread	7	47
Whole Wheat Pita	10	55
White Pita	9	56
French Bread	12	57

Table 27. Incomplete Proteins Rich in Fat

FOODS	Protein (g)	Fat (g)
Chestnuts	2	3
Pistachio Nuts (with Shells)	10	30
Peanuts	25	46
Cashew Nuts	20	50
Peanut Butter	22	54
Almond	21	56
Hazelnut	14	64
Coconut	6	65
Brazils Nuts	14	68
Pine Nuts	14	69
Walnuts	6	69
Pecan Nuts	9	70

Sources of Proteins

More and more often we start seeing on the shelves of our supermarkets sections or packages with Organic labels on them. What does it mean in terms of quality of the proteins?

Chickens grown on *free-range* farms and fed with natural food—grains and grass instead of regular chow—produce much better eggs, and their meat is also of better quality—more nutritious and without anabolic steroids.

Unfortunately, some nonorganic chicken farms still practice steroid injections. Steroid shots are given for obvious reason—to speed up the growth. These shots are usually given at the chicken's necks or wings. Therefore, these places are with the highest concentration of steroids.

Hormones and steroid use in Canada has been illegal since the 1960s, and chickens are not supposed to be given any hormones or steroids.

Moreover, chicken meat should be tested by the Canadian Food Inspection Agency to ensure that there are absolutely no medication residues that could cause any risk to human health.

Poultry-related fears in United States about this nature are misplaced. As the US Food and Drug Administration (FDA) notes, "Residue levels of hormones in food have been demonstrated to be safe, as they are well below any level that would have a known effect in human." The rules governing cattle are different, though. "Certain steroid hormones have been approved for use at very low concentrations to increase the rate of weight gain and/or improve feed efficiency in beef cattle," says the FDA.

Even though the meats produced in the USA and Canada may (to only a certain degree) be considered as safe, keep in mind that there is also meat import from other countries. For example, samples of meat and chicken from Puerto Rico were tested for steroid hormone residues. Always check where your supermarket buys meat. This information must be provided to you as a consumer.

Early puberty in girls has been found to be associated with a higher risk for breast cancer. Steroid hormones in food were suspected to cause early puberty in girls in some reports. These steroids have terrifying effects on the body as it accelerates growth. It has an even more dangerous effect in the presence of female hormones; this leads to women being more prone to the growth of a cyst in the womb.

Another precaution we should consider with buying *cheap* chicken meat is that those chickens are grown standing in their own waste. That waste develops to two very dangerous diseases associated with chickens: campylobacter and salmonellosis. Campylobacter's symptoms are dizziness or headaches, diarrhea, and vomiting. It takes an average ten days to develop it, and it usually lasts for approximately seven days. Salmonella is stronger and has similar symptoms, and it takes about four days to develop it, and it can last up to four weeks. Usually patients with salmonellosis need to be hospitalized. In some cases, infections by salmonella can lead to fatal consequences. Both of these diseases can be caught by eating undercooked chicken and other poultry. Cooking until the meat is *white with no pink at all* can greatly reduce the chances of catching these dangerous diseases.

Also ensuring that all cooking surfaces are thoroughly cleaned after preparing the meat is crucial because the infection can be spread around all other working surfaces of your kitchen. Hands must be thoroughly washed after preparation with soap, or protective gloves should be worn before the meat preparation.

The problem usually lies in how the meat is processed once the birds are killed, how long that meat remains in the ambient temperature at those farms, and also how quickly the food stores refrigerate the meat. Not all farm and store workers are responsible enough to minimize that time, so ensure your own safety before you put anything on your table.

In organic systems, chickens are free range. Organic chickens are slower growing, more of the traditional breeds, and live typically for around eighty-one days. They grow at half the rate of intensive chickens. They have a larger space allowance outside (at least two square meters and sometimes up to ten square meters per bird).

What about beef meat? Is the meat we buy in supermarkets safe?

Almost all beef cattle entering feedlots in the United States are given hormone implants to promote faster growth. The first product used for this purpose, DES (diethylstilbestrol), was approved for use in beef cattle in 1954. An estimated two-thirds of the nation's beef cattle were treated with DES in 1956 (Marcus 1994, cited in Swan et al. 2007).

Today, there are six anabolic steroids given to nearly all animals entering conventional beef feedlots in the United States and Canada:

- Three natural steroids (estradiol, testosterone, and progesterone), and
- Three synthetic hormones (the estrogen compound zeranol, the androgen trenbolone acetate, and progestin melengestrol acetate).

Anabolic steroids are typically used in combinations. Measurable levels of all the above growth-promoting hormones are found in the muscle, fat, liver, kidneys, and other organ meats. The Food and Drug Administration has set "acceptable daily intakes" (ADIs) for these animal drugs.

Questions and controversies over the impacts of these added hormones on human development and health have lingered for four decades. In 1988, the European Union banned the use of all hormone growth promoters. The "acceptable daily intakes" are based on traditional toxicity testing methods and do not reflect the capacity of these drugs, which are potent endocrine disruptors, to alter fetal and childhood development.

According to Swan, *"The possible effects on human populations exposed to residues of anabolic sex hormones through meat consumption **have never, to our knowledge, been studied**."*

How "great"! We go to a nice restaurant, order a fifty-dollar steak, slowly and enjoyably eat it, and will never find out whether that steak will develop a tumor in our body at our own cost!

This gap in research is remarkable, given that every beef-eating American for over fifty years has been exposed to these hormones on a regular basis.

The study team assessed sperm quantity and quality of 387 men who were born to mothers who consumed beef during pregnancy. These mothers were divided into a high beef consumption group (more than seven meals per week) and a low-consumption group (less than seven per week).

The scientists compared sperm concentrations and quality among the men born to women in the high and low beef consumption groups, and they found the following:

- Sperm concentration (volume) was 24.3 percent higher in the sons of mothers in the "low" beef consumption group.

- Almost 18 percent of the sons born to women in the high beef consumption group had sperm concentrations below the World Health Organization threshold for subfertility.

The authors of the study concluded that *"these findings suggest that maternal beef consumption is associated with lower sperm concentration and possible sub-fertility, associations that may be related to the presence of anabolic steroids and other xenobiotics in beef."*

This study lends urgency to the long-recognized need for the FDA to reconsider the acceptable daily intakes of hormones used to promote growth in beef feedlots. This reassessment will, in all likelihood, be resisted by the animal drug and beef industries, and once begun, will take many years to be carried out. In the interim, *families wanting to avoid the risk of developmental problems in their **male children** can do so by choosing organic beef or no beef at all.*

Source: "Semen Quality of Fertile US Males in Relation to Their Mothers' Beef Consumption During Pregnancy"
Authors: S. H. Swan, F. Liu, J. W. Overstreet, C. Brazil, and N. E. Skakkebaek
Journal: Human Reproduction, Advance Access published online March 28, 2007
http://humrep.oxfordjournals.org/content/22/8/2325.short

Preparation of Proteins

Meats properly prepared provide better protein and are also safer to eat. In contrary to a popular belief, ***overcooked** meat can be **more unsafe** to consume than undercooked.* Regular consumption of well-done or panfried meat is associated with increased risk for *colorectal* or *rectal* cancer. Some published reports suggest that risk of *colorectal cancer* or *adenoma* may be increased among individuals who consume meat with a heavily browned surface, but not among those who consume meat with a medium or lightly browned surface. Studies have also demonstrated that meats cooked at high temperatures for a long time is not healthy. Further, the process of *grilling* of certain meats over a *direct flame* has been associated with greater production of the carcinogens—cancer elements.

Freshness of Proteins

It is very important to inform yourself of how to find the freshest and safest ingredients to feed yourself and your family. Fresh meat, in particular, is worth learning about, as bad meat can make you and your loved ones very sick. How do you recognize the freshness of the meat?

1. *Date.* Look at the date on the meat label. Usually those labels display when the meat was packaged and when it expires. Remember that the shelf life of meat is shorter than for poultry. For ground beef, sale date, for example, is just one day because it is highly perishable. For chops and steaks, the sale period is 3 to 5 days. For vacuum-packed cuts of meat, the sale period is much longer—21 to 28 days.
2. *Color.* Look at the meat's color. Beef and lamb should be a bright cherry red. Pork has a pale color. Ground beef could be red on the outside and purplish inside—that is OK and only means that the meat was exposed to very little oxygen. It is normal for vacuum-packed cuts of meat to have a dark color.
3. *Firmness.* This works mostly for steaks and pork chops. Press firmly on the meat, and if the meat is fresh, it should spring right back.
4. *Smell.* You might not be able to open the vacuum-packed meats at the store, but you must do it right before cooking. This is a matter of experience and is probably the most reliable method if you aren't working with intentionally aged beef. As meat ages, it will develop a characteristic odor. The stronger the odor, the more bacteria has been at work in degrading the meat.

Processing of the Meats

Most fast-food restaurants offer only highly processed meat, which is made out of very low-quality source.

Consuming processed meats increases the risk of pancreatic cancer, says new research conducted at the University of Hawaii that followed nearly 200,000 men and women for seven years. According to lead study author, Ute Nöthlings, people who consumed the most processed meats (hot dogs and sausage) showed a 67 percent increased risk of pancreatic cancer over those who consumed little or no of those meat products.

"Nearly all processed meats are made with sodium nitrite: breakfast sausage, hot dogs, jerkies, bacon, lunch meat, and even meats in canned soup products. Yet this ingredient is a precursor to highly carcinogenic nitrosamines—potent cancer-causing chemicals that accelerate the formation and growth of cancer cells throughout the body. When consumers eat sodium nitrite in popular meat products, nitrosamines are formed in the body where they promote the growth of various cancers, including colorectal cancer and pancreatic cancer," says nutritionist Mike Adams, author of the *Grocery Warning*.

"Sodium nitrite is a dangerous, cancer-causing ingredient that has no place in the human food supply," he explains. The USDA tried to ban sodium nitrite in the 1970s, but was preempted by the meat processing industry, which relies on the ingredient as a color fixer to make foods look more visually appealing. *"The meat industry uses sodium nitrite to sell more meat products at the expense of public health, and this new research clearly demonstrates the link between the consumption of processed meats and cancer."*

Pancreatic cancer isn't the only negative side effect of consuming processed meats such as hot dogs. Leukemia also skyrockets by 700 percent following the consumption of hot dogs.

Sadly, nearly all school lunch programs currently serve schoolchildren meat products containing sodium nitrite. Hospital cafeterias also serve this cancer-causing ingredient to patients. Sodium nitrite is found in literally thousands of different menu items at fast-food restaurants and dining establishments. *"The use of this ingredient is widespread,"* says Adams. *"And it's part of the reason we're seeing skyrocketing rates of cancer in every society that consumes large quantities of processed meats."*

CHAPTER 32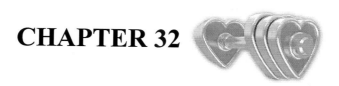

BALANCED DIET—KEY TO HUMAN'S HEALTH

A balanced diet *provides everything that the body needs for optimum health, normal growth, and development.*

But what does this really mean for a regular person who doesn't know much about nutrition or physiology? Even studying at the university, I didn't quite understand what I exactly need to balance to make my diet balanced. Is it amounts of different foods we eat? Or is it the content of each food and their combinations?

Here are some major aspects to consider:

1. Nutritional balance

All the nutrients in our body are interconnected with each other, and many of them depend on each other. Try eating something salty or sweet, and you will notice how your body will "ask" for water by making you thirsty. This is how the body balances itself to stay alive—all the nutrients must be present in the right combination. Very often, when something is missing, something else is missing too. Most vitamins, for example, work in combination of certain minerals, and each mineral is a "partner" of that vitamin. If that mineral is missing, the vitamin will not work no matter how much of it we will consume.

The nutrients in foods created by Mother Nature are combined in their best possible way. Most supplements, on the contrary, don't contain proper combinations of those nutrients. This makes them indigestible even if they contain the same ingredients as natural foods. Most supplements don't have a controlling industry, so the manufacturers can put inside of their containers whatever they want, and they can write on those containers also whatever they want to grab your attention. Of course they will say that their protein shake is natural and contains all the essential and even nonessential amino acids; and, of course, they will tell you that their calcium supplements are the best, absolutely natural, and amazingly effective. But who knows if any of these products have ever been researched or tested? Practically anyone these days can open his own company to sell supplements—grind the eggshell after you eat your boiled eggs, put that powder in capsules, and here you are—in the business selling calcium supplements.

To get a proper nutritional balance in your diet, you can take two approaches: a complicated one—trying to learn how to properly combine nutrients, or the simple one—trusting Mother Nature and eating food as close as it is possible to their original form and also having a vast variety of it.

2. Balance of carbohydrates, proteins, and fats

Carbohydrates are the most important *source of energy*. The most recent dietary guidelines for Americans suggest that about 50 percent of our daily calories come from carbohydrates.

Proteins are required for *growth and repair*. Most experts recommend that your protein intake be approximately 20 percent.

Fats are a valuable *source of energy* and are also *vital for many other functionalities* in our body. The USDA suggests that about 30-35 percent of your calories come from fat. See figure 27.

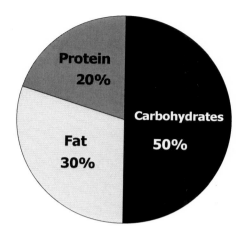

Figure 27. Balance of Carbohydrates, Proteins and Fat

How do you balance your diet based on these numbers?

First of all, you need to know how to identify carbohydrates, proteins, and fats. If you don't completely understand what they are, you will not be able to balance them.

Second, you need to understand *metabolism* and what your daily metabolic rate is.

Metabolism, in simple words, is the amount of calories that your body burns per day.

There are *resting* and *daily metabolic rates*. The main contributor of the energy in your body is resting metabolic rate. It takes about 70 percent of the energy.

Resting metabolic rate is *how many calories your body burns at absolute rest*, when you are doing absolutely nothing—not even eating. Digestion, mental and physical activities require additional energy.

Resting metabolic rate depends on four major factors: weight, height, age, and gender.

Resting metabolic rate formula for men is calculated as follows:

66 + (6.22 × weight [lb.]) + (12.7 × height [in.]) - (6.8 × age)

Example: Resting metabolic rate of a thirty-year-old man with 190 lb. weight and 72 in. height will be calculated as follows:

66 + (6.22 × 190) + (12.7 × 72) - (6.8 × 30) = 66 + 1181.8 + 914.4 - 204 = 1,958.2 calories

Calculate yours: 66 + (6.22 × ___) + (12.7 × ___) - (6.8 × ___) =

= 66 +_____+_____-_____=_____

Resting metabolic rate formula for women is calculated as follows:

655 + (4.36 × weight [lb.]) + (4.32 × height [in.]) - (4.7 × age)

Example: Resting metabolic rate of a thirty-year-old woman, 130 lb. weight and 67 in. height will be calculated as follows:

655 + (4.36 × 130) + (4.32 × 67) - (4.7 × 30) = 655 + 566.8 + 289.44 - 141 = 1,370.24 calories

Calculate yours: 655 + (4.36 × ___) + (4.32 × ___) - (4.7 × ___) =

= 655 + _____+_____-_____=_____

The *daily* metabolic rate includes resting metabolic rate and all other activities. For example, daily food digestion takes approximately 100 calories, workouts about 200 to 400 and more per half hour. If you are a hyper person, add another 100 calories. If you are exercising regularly, your resting metabolism is higher by 10-15 percent at rest.

Let's take the resting metabolic rate of the female from calculations above to estimate a sample *daily metabolic rate* based on some of the activities and human factors. Let's give the female from example above a name, Miss A, for easier explanations.

Miss A's *resting* metabolic rate from the calculations above was 1,370.24 calories. Let's first add 100 calories for her digestion, and then assume that Miss A will work out today and will burn 250 calories during her workout. Then the calculations will be as follows:

1,370.24 + 100 + 250 = 1,720.24 calories per day

But let's now also assume that Miss A is a hyper person and add another 100 calories to her daily metabolic rate, and let's also assume that she regularly exercises, thus her resting metabolism is higher than normal by approximately 10 percent which will equal to approximately 137 calories. The final calculations of the total daily metabolic rate of Miss A will be as follows:

1,720.24 + 100 + 137 = 1,957.24 calories per day

Let's round this number out to 2,000 calories and calculate how many calories this female should consume from carbohydrates, proteins, and fats.

Based on the above percentages for carbohydrates, protein, and fats, these calculations will be as follows:

carbohydrates (50%) 2,000 × 50% = 1,000 calories per day
proteins (20%) 2,000 × 20% = 400 calories per day
fats (30%) 2,000 × 30% = 600 calories per day

"This is all great," you might say. "But how do I apply these numbers to the food that I eat?"

It is simpler than you think—by reading labels on the products you buy, you can quickly estimate all these values. You don't need to be precise in your calculations because no one can predict with what kind of efficiency food burns in our body, but food labels can give you an excellent guideline how to balance your carbohydrates, proteins, and fats.

Not all the products have labels on them directly at the store where you buy your food, but with today's Internet technology, you can easily find any label information for practically any product.

Let's learn how to read labels.

Most food labels are designed for an average customer who consumes 2,000 calories per day (conveniently for Miss A), and all the percentages of carbohydrates, proteins, and fats on those labels are calculated based on that. **"Percent daily values are based on a 2,000 calorie diet"** is what you will see on many labels.

Take a look at figure 28. This is the label of an organic yogurt.

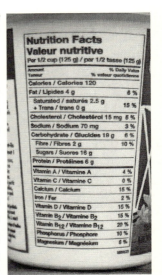

Per ½ cup (125 g). This is the portion size. Everything listed on this label all the way down is based on the portion size of ½ cup or 125 g of yogurt, and not on the size of the whole container. Some labels may display their portion sizes in grams, some in ounces, and some in cups, but whatever it is, make sure that you understand that this is the portion size. If, for example, you were planning to eat the whole container of this yogurt, you would need to look at the total weight of this container, which is usually displayed in front of it, and then recalculate accordingly.

Figure 28. Reading food labels

Amount and % daily value. Under "amount," you will see all the listed ingredients displayed in grams per given portion size (in this case ½ cup).

Daily value. This indicates the percentage amount of a nutrient that is provided by a single serving. Again, this is based on 2,000 calories per day. For example, if you eat ½ cup of this yogurt, you will consume 4 g of fat (look at the label), and if your daily metabolic rate is 2,000 calories per day, this will be equal to 6 percent of your total fat intake for today.

These percentages may not work for you if your metabolic rate is higher or lower than 2,000 calories, and you will need to recalculate them. **See how to calculate page 366.**

Calories. Number of calories displayed is the number of calories per portion size.

Fat. See above.

Saturated. This line describes the total amount of saturated fats *within the portion size.*

Cholesterol. The percentage calculations are based on recommended cholesterol intake of 300 mg per day. Fifteen milligrams of cholesterol, as the label displays, equals to 5 percent of daily allowance based on the following calculations:

$$/ 300 \times 100 = 5\%$$

Sodium. The total daily recommended allowance for sodium is approximately 2,300 mg per day, so the calculations of percentages based on the displayed 70 mg amount will be as follows:

$$70 \text{ mg} / 2,300 \times 100 = 3\% \text{ of daily value}$$

Carbohydrate. Chemically, carbohydrates are the sum of the sugars, starches, and fiber. But the label regulations require calculating total carbohydrates by the difference rather than by measuring them directly. When the calculations are done, those who calculate subtract the insoluble fiber from this calculation. So the calculations below are based not on 19 g of total carbohydrate, but on 16 g of only sugar carbohydrate.

Protein. The recommended daily allowance for protein according to US government standards is 0.8 g/kg (2.2 lb.) of ideal body weight for the adult. However, if you exercise, your protein needs may increase since resistance training and endurance workouts can rapidly break down muscle protein. That means that those who exercise may need to increase protein intake from the RDA's recommendation of

0.8 g/kg to 1.2-1.8 g/kg. This is the reason why most labels do not display the value percentages for protein per day, but only present these numbers in grams.

Vitamins and minerals. The daily values of the most vital vitamins and minerals are also listed on labels but only in percentages (not in grams). Those percentages are based on the recommended daily allowance for each vitamin or mineral (see table 28).

Table 28. Daily Allowance for Vitamins and Minerals

Nutrient	Daily Value
Vitamin A	5000 IU
Vitamin C	60 milligrams
Vitamin D	400 IU
Vitamin E	30 IU
Thiamin	1.5 milligrams
Riboflavin	1.7 milligrams
Niacin	20 milligrams
Vitamin B6	2 milligrams
Vitamin B12	6 micrograms
Folic Acid	0.4 milligrams
Biotin	0.3 milligrams
Pantothenic Acid	10 milligrams
Calcium	1000 milligrams
Iron	18 milligrams
Phosphorus	1000 milligrams
Iodine	150 micrograms
Magnesium	400 milligrams
Zinc	15 milligrams
Copper	2 milligrams

Ingredients. It is crucial to read this part of any label because this is where all the dangerous and harmful elements are listed. Most people don't read this part or skip unknown names, but repetitive consumption of those unknown elements may lead to developing degenerative diseases. Always research them before swallowing.

3.   *Making of better choices*

Manufacturers keep producing products with dangerous ingredients in them; people don't read labels because they are too busy, and the Food and Drug Administration keeps approving dangerous products due to not having better alternatives. People need to eat, and the economy must be growing.

Meanwhile, the drug industry is prospering too. People get sick because they eat those dangerous products, then they visit their doctors, buy medicine, do surgeries, etc.—this is all really good for the economy. But what about us?

Maybe we should be thinking differently? But I guess this is everybody's choice. Major food manufacturers are hoping that we are just going to trust their big names, their history of staying in business, or their cute commercials on the radio and TV.

But luckily, people's awareness is growing, and the number of enthusiasts who deliver that awareness is growing too. I hope that soon most of the poisoned food sold in our supermarkets will be eliminated from their shelves, Food and Drug Administration will raise nation standards, and we will stop separating our food as organic and nonorganic and we will just have normal food.

To set yourself up for success, think about planning a *healthy and balanced diet* as a number of small, manageable steps rather than one big drastic change. If you approach the changes gradually and with commitment, you will have a healthy diet sooner than you think.

   1.   ***Quality first.*** Instead of being overly concerned with counting calories or measuring portion sizes, think first of making healthier choices. For example, replacing margarine on your

toast with avocado may not cut down your total calories, but it will definitely make you healthier and more agile which, in the end, will still make you burn more calories.

2. **Improve slowly.** You have to feel comfortable with every step you take to change your diet. Don't look at other people on how they progress. Go at your own speed.

3. **Appreciate all small steps.** You may fail many times while trying to improve your diet, but don't get discouraged. Keep trying and appreciate every single small change you make.

4. **Substitute, substitute, substitute.** Do not eliminate your favorite foods immediately from your diet. Try to substitute them with better choices, or start slowly reducing sizes that is comfortable for your level.

For example, a frozen yogurt or a piece of dark chocolate is a good substitute for an ice cream.

5. **Prepare your food in advance.** When we get hungry, very often we fall for eating whatever is available at that moment. As we get used to eating *whatever is available*, we develop habits which later can be very difficult to change.

Prepare your food in advance before you get hungry and bring it with you to work, school, sports game, or a concert. Most of those places usually sell only unhealthy choices.

6. **Break your meals into smaller portions and sizes.** Instead of standard three large meals, break down your food into more often smaller portions. This will speed up your metabolism and help you lose weight. Buy small food containers and fill them up when you are *not hungry.* Always thoroughly analyze what you are putting in and write down on each container what it is for—*breakfast, lunch, snack,* etc.

7. **Cook whenever you can.** You can incorporate preparing your meals while watching TV, talking on the phone, etc. Organize yourself and use your time wisely, and remember that planning is everything.

8. **Learn to enjoy your food.** Your healthier food choices must taste and smell good. Learn how to cook healthy and delicious;

chances that you will fall for unhealthy alternatives will be much lower.

9. ***Do smart grocery shopping.*** Plan your shopping list in advance and don't bring home foods that you are trying to avoid.

10. ***Drink plenty of water.*** Drinking at least eight glasses per day helps fat and muscle metabolism in many ways. Train your body to drink more water even if sometimes you don't feel thirsty. The reason why your body is not asking for more water is often because it has adopted to survive this way and not because it doesn't need more water.

When your body is fighting toxins it is too busy to burn fat. Supply enough water to make it easier for your body to flash out those toxins. Put reminders on your phone or computer to drink more water.

The only times when it is not suggestible to drink water is during your meals or immediately after them because this way you will be diluting the juices in your stomach making your digestion problematic. Also be careful with drinking too much water close to your bed time for obvious reason.

Tap filtered water is safest because it is getting periodically tested. Bottled water is toxic by plastic.

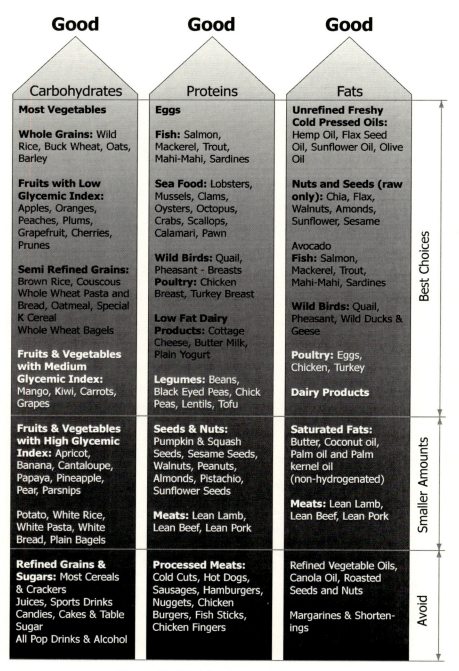

Good — Carbohydrates

Best Choices

Most Vegetables

Whole Grains: Wild Rice, Buck Wheat, Oats, Barley

Fruits with Low Glycemic Index: Apples, Oranges, Peaches, Plums, Grapefruit, Cherries, Prunes

Semi Refined Grains: Brown Rice, Couscous Whole Wheat Pasta and Bread, Oatmeal, Special K Cereal Whole Wheat Bagels

Fruits & Vegetables with Medium Glycemic Index: Mango, Kiwi, Carrots, Grapes

Smaller Amounts

Fruits & Vegetables with High Glycemic Index: Apricot, Banana, Cantaloupe, Papaya, Pineapple, Pear, Parsnips

Potato, White Rice, White Pasta, White Bread, Plain Bagels

Avoid

Refined Grains & Sugars: Most Cereals & Crackers Juices, Sports Drinks Candies, Cakes & Table Sugar All Pop Drinks & Alcohol

Good — Proteins

Best Choices

Eggs

Fish: Salmon, Mackerel, Trout, Mahi-Mahi, Sardines

Sea Food: Lobsters, Mussels, Clams, Oysters, Octopus, Crabs, Scallops, Calamari, Pawn

Wild Birds: Quail, Pheasant - Breasts
Poultry: Chicken Breast, Turkey Breast

Low Fat Dairy Products: Cottage Cheese, Butter Milk, Plain Yogurt

Legumes: Beans, Black Eyed Peas, Chick Peas, Lentils, Tofu

Smaller Amounts

Seeds & Nuts: Pumpkin & Squash Seeds, Sesame Seeds, Walnuts, Peanuts, Almonds, Pistachio, Sunflower Seeds

Meats: Lean Lamb, Lean Beef, Lean Pork

Avoid

Processed Meats: Cold Cuts, Hot Dogs, Sausages, Hamburgers, Nuggets, Chicken Burgers, Fish Sticks, Chicken Fingers

Good — Fats

Best Choices

Unrefined Freshy Cold Pressed Oils: Hemp Oil, Flax Seed Oil, Sunflower Oil, Olive Oil

Nuts and Seeds (raw only): Chia, Flax, Walnuts, Amonds, Sunflower, Sesame

Avocado
Fish: Salmon, Mackerel, Trout, Mahi-Mahi, Sardines

Wild Birds: Quail, Pheasant, Wild Ducks & Geese

Poultry: Eggs, Chicken, Turkey

Dairy Products

Smaller Amounts

Saturated Fats: Butter, Coconut oil, Palm oil and Palm kernel oil (non-hydrogenated)

Meats: Lean Lamb, Lean Beef, Lean Pork

Avoid

Refined Vegetable Oils, Canola Oil, Roasted Seeds and Nuts

Margarines & Shortenings

Figure 29. Making better food choices

4. *Proper food combining*

Many of those who invent popular recipes know a lot about taste but very little about digestion. Our food should taste delicious, but it also has to be combined in the best possible way to help our body to digest it.

Proper food combination is not just a theory. This is a practical approach supported by many medical experiments.

When I was about twenty-five, I was diagnosed with *gastritis*—a stomach inflammation. To find out what was exactly wrong with my stomach I had to go through a very repulsive process called *gastroscopy*. This is how it's done:

A flexible pipe with a small camera and a light is inserted through your mouth right down to your stomach. Through the camera, the examiner can see on his monitor what is happening in your stomach. First he checks if your stomach is structurally OK—if there are no ulcers or tumors. Then he starts giving you different liquid solutions to test your digestion. Those solutions produce different results, and the examiner can see how your stomach reacts to each of them. During that process, the examiner takes a sample of each stomach juice by sucking them out of your stomach through an inserted pipe.

Proper food combination is based on similar experiments. When an examined person was given protein to eat, his stomach formed *acidic* gastric juices, but when he was given carbohydrates, his stomach formed *alkali* juices.

Some of you might say, "Who cares, let the body deal with it. We don't have to think about it!"

But before we say it, let's think about it.

If you do a chemical experiment mixing an acid with alkaline in equal proportions, these two substances neutralize each other producing salt and water. Take a look at the sample chemical formula below.

$NaOH + HCl \longrightarrow NaCl + H_2O$

NaOH is an *acid*, and HCl is an *alkali*. When these two are mixed together, they produce NaCl—salt, and H_2O—water.

How significant is this?

Remember that bloated feeling in your stomach sometimes? When you mix proteins and starchy carbohydrates in proportion close to 1:1, your stomach juices will produce similar reaction, and your acid and alkali gastric juices will neutralize each other. What happens with the food you just ate? It simply does not get digested and sits in your stomach waiting for your body to readjust your stomach juices.

Your body will keep trying to produce proper combination of digesting juices, but it will take longer time than it should, and part of the food you just ate will be left undigested. Then, this undigested food will pass through the rest of your digestive tract creating unhealthy bacteria and clogging your guts with dangerous elements. Of course, your body will try fighting those bacteria, but who needs that extra unnecessary energy spent on something that could have been prevented? We then could have used that energy to do things that we enjoy instead of always feeling run-down.

Let's take a look at some of the foods to see how they are naturally created and what their natural ratios between carbohydrates and proteins are. See table 29.

Table 29. Carbohydrate to protein ratio of some foods

Food	Total g	Carbohydrates g	Protein g	Ratio
Brown Rice	195	45	5	9/1
Barley	157	44	4	11/1
Apple	125	17	0.3	>17/1
Orange	96	11	0.9	>11/1
Beef	85	0	26	>0/26
Chicken	86	0	26	>0/26
Beans	171	45	15	3/1

The more carbohydrates are in the food, the more *alkali* gastric juices will be produced, and the more proteins are in the food, the more the *acidic* juices. Most foods in nature have either more of the carbohydrates or more of the protein, and very few foods have ratio closer than 5:1 between their carbohydrates and proteins. You may have already noticed from the table that beans are the only ones that have closer than the usual ratio, and we know how many people experience stomach gas when they eat beans. The main reason for that gas is the wrong mixture of the alkali and acid—too close to 1:1.

If you are going to eat more than one food at a meal, you can greatly improve digestion by eating foods that require the same gastric juices. Proper food combination leads to a good digestion and to better health. *Having a wide variety of food doesn't mean eating it all at a single meal.* See figure 30.

Proper Food Combining Chart

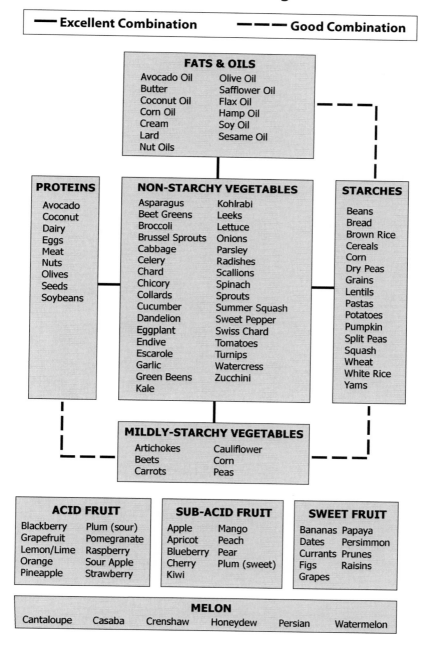

Figure 30. Proper food combining

CHAPTER 33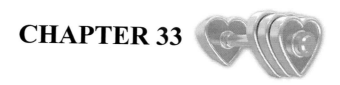

FAT-BURNING "MACHINE"

The *in-body reactions* described in chapter 17, "Why We Gain Weight," might discourage some of you to lose weight, but the more you know about your body, the more chances that you will succeed.

The human body burns body fat *only one way*. This is how it is thousands of years ago, and this is how it will be many thousands in the future. The way our body works is never going to change, and no matter how many different programs or exercises will be invented, our body will still burn body fat the same way. This process is based on human body physiology and not on some kind of magic.

But burning body fat is not just about exercise. It is a combination of different things. We can utilize those things to get maximum results with minimum time and spend that extra time on doing other things that we love to do. We don't live to exercise, and most of us don't want their exercise program to be too long. Eating better, for example, can dramatically reduce the time spent at the gym.

I have witnessed many people who exercised very hard but still could not improve their bodies for many years. How disappointing this might be, and who wants to spend years and years running on treadmill or lifting weights without visible results?

While this is true that some people utilize dietary fat and burn their body fat more efficiently, anyone can reinforce this process by providing certain circumstances.

For easier explanations, let's imagine body-fat-burning process as a machine, and let's see what we need to turn that machine on (see figure 31).

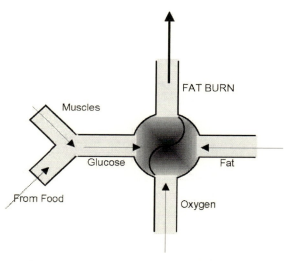

Figure 31. Body's fat burning Machine

1. **Dietary fat.** The essential fatty acids (omega-6 and omega-3) are always preferred when it comes to support life. Other fats are usually used for energy, and if that energy is not needed immediately, they are used for fat storage. Saturated fats are great sources of energy but only if we spend that energy. If we are inactive and eat saturated fats, our body stores them as body fat. Breaking down solid fats takes more time than essential fatty acids because the essential fatty acids are liquid and have lower melting temperatures.

   Fat-burning process requires essential fatty acids. It may sound paradox, but *we need fat to burn body fat* (figure 31, right). The only trick is that for this purpose, we need very specific fats—omega-6 and omega-3 *in their proper ratio 3:1.* (Read more in "EFAs Balance," page 313.)

2. **Glucose.** Glucose is always needed to support life. All body processes require it, and the fat-burning process is not an exception. No matter what we eat, our body will always "find" glucose within itself.

   Glucose, during the burning of fat, can be provided from two sources—from the food we eat or from muscle deposits (figure 31, left). The body will always try to get glucose from food first, "saving" muscle deposits for later—when we don't eat at all or need more glucose than the food can provide.

   Some people, when trying to lose body fat, reduce their carbohydrate intakes hoping for fat loss but end up with muscle loss instead. If we don't supply enough carbohydrates through our food, the body may end up manufacturing glucose out of our muscles.

   Providing proper amount of glucose is crucial for fat-burning process because *gaining muscles and losing fat* is the way to go.

   Depleting muscle storages of glucose, if not over exceeded, is a good idea because the more often we use those storages, the more our body "trains" to expand them and store more sugar as glycogen rather than fat. Only by exercising regularly can you develop this capacity. The type of exercise is not as important as its *consistency*, *duration*, and *intensity*.

3. **Oxygen.** The body burns body fat most efficiently in the presence of a lot of oxygen (figure 31, bottom).

   Let's look at the fat-burning process as something else to understand it better.

   Picture yourself making a barbecue: First thing you need is a *starter fluid* to start the fire and then the *charcoal* to keep the fire burning longer and steadier. In the fat-burning process, the glucose plays the role of a starter fluid, and the fat plays role of the charcoal. For short-time physical activities such as sprints, our body uses mostly glucose because glucose burns faster just like starter fluid in the fire, but for slow and prolonged activities, our body prefers fat because the amount of glucose stored in our body is very limited. When we go for a *nonstop physical activity*, our body tries to save glucose by switching to the burning of fat. Those physical activities are what we call *aerobic* or *cardio* exercise.

The amount of oxygen you receive during your aerobic exercise is crucial. You should always try to exercise harder, but as soon as you go out of breath, the oxygen reduction caused by the shortage of your breath will slow down the fat-burning process, just like if you would close oxygen to your fire when making your barbecue—the charcoal would stop burning.

4. **Aerobic activity** (figure 31, center). When people think of aerobic activity, first what comes into their minds is running, cycling, or doing cardio machines. But to get aerobic effect and to burn body fat, you can do practically anything. As long as your exercise is nonstop for at least 10-15 minutes, and the intensity is high enough, you can do whatever you want—dance, jump, hike, do resistance training, etc. Of course, the longer the time, the more body fat you will burn.

Regular aerobic activity "trains" the body to burn more fat per minute. Three months down the road, you will be burning more body fat during the same twenty minutes than today because regular aerobic activity promotes the growth of so-called fat-burning enzymes. As the quantity of those enzymes grow, more work gets done for the same amount of time. It's like hiring hundreds of people instead of only ten to do the same job.

How intense should the aerobic exercise be?

You can figure it out by three methods—your *heart rate*, *talk test*, and *Borg's scale*.

Heart rate monitoring method works for most people and is being widely used in fitness. It is done in two simple steps: first, calculating your *maximum heart rate*, and second, calculating your *training heart rates* based on your maximum heart rate.

Maximum heart rate calculations depend on one's age. The formula is very simple—220 minus your age. For example, a forty-year-old person's maximum heart rate calculations will be as follows: 220 - 40 = 180 beats per minute.

Training intensities are calculated based on your maximum heart rate number. Table 30 displays those calculations.

Table 30. Aerobic Training Intensities

Target Heart Rate Chart							
	Intensity						
Age	60%	70%	75%	80%	85%	90%	Max.
20	120	140	150	160	170	180	200
25	117	137	146	156	166	176	195
30	114	133	143	152	162	171	190
35	111	130	139	148	157	167	185
40	108	126	135	144	153	162	180
45	105	123	131	140	149	158	175
50	102	119	128	136	145	153	170
55	99	116	124	132	140	149	165
60	96	112	120	128	136	144	160
65	93	109	116	124	132	140	155
70	90	105	113	120	128	135	150
75	87	102	109	116	123	131	145

Red Zone

Anaerobic Zone

Aerobic Zone

Fat Burning Zone

Healthy Heart Zone

Healthy heart zone—Sixty percent of your maximum is the easiest and most comfortable zone and is best for people who are just starting an exercise program or have physical limitations. Although this zone has been criticized for not burning enough total calories and for not being intense enough to get great cardio respiratory benefits, it has been shown to help decrease body fat, blood pressure, and cholesterol. It also decreases the risk of degenerative diseases and has a low risk of injury.

Fat-burning zone—Approximately 70 percent of your maximum heart rate. This zone can also be used by beginners unless there are physical limitations—heart conditions, knee problems, lower back problems, etc. Precautions should be taken. Studies have shown that in this zone you can get fat out of your cells most efficiently, and you are also training your fat cells to increase the rate of fat release (increasing the number of fat-burning enzymes) while still providing cardiorespiratory benefits.

Aerobic zone—approximately 75-80 percent of your maximum heart rate. This is the preferred zone if you are training for endurance. Your functional capacity will improve, the number and size of blood vessels will increase, and the resting heart rate will decrease. Your cardiovascular and respiratory system will improve, and you will increase the size and strength of your heart. This zone is for intermediate or advanced cardio training.

Anaerobic zone—Eighty to 90 percent of your maximum heart rate. Since the intensity is high, more calories will be burned, but 85 percent of the calories are burned from glucose, and only 15 percent from fat because of lack of oxygen. This zone is recommended for advanced training.

Red zone—Ninety to 100 percent of your maximum heart rate. This zone burns the highest total number of calories but the lowest percentage of fat calories: 90 percent glucose. This zone is very intense, and in fitness training, it is recommended only for interval training at advanced levels. For example, you might do a sprint of thirty seconds in this zone and then go back to any of the lower zones.

The zone training method may not work for all people because some people have smaller or bigger heart sizes. Bigger heart pumps more blood with every stroke, smaller heart, less.

If you find yourself not fitting into calculations above, use the *talk test*. The reasons for not fitting could be that your heart rates do not match with how you feel. For example, people with bigger heart size may feel the fat-burning zone as anaerobic zone and go out of breath while their heart is still pumping low; people with smaller heart size may have skyrocketing heart rates while they still don't feel any resistance.

Talk test is the method when you are exercising at the intensity to be able to handle a conversation with short sentences. As it becomes harder to talk, the intensity should be reduced. If long sentences can be made during your exercise, the intensity should be increased.

Borg's scale is the third method of tracking your heart rate level, and it provides a rough guideline to measure intensity that quick and easy. While training, you have to determine by yourself how difficult it is for you to do the exercise. It can be done in two different ways:

1. Scale 6-20

Think of a number between 6 and 20. The harder it is to exercise, the higher the number you should be thinking of. Adding 0 to the number you picked will determine your approximate heart rate. For example, if performing the exercise is hard for you, pick the number 15 (hard). This would correspond to approximately 150 beats per minute. Refer to the chart below for more details.

6 7 - very, very light 8 9 - very light 10 11- fairly light 12 13-somewhat hard	14 15-hard 16 17-very hard 18 19- very very hard 20

2. Scale 0-10

Think of a number between 0 and 10. The harder it is to exercise, the higher the number you should be thinking of. Adding 0 to the number you picked will determine your approximate *percentage* of your maximum heart rate and belonging to the training zones described earlier. For example, if performing the exercise is hard for you, pick the number 7 (very strong). This would correspond to 70 percent of maximum heart rate. Refer to the chart below for more details.

```
0
0.5 - very, very weak
1 - very weak
2 - weak
3 - moderate
4 - somewhat strong
5 - strong
6
7 - very strong
8
9
10 - maximal
```

CHAPTER 34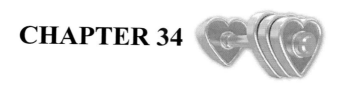

THE PSYCHOLOGY OF PIGGING OUT

People like to eat; there is no doubt about that. If there is no other pleasure to fulfill life—there is always food. For many of us, getting together on the weekends never ends up with just a cup of coffee or tea. Very often tables are "bending" from food, all sorts of alcohol, pops, juices, meats, potatoes, pastas, salads, cakes, cookies, puddings—you name it.

This is the reason why in all countries all over the world, gyms are packed with people on Mondays and Tuesdays—people feel guilty after their weekends.

At a regular party with 3-5 course meal and alcohol, you can easily consume between 2,000 and 5,000 calories. This is not very hard to calculate:

- 3 drinks—450 calories (150 cal. each)
- 3 courses—900 calories (300 cal. each course)
- 1 midsize desert—450 calories.

Here you go, the total is approximately 2,000 calories. But at a single party, some people drink more than 3 drinks, eat more that 300 calories per course, and have more than 1 desert.

How can we enjoy our parties but still prevent from gaining fat? In order to understand that, let's first see how our body stores the energy.

Imagine your body storages as containers. There are containers for sugar and also containers for fat. Our body always tries to keep those containers full for future use. When we exercise, our body uses energy from those containers. Later when we eat again, the body fills them up.

The fat containers are the ones that cause us to get bigger because the body has the ability to build more of them. It does it by building more of the fat cells. Later, when we try to lose body fat, the unpleasant thing happens—the body gets too "comfortable" with the new number of fat cells because these new fat cells are like a bank account for the body and are not considered as a bad thing. The body always tries to hold on to that new "account"—number of fat cells—and empty them only temporarily. When we overeat again, the body will try to fill them up just like we would try to recover money we spent from our account. Once new fat cells are built, they never get removed from the body, and those "accounts" never get closed. This is one of the main reasons why people "go back and forth" on the weight loss progress—their bodies don't like the idea of keeping the new fat cells empty.

Preventing building new fat cells is the main trick to always stay in good shape. Keeping fat cells empty is harder, and those who previously lost weight know how hard it can be to lose body fat and how easy it is to gain it back.

But there is a trick to prevent yourself from generating new fat cells when going to parties, and that trick is called "paying it forward."

If you do intensive workout right before your party, you will partially empty your storing containers, and before your body builds new fat cells, it will try to fill them up, converting sugar from your cake into glycogen instead of fat, using your meat protein from your steak to rebuild your muscles, and using fat from your sauces and salad dressings to help your body recover after the workout. If during your party you move, dance, or play instead of sitting around, some more energy will be spent, leading to even less chances for a new fat cell generation.

People who don't exercise during their weekends and go to their gyms after their parties are doing it too late. While they are still burning some body fat, that fat comes from fat cells newly generated over their weekends.

In order to prevent building new fat cells, exercise before your party, not after, and <u>pay it forward.</u>

CHAPTER 35

WHY WOMEN LOSE WEIGHT SLOWER THAN MEN

When it comes to losing weight, women face a disadvantage compared to men. Research involving two groups of people—60 men and 60 women—confirmed that women not only lose weight slower but also gain it faster. The participants of both groups who were at approximately the same age and had the same lifestyle were asked to perform 30 minutes of jogging every day for 6 months. At the end of the experiment, the men reduced their body fat percentage while the women did not notice any dramatic changes.

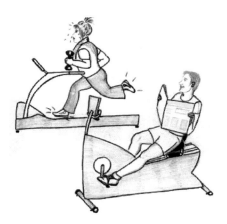

Women have lower resting metabolism than men, and fat settles differently on men and women. Men usually tend to store fat around their bellies. Women store fat on their hips and thighs. These areas are comprised of mostly brown fat, which is harder to lose. Women have smaller muscles.

But if a woman involves in a complete program that includes not only cardiovascular activity but also resistance training, she can burn fat just as effective as men. Combined with balanced eating, these two exercises speed up metabolism and enhance the fat loss, give the skin and the body a tone and tight appearance.

Resistance training increases metabolism at rest. When muscles break down during training, the body still works after you finish your workout to repair your muscles. This repair can take up to forty-eight hours, and the rate of elevation of your metabolism can be between 5 to 15 percent. So after a good resistance-training workout, you can burn up to 200 extra calories while watching your TV.

Tips

- If you are pregnant, your metabolism is faster.
- Breast-feeding is one of the best ways to get rid of brown fat on your thighs and hips.

CHAPTER 36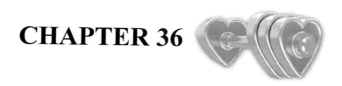

RESISTANCE TRAINING

Just a few decades ago, only some people were involved in resistance training. Those were mostly bodybuilders and athletes. The rest used muscles otherwise—playing games, doing home duties, walking, gardening, or some other physical jobs.

Most of the jobs today are in comfortable chairs, and there is no physical activity at home either. We stopped going out because we have large TVs and computers. We limited our conversations with each other by e-mail, text messaging, or by phone. Phones have gotten so sophisticated that we can see each other live when talking. Why bother going anywhere when you can do it right on the spot?

Our brain always tries to find easier and easier solutions. This is just human nature. But what about the muscles? Don't they have a purpose?

The more I watch technology developing, the more I get inclined into thinking that maybe the producers of kids movie *WALL-E* somehow envisioned our future, and one day, we all will be fat and lazy and wouldn't have to get out of our chairs at all. The tendency of this happening unfortunately is there.

Muscles provide us life. They are not just for beauty and strength, but they are also for everything else that makes us live. Well-developed muscles help to stay in good health, and they actively help our organs and systems. Muscles are tightly connected with the work of our heart, and they are often called a *second heart*. If muscles don't work enough, the heart has to do double work, overloading itself. This is why the resting heart rate of those who exercise is lower—their hearts don't have to work as hard since muscles are taking over the part of that work.

Research conducted almost a century ago demonstrated the absolute vitality for us to move our bodies—healthy men between twenty to twenty-eight years old were put in casts below their waist and for seven weeks were not able to move their lower bodies. With loss of physical activity, the men started to develop some serious health conditions including heart problems. As soon as the casts were removed and the men could move again, all their health problems disappeared.

If we don't use our muscles, they get smaller, blood circulation gets worse, capillaries narrow, muscles get flabby and eventually atrophy leading to degenerative diseases.

Regular weight-resistance exercise enhances blood circulation, widening the capillaries. Muscle tension during resistance training is also the best way to enhance bone growth and stop bone loss because bone is also a living tissue. It reacts to such exercises by becoming stronger and denser. Well-developed muscles provide good appearance and, as a result, also provide self-confidence.

Basic Terminology

agility
Ability to change the body's position. Agility is a combination of balance, coordination, speed, reflexes, and strength. *Agility* can also be defined as a power of moving the limbs quickly and easily. Basic example of agility training is skipping rope.

anaerobic training
Training that uses movements requiring very little oxygen. These are quick explosive actions that last a short time such as sprinting.

balance
Body's ability to remain upright with minimal postural sway. Gymnasts performing exercises on the beam is a good example of balance training.

cool down
A form of light training or stretching that allows your body to gradually slow down after exercise.

coordination
Someone's ability to synchronize few different tasks or body movements. Gymnasts are examples of persons with good coordination.

flexibility
Range of movement in joints. Stretching exercises develop flexibility.

lactic acid
A liquid that is produced in muscles as a result of anaerobic training. It slows down the body movements if it builds up too much.

rep (repetition)
A single complete action of any one given exercise beginning from its starting position, progressing to its ending position, and then returning back to starting position. For example, raising your hands above your head and then returning them back is 1 rep.

set
A given number of repetitions performed continuously and consequently without rest. For example, eight repetitions of any exercise will make one set.

stamina
Someone's ability to withstand activity for a long time. Marathon runners have a lot of stamina.

strength
Ability of muscles to produce force on physical objects.

VO2 max
The maximum amount of oxygen a person can use in a one-minute workout. A high V02 max makes the body more efficient for performance.

warm-up
A preparation time before workout begins.

CHAPTER 37

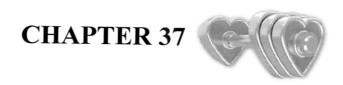

FUNDAMENTAL PRINCIPLES OF RESISTANCE TRAINING

Set system. In order to completely exhaust a muscle or muscle group within resistance training, multiple sets must be completed. Number of sets may vary depending on one's goal. If your goal is general health or you are a beginner, perform 2-3 sets for each exercise with 30-90 seconds rest in between, or go to the next set only after your breathing becomes normal or your heart rate drops to 90 beats per minute.

Repetition system. In order to achieve different results, different number of repetitions must be performed in each set. If your goal is to build muscle mass, your weight must be heavy, allowing you to perform only 6-9 repetitions in each set. But if your goal is general health or muscle tone, your weight must be moderate to light allowing you to perform 12-25 repetitions in each set.

Muscle flush. Completing multiple sets causes the muscle to be flushed with blood, which provokes the feeling of a "*satisfying pump*" signifying that the muscle has been *adequately* stressed.

Cycle system. Throughout the year, different routines and phases should be implemented in resistance training (cycles). This prevents boredom and helps to avoid overuse injuries while still achieving continued training effect.

Muscle isolation. This method is used when you wish to target (isolate) a specific muscle, *purposely* leaving other muscles out of the exercise. For example, if you bend your arms at your elbows, holding elbows tight to the body (bicep curl exercise), you will isolate your bicep muscles.

Muscle isolation is also referred as *single joint* exercises, which means that you use only one joint of your body for each particular exercise. Muscle isolation is the safest way of resistance training for beginners due to this fact because it reduces chances of injuries.

Muscle isolation is achieved best on exercising machines and using free weights. Usually, the exerciser performs a number of repetitions and sets with appropriate rest in between.

During any exercise when using the muscle isolation method, you can purposely decrease or increase the isolation by allowing or disallowing other muscles to get involved. What helps to achieve that?

Body positioning is extremely important for muscle isolation. Which muscles you will use during the exercise depends on how your muscles are aligned. For example, if you raise your hands directly over your head when your body is vertical, most of the pressure comes on your shoulders, but when you are raising your hands lying on the forty-five-degree bench, half of that pressure comes to your chest.

The *speed* of performing the exercise can influence the isolation. For example, if you perform exercise too fast, other muscles may get involved, and you will not feel the muscle that you want. Slow-movement weight training is a new trend in some gyms. The idea is to lift weights very slowly. This method will assist in isolating the muscle group being worked on. However, there is no scientific magic behind slow-movement lifting. Moderate tempo of two seconds one way and two seconds the other way works well for most exercises.

Concentration is important in muscle isolation, and it simply means thinking about the muscle you train in order to make it work harder. When you consciously focus your attention on the muscle you are training, other muscles stop assisting the exercise. You can experiment this trick with your fist by "telling" your fist to squeeze harder and harder. This can be done in two ways: (1) squeezing your whole body as you squeeze your fist, or (2) concentrating only on your forearm. You may notice how when you don't use the rest of your body, you can actually apply more strength within your forearm, making it squeeze the fist harder. Achieving the same results with your other muscles will take some time, but if you practice *concentration*, you will be able to control any of your muscles the same way. You will see how easily you can direct the tension just by thinking about it.

Compound exercises. This type of resistance training is requiring use of more than one muscle group. Compound exercises are also referred to as "multijoint exercises." For example, when you are performing a squat, you are involving many muscles of your lower body: quadriceps (fronts of your legs), hamstrings (backs of your legs), your buttocks and your calves, and you are also using multiple joints—knees, hips, and your lower back.

Circuit training. With this type of training, several different exercises are completed, one immediately after another. The purpose of the circuit training is to save time while achieving muscle toning and cardiovascular benefits all at once. Circuit training is recommended for intermediate or advanced training since it requires basic knowledge of exercises to be performed and also certain level of cardiovascular performance.

Muscle confusion. This method is based on constant variation of the exercises, using their *volume, intensity, angles of motion, positions,* and exercises' *sequences*. This prevents muscles from adaptation to a specific training routine, which ensures a continuing training effect, and also burns more calories. Muscle confusion is also beneficial for those who get easily bored with exercise routines to maintain their enthusiasm.

There is no particular secret or trick about muscle confusion training, as it may be presented in some advertisements, as there is no such a particular combination of exercises that will constantly maintain the confusion. *As long as the variation of exercises is maintained, the muscle confusion is achieved.*

Split training system. Instead of training all body parts in the same day (whole body system), the stress can be placed on only one or few body parts at a time. The purpose of split system is to maximize the effectiveness of training for each specific muscle or a muscle group. The total number of training sessions per week is usually increased. For example, instead of training every other day, sessions can be scheduled every day, sometimes few times a day, since different muscle groups are trained those times. The time of each training session is usually reduced due to fewer number of muscles trained.

Different goals can be achieved with split system. Those who strive for muscle gain and strength can greatly benefit from this system, as well as those who are just looking for general health.

Muscle priority. Different muscles are developed differently in different people. The weaker muscles need to be trained first within a single training session while energy levels are high.

Functional training. This method is used to stimulate the individual's everyday life, work, or sports actions. Exercises to be performed are selected *to imitate* those activities or functions.

CHAPTER 38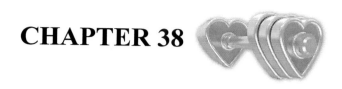

WHAT'S IN THAT NAME?

A ll exercises can be done using five major starting body
   positions:

1. **Upright** position—when your upper body is *perpendicular to the floor <u>head up</u>*.
2. **Flat** position—when your upper body is *parallel to the floor*.
3. **Upside down** position—when your body is *perpendicular to the floor <u>head down</u>*.
4. **Incline** position—when your upper body is at *any angle between upright and flat position*.
5. **Decline** position—when your body is at *any angle between upside down and flat position*.

Many exercises are named after these positions. For example, bench press exercise lying *flat* on the bench is called *flat bench press*, when the same exercise with your body leaned at 45 degrees is called *incline bench press*, and when your body is at forty-five degrees upside down, the exercise is called *decline bench press*.

Exercises performed from *standing*, *seating*, or *lying* positions are often named that way. For example, *seated bench press*, *standing dumbbell curl*, or *lying triceps extension* are the exercises specified by those positions.

Sometimes, exercises are called with combinations of few different words to make it clearer what type of equipment and what position are being used. For example, when using free weights, it is hard to understand what type of free weight you are using unless you specify it. *Incline dumbbell press* makes it obvious that this press is performed at incline position using dumbbells.

Exercises' names may also include words that are used for describing specific fitness motions:

Press—pushing machine handles or free weights away from your body

Pull—bringing the object toward you

Curl—bending your arms or legs

Extension—straightening arms or legs

Pullover—bringing the weights from behind of your neck with arms slightly bent

Dead lift—lifting the weight from the floor

Whenever you read the name of the exercise, think of the words that are put in that name. This will always help you to understand what to do.

CHAPTER 39

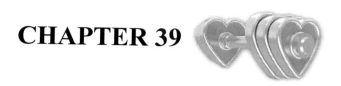

THE SIMPLE ANATOMY

Learning anatomy is never easy because names of the muscles, bones, and all the connections don't make sense; you just have to memorize them. *Chest, shoulder, leg* are the easy names, but when it comes to proper anatomy, this can get challenging.

At the beginning of my fitness career, I tried to use proper names when explaining about muscles to my clients, but was discouraged using them for a simple reason that my clients could never remember those names. Just to give you an idea about those names, I will give you few examples: If I had to explain about calves, the muscles between your kneecap and your ankles, I would have to use few of the following names: *gastrocnemius, peroneus longus, extensor digitorium longus, tibialis anterior*, and *soleus*.

On my anatomy diagrams on figures 32 and 33, I used what is called *slang* fitness terminology. You will not find most of these names in any anatomy books, but these are the abbreviations commonly used in gyms, and if you say these words, you will be understood. Proper full names of the muscles are used mostly only for passing the anatomy exams. Behind doors, even most trainers use the terminology mentioned below.

BODY

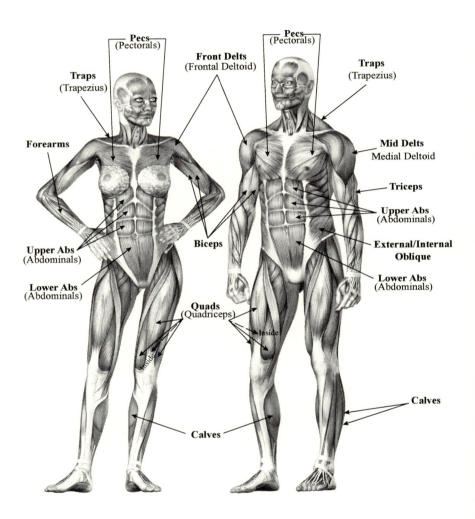

Figure 32. Anterior human anatomy (gym terminology)

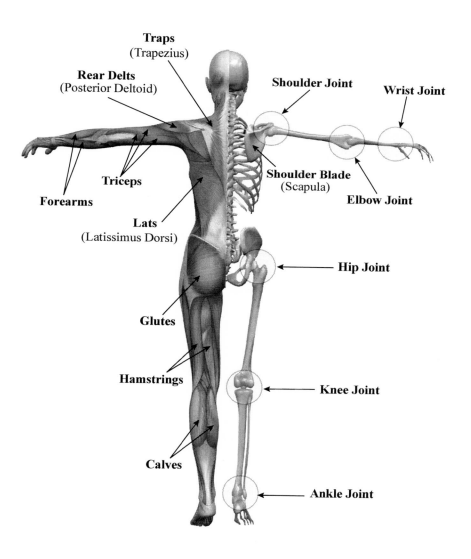

Figure 33. Posterior human anatomy (gym terminology)

CHAPTER 40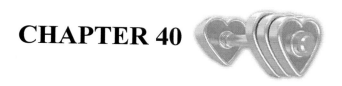

RESISTANCE TRAINING PROGRAMS

"I just don't want to look like macho"

Very often, when I interviewed women or even some men and tried to convince them to build muscles, I heard these words: "Oh, I just don't want to look like macho!"

"I wish it was that easy," I thought to myself. "I'll take all the muscles that you don't want."

In today's world, we should be concerned more about having too little muscles rather than too much especially when you are exercising with moderate to light weights—chances that you will bulk up this way are almost zero.

To understand better how muscles change when you train with moderate to light weights, let's picture something else. Imagine a bus that has no people in it, and then imagine the same bus in traffic time—full of people. After people got in, the size of the bus didn't change, right? But the density inside of it did. The same happens with your muscles when you train them with moderate to light weights—they don't change in size, but become denser and fuller, providing you nice appearance and great health.

Try Before You Buy

Learning how to use exercising machines before exercising on them is the same as reading the manual for your new computer or TV before turning it on—it will help you to avoid problems. Come to your gym at the least-busy time, when there are not that many people on the gym floor. Those times are the following:

- 1:00 p.m.-3:00 p.m. Monday through Thursday
- Any time on Friday (especially in the evening)
- Saturday afternoon and Sunday afternoon.

Choose one machine at a time and make sure that you understand everything about it. What you need to know you will find out from reading further.

Most gyms offer three-day, one-week, or two-week trials. Use these trials *before joining* to make sure that you are fully comfortable with all the equipment that your gym offers.

How do you determine your exercising weight?
There are two ways, and they are the following:

1. **Maximum weight**. This method is done by performing an exercise with only one repetition at your maximum capability and then calculating an exercising weight based on your goal.

   Here is how it is done:
   You perform few tryouts, increasing the weight until you can only perform one repetition in a set (with still the correct technique). This number will determine your calculations.

   Let's assume that your weight with one repetition came up to be 100 lb. Depending on what you are trying to achieve, your *exercising* weight will be as follows:

pure strength and power /little mass—80%-100% (or in this case 80-100 lb.)
strength and mass—70%-80% (or 70-80 lb.)
some strength and mass—65%-75% (or 65-75 lb.)
endurance/little strength and mass—less than 70% (or less than 70 lb.)

Source: CPTN—The Art and Science of Personal Training

This method is not advisable for beginners because it could lead to muscle and joints damage. When someone is not experienced and doesn't know proper technique and their muscles and joints are not prepared for maximum overload tryouts, the risk of injury is greatly higher.

2. **Repetitions**. This method is done by gradually increasing the weight until you reach the maximum load to perform the number of repetitions based on your goal.

   Here is how it is done:
   You perform a few tryouts where with every next set you gradually increase the weight until you complete the following number of repetitions (with still a correct technique):

   pure strength and power/little mass—1-5 reps
   strength and mass—6-9 reps
   some strength and mass—10-15 reps
   endurance/little strength and mass—12-20 reps

   Source: CPTN—The Art and Science of Personal Training

Let's say you have loaded your machine with 100 lb. and performed a maximum of 17 repetitions with that weight. If your goal is to tone your muscles or develop endurance (see above), this weight might be exactly what you need. But if your goal is to bulk up or develop strength, you need to keep on loading more weight until you can only perform 6-9 repetitions.

Walking around the gym, I have noticed many times how some people "getting sold" on the idea of using lightweights, use no weight at all. Even if your goal is not to bulk up, performing 12-20 repetitions doesn't mean doing them effortlessly. This will only waste your time. Your last 3 repetitions must always be performed with a struggle no matter what your goal is. When I was explaining my clients how many repetitions they have to do, I had my saying: "Do as many as you can, and then 3 more." What this means is that whatever the number of repetitions you need to perform to achieve your goal, the last three must be almost impossible to do. You have to experience great blood flash within the muscles you train.

Whole Body Program

The whole body program includes exercises for all major body parts performed within a single workout, and it is recommended for those who want to lose weight, tone muscles, or maintain the weight. Workouts are usually scheduled three times per week every other day, giving a forty-eight-hour break in between. The number of exercises varies from 5 to 15 depending on the time availability. Large muscle groups, such as chest, back, or legs are usually trained first due to their multijoint functionalities—when other muscles and joints assist the exercise, the risk of injury is lower. When your body is warmed up by these large muscle group exercises at the beginning of your program, you can start training small muscles such as shoulders, biceps, triceps, forearms, and calves. Abdominal muscles can be trained anytime. Table 31 displays some samples how you can structure your whole body program.

Table 31. Whole Body Program Variations

Chest	Back	Legs	Legs
Back	Chest	Chest	Back
Shoulders	Shoulders	Back	Chest
Biceps	Biceps	Shoulders	Shoulders
Triceps	Triceps	Biceps	Biceps
Legs	Legs	Triceps	Triceps
Abdominals	Abdominals	Abdominals	Abdominals
* Offered in this book.			

Split Body Program

This type of program is widely used by those who want to build muscle mass and strength, but it can also be recommended to anyone who wants to make their workouts shorter but do them more often. Only few muscles are being trained during each workout, but those workouts can be as short as 15-20 minutes.

Splits can be done in various ways. You can choose to train one muscle of your upper body with one muscle of your lower body, or you can combine two upper body parts together, but what is usually recommended for the upper body is to combine muscles on *"one push"* with *"one pull"*—some muscle groups, when you train them, do *pull* motion (toward your body), and some *push* (away from your body). For example, *push* motions are chest and triceps, and pull motions are back or biceps. So in your split program, you can choose to train together chest (*push*) with biceps (*pull*), or back (*pull*) with triceps (*push*), or chest (*push*) with back (*pull*). You can also combine any of these muscles with muscles of your lower body.

When planning your workout, make sure to give forty-eight hours for each muscle group to recover.

As you get more experienced, you may also try ignoring this rule to bring more confusion to your muscles, but be careful how you perceive it. Large muscle groups are preferred to be trained first. For example, if you choose to train your chest with your biceps, chest comes first.

The *number of sets* prescribed for each exercise varies depending on your goal and fitness level. Usually 12-36 sets are recommended for an entire given session. For example, if your whole body program consists of 12 exercises, the maximum number of sets for each exercise will be 3 (12 × 3 = 36 sets). Beginners should start with fewer sets. The average number of sets for beginners is recommended 12-24, which could be either 6-12 exercises with 2 sets, or 4-8 exercises with 3 sets, or 3-6 exercises with 4 sets. More sets can be added later with experience.

Rest between sets depends on your fitness level, intensity of exercise, or specific goal, and it varies from few seconds to few minutes. If your training for endurance rest is shorter, but if your goal is to build strength or a muscle mass, it is longer. Beginners should track their heart rate in order to learn how much time they need to rest between sets—as soon as your heart rate drops to 90 beats per minute, this is usually the time for a new set.

Types of Equipment

There are four most popular ways to do resistance training in any gym. They are the following:

- *Selectorized machines*
- *Plate-loaded machines*
- *Free-motion machines,* and
- *Free weights*.

The training programs described in this book are intended for learning how to use various gym machines and free weights. They are the following:

program 1—selectorized machines

program 2—plate-loaded machines
program 3—free-motion machines
program 4—free weights

If you are a beginner, learn these programs in the same sequence. Program with selectorized machines is placed first because these machines are safer and simpler to understand, and they will teach you basic body movements. Once you learn those movements, it will be easier for you to understand the rest of the machines and the free weights.

Do not rush to the next level if you still don't completely understand all exercises from previous program because explanations are universal. Learn the proper technique first.

Always write machine settings down. On the pages where each exercise is explained, there are specific slots for each of those settings. There are also slots for your starting weight and number of the machine. In the future when you get stronger, the weight will change, but keep this record. This will be your history. If you are still young and your body is growing, settings for each machine may also change.

Program 1 (Selectorized Machines)

Note: <u>**Machines displayed on the pictures in this book may not be exactly as the ones in your gym, but don't get discouraged—all machines are similar in use.**</u>

Selectorized machines are the ones that are with preloaded stacks of weights where you can easily adjust your weight just by reinserting the pin. The main advantages of selectorized machines are the following:

- **They are supportive**, which is great for people who need help when learning new movements. They are also good for people rehabbing injuries or those who want to lift heavy weights without anyone's help.

- **They are easy to use** because they work on a fixed path and have instructions and diagrams posted.
- **They save time** when changing weights.
- **They are less intimidating** because you know exactly what muscles you're working on and how to do the exercise correctly.

Selectorized machines have some adjustments—*seat adjustment, range of motion adjustment,* and some others. Let's take a look at some of these machines to understand better how they work.

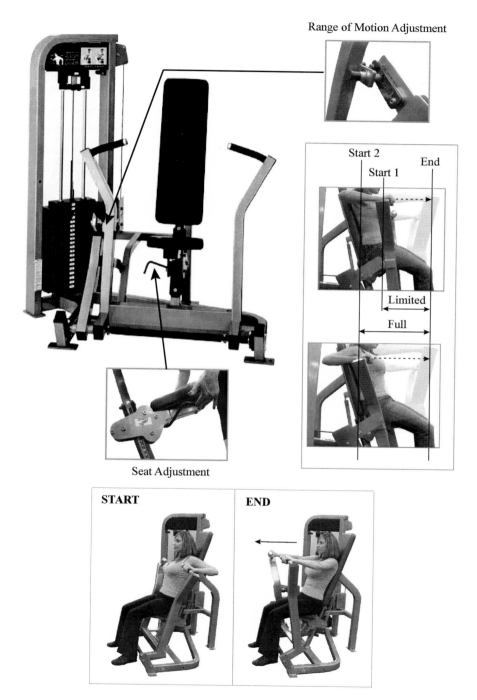

Figure 34. Chest Press machine

This machine is designed to perform the *push* (away for body) motion, and it has the following adjustments:

Weight adjustment

Every selectorized machine is designed for anyone's use. Weights on them may vary from 5 lb. to 300 lb. or more, but any beginner can work out together with an experienced person on the same machine. The weight is changed quickly by reinserting the pin in a different hole.

Most recent machines display weights in pounds (or kilograms in Europe), but some older models display by numbers on the plates (1, 2, 3, etc.).

When you are learning exercises, it is important to write your working weight down so you can track your progress.

Seat adjustment

Seat adjustment is an absolute necessity for proper machine use. If you are not correctly positioned on the machine, you are not only going to be using wrong muscles but also may injure yourself.

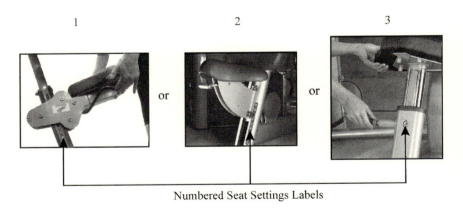

Numbered Seat Settings Labels

Figure 35. Most common seat adjustments on Selectorized Machines

Figure 35 displays some of the seat adjustments. Throughout my working experience I have noticed women struggling with seat adjustment number 3. The adjustments number 1 and 2 are very easy.

If you are a woman, you should definitely try all the seat adjustments to see how comfortable you are with them because struggling with machines can later discourage you from exercising. Always shop around to choose your gym.

Range of Motion Adjustment

What is range of motion?

In simple words, range of motion is the distance at which each joint in your body can move to its full potential.

Exercising at *full range of motion* gives you ability to move your body freely in any direction, reduce stiffness, prevent deformities, and help keep your joints flexible.

Daily activities, such as housework, climbing stairs, dressing, bathing, cooking, lifting, or bending do *not* move your joints through their full range of motion, thus they cannot replace the exercises.

Flexibility training helps to increase the range of motion in each joint by specific exercises. Further, in this book, when you learn exercises, you will also learn stretches for those exercises. Stretching between sets will help you develop flexibility, relax your muscles, and recover faster.

There are four types of stretching: *ballistic, dynamic, static,* and *PNF* (usually partner assistant)

Ballistic stretch is bouncing exercises where the end position is not held. This stretch is believed to inconsistently stretch the tissue, which *may lead to injury*. Example of ballistic stretch is swinging your legs or arms.

Dynamic stretch is a *controlled ballistic* stretch where movement gradually proceeds from one body position to another and then returns slowly and smoothly to the starting position. Dynamic stretch avoids bouncing and usually involves motions specific to sports or movements patterns. Example of dynamic stretch is repeatedly performing a motion and *gradually increasing the reaching point.*

Static stretch is a fully controlled stretch. It is initiated by the movement of a joint through its *full range of motion* and held in this position for a given period of time. During the holding time, the muscle being lengthened is relaxed. Example of static stretch is sitting on the floor with your legs straight trying to reach your toes without bouncing or any dynamic motion. *Static stretches are recommended between sets of exercises and described further in this book in more details in exercising programs.*

PNF (full name *proprioceptive neuromuscular facilitation*) involves lengthening the stretching muscle by static movement *until the end of its range of motion*, usually to the point of slight discomfort. PNF is achieved best with a partner who pushes on various body parts to maximize the stretching effect.

Note: Never stretch cold muscles (before workouts). Warm them up first by performing at least 8-10 minutes of nonstop physical activity.

Range of motion adjustments on exercising machines are designed to customize each machine for you. This is done for two main purposes:

1. To avoid injuries
2. To target a specific part of your muscle. Shorter range of motion targets more of the middle of each muscle while wider range of motion exercises the muscle's full length.

If your goal is to have long and flexible muscles, you should always try exercising at full range of motion, but if your goal is to bulk up, you might benefit from exercises with limited range of motion.

Range of motion adjustments on exercising determines at which point exercise starts. Take a look at figure 34 again and notice how you can begin the exercise using different starting points (ranges of motion). You can adjust this machine to begin the exercise further from your chest (start 1—*limited* range of motion), or you can use *full* range of motion (start 2) by beginning the exercise closer to your chest.

You can also limit your range of motion by not completing the exercise until the end.

Different manufacturers use different ways for their range of motion adjustments. Different machines also have various ways to adjust. Figure 36 displays some examples:

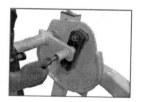 or 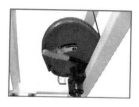 or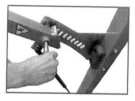

Figure 36. Most common Range of Motion adjustments
on Selectorized Machines

Before using any of the machines in your gym, make sure that you understand how to set your range of motion. This is very important because using somebody else's settings may cause you damaging your muscles or joints. All range of motion adjustment settings are labeled by numbers. Always write down or remember your adjustments.

Note: Not all machines have range of motion adjustments.

Let's now look at some leg machines.

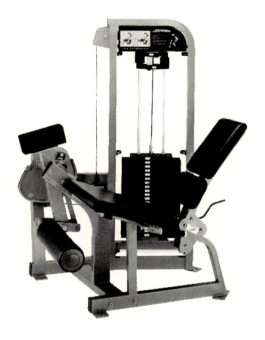

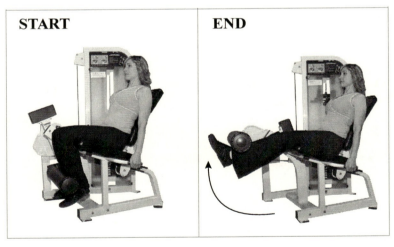

Figure 37. Leg Extension machine

This machine is for the front of your thighs, and its motion is to straighten (extend) your legs from their bent position. Let's now move to figure 38 to learn more about this machine.

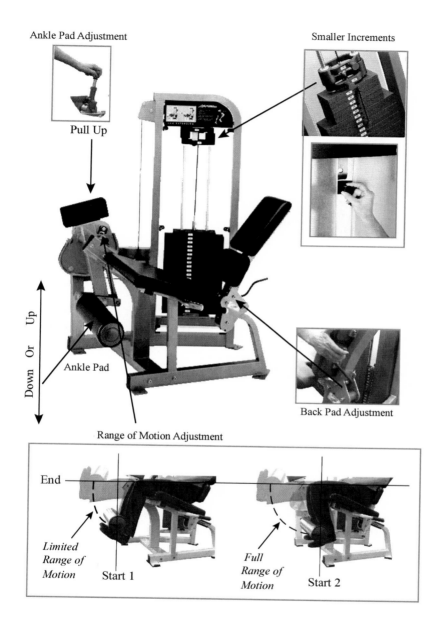

Figure 38. Leg Extension machine adjustments

As you can see, this machine has some similar and some additional adjustments.

RulesRules:

Smaller Weight Increments

Smaller increments are designed for more precise adjustments. If your working weight becomes too light for you but the next selection from the main weight stack is still too heavy, you can adjust your weight by smaller increments. For example, if the increments on the main weight stack are every 15 lb., which is displayed as 10 lb., 25 lb., 40 lb., etc., you can make your exercising weight something in between by adding one or two smaller increments of 5 lb.

Not all the machines have smaller increments. Different manufacturers use different designs. Figure 39 displays some of them.

Smaller Increments

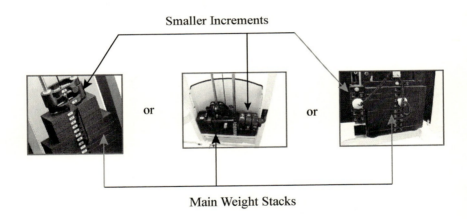

or   or

Main Weight Stacks

Figure 39. Most common smaller increments adjustments

Ankle Pad Adjustment

This adjustment makes the machine to fit any leg length. You can release the ankle pad by pulling the pin up and then moving the pad accordingly based on your leg length (some designs are different).

Range of Motion Adjustment

Take a look at the figure 38, bottom, and notice how ranges of motion can be adjusted—on the left picture, *limited range of motion* (start 1), and on the right picture, *full range of motion*, legs are bent more (start 2).

Back Pad Adjustment

The back pad is designed for comfortable support when performing exercise. The longer your thighs are, the further behind the back pad should be moved, but keep in mind that the back pad is to provide back support, so it cannot be moved too far back to lose contact with your lower back.

Seated Leg Curl Machine (Figure 40)

If you look carefully, you may find this machine similar to the previous one, the leg extension machine. The only difference here is that you don't extend your legs up but bend them down, and obviously the ankle pad should be located on the *back* of your ankles and *not in front* of them as on the leg extension machine.

Ankle Pad Adjustment

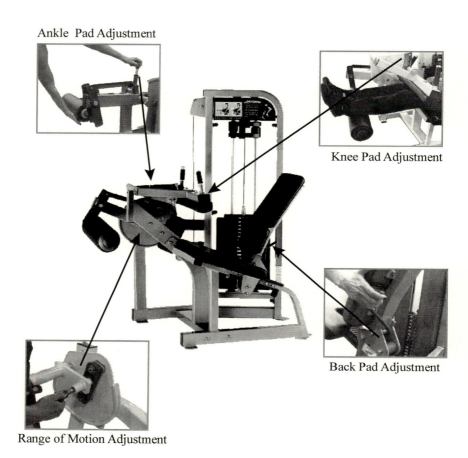

Knee Pad Adjustment

Back Pad Adjustment

Range of Motion Adjustment

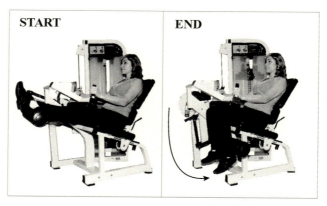

Figure 40. Seated Leg Curl machine adjustments

RESISTANCE TRAINING PROGRAMS

Besides other similar adjustments, this machine has one more—*knee pad adjustment*. This adjustment is set to lock your knees, preventing them from going up when you bend your legs—the motion will always force your knees to go up. Many people when using this machine let their knees to go off the knee pad. Usually, this happens due to lack of *concentration*. Naturally our body will try to use other muscles, and when you bend your legs down on this machine, you might even involve your back, arms, and abdominal muscles. But try to concentrate and learn how to "stay still" with the rest of your body, while putting maximum pressure on the muscles that this machine is designed for—hamstrings (back of your thigh). If you concentrate, you may immediately notice how your knees will "stick" up to the knee pad.

Try also not to slide forward on the seat while performing this exercise. This happens due to lack of concentration as well.

Range of motion adjustment is very important on this machine especially for those who have knee problems. If the ankle pad is moved too high up, you will be in the position of locking your knee joint. Do a few experiments using very light weight before exercising on this machine.

*　　*　　*

I hope that these three demos gave you enough of understanding about selectorized machines. But before you jump into using them, I want to encourage you again and again on learning each of the machines first. This will help you to feel like a pro every time you come to the gym.

PROGRAM 1 - Selectorized Machines

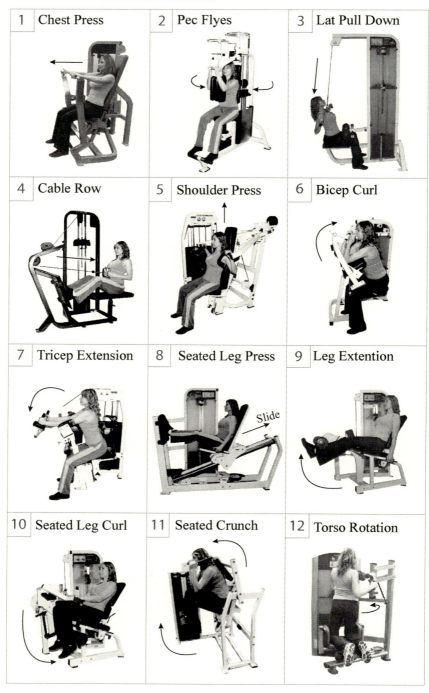

1 Chest Press	2 Pec Flyes	3 Lat Pull Down
4 Cable Row	5 Shoulder Press	6 Bicep Curl
7 Tricep Extension	8 Seated Leg Press	9 Leg Extention
10 Seated Leg Curl	11 Seated Crunch	12 Torso Rotation

1. Chest Press

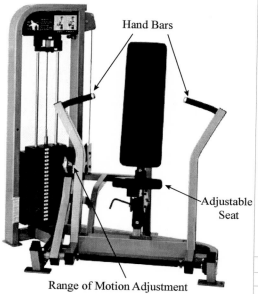

Hand Bars

Adjustable Seat

Range of Motion Adjustment

Muscles Used

Primary:

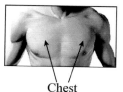

Chest

Secondary:

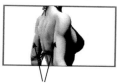

Triceps

Machine number:	
Weight:	
Seat:	
Range of Motion:	

Start

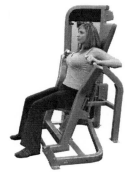

1. Adjust the weight using the pin.

2. Adjust the seat so the hand bars are at your chest level when you sit.

3. Adjust preferred range of motion.

End

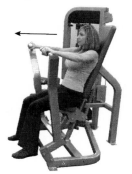

4. Place your hands on the hand bars and push them forward in a controlled manner. Do not lock your elbows or move your body forward.

5. Slowly return to the starting position and stop just before the weights touch the stack.

Stretch

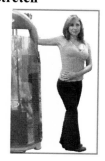

1. Bend your arm at a right angle and place elbow against machine.
2. Turn your body and feet away from machine so that your elbow is behind you.
3. Twist your body until you feel the stretch in your chest. Hold for 10–15 seconds.
Repeat for the other side.

Keep away from moving parts.

431

2. Pectoral Flyes

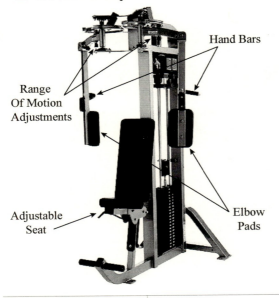

Hand Bars

Range
Of Motion
Adjustments

Adjustable
Seat

Elbow
Pads

Muscles Used

Primary:

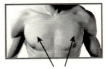

Chest

Secondary:

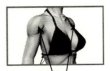

Front Shoulder

Machine number:	
Weight:	
Seat:	
Range of Motion:	

Start

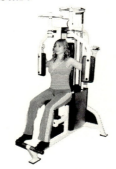

1. Adjust the weight using the pin.

2. Adjust the seat height so that when you place your hands on the hand bars, your elbows are at your chest level.

3. Adjust the range of motion for each arm.

End

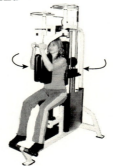

4. Place forearms on the elbow pads and grip the hand bars.

5. Using a slow, steady movement, push elbows together while keeping shoulders against the back pad.

6. Slowly return to the starting position and stop just before the weights touch the stack.

Stretch

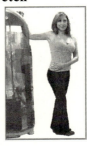

1. Bend your arm at a right angle and place elbow against machine.

2. Turn your body and feet away from machine so that your elbow is behind you.

3. Twist your body until you feel the stretch in your chest. Hold for 10–15 seconds.
Repeat for the other side.

Keep away from moving parts.

3. Lat Pulldown

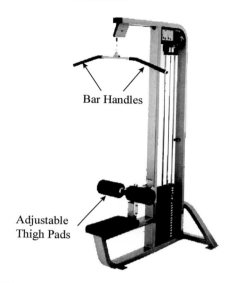

Bar Handles

Adjustable
Thigh Pads

Muscles Used

Primary:

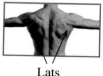

Lats

Secondary:

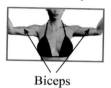

Biceps

Machine number:	
Weight:	
Thigh Pads:	

Start

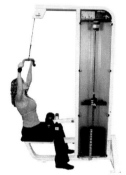

1. Adjust the weight using the pin.
2. Sit and adjust the high pads so that your knees are locked.
3. Stand up and grip the bar handles wide evenly on both sides. Sit pulling the bar down with your body weight and slide thighs under the thigh pads.
4. Slightly lean back and look up on the bar.

End

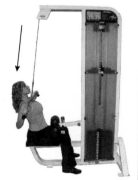

5. Pull the bar down to the front of your chest, keeping the chest up.
6. Slowly return bar up to the starting position, keeping the body stable.
7. When finished, straighten arms and carefully stand up until weight stack comes to a rest.

Stretch

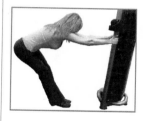

1. Stand facing any tall part of the machine approximately two feet away.

2. Grab the machine with both hands at your hips level.

3. Keeping your knees slightly bent, drop your hips backward to elongate and stretch your back muscles. Hold for 10–15 seconds.

Keep away from moving parts.

4. Cable Row

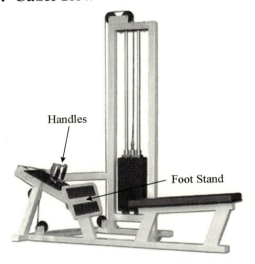

Handles

Foot Stand

Muscles Used

Primary

Upper and Mid Back

Secondary:

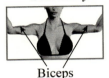

Biceps

Machine number:	
Weight:	

Start

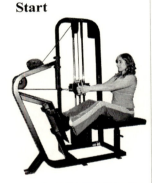

1. Adjust the weight using the pin.

2. Sit and place one foot on the foot stand.

3. Reach for the handles, and while pulling them toward yourself, place second foot on the foot stand to get to starting position as shown above—body straight and tight, knees slightly bent.

Do not lean over at the waist.

End

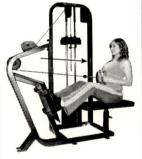

4. Pull handles toward your abdomen, drawing your shoulders back first. Concentrate on pulling from your elbows. Arch your lower back and puff your chest out.

5. Slowly return to starting position, allowing shoulders to stretch forward without losing tension on your back.

Stretch

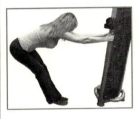

1. Stand facing any tall part of the machine approximately two feet away.

2. Grab the machine with both hands at your hips level.

3. Keeping your knees slightly bent, drop your hips backward to elongate and stretch your back muscles. Hold for 10–15 seconds.

Keep away from moving parts.

5. Shoulder Press

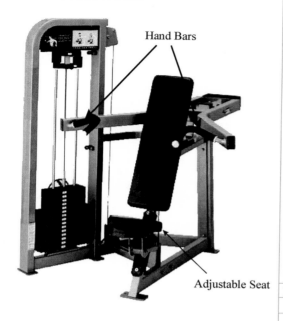

Hand Bars

Adjustable Seat

Muscles Used

Primary:

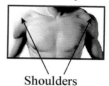

Shoulders

Secondary:

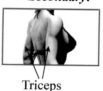

Triceps

Machine number:	
Weight:	
Seat:	

Start

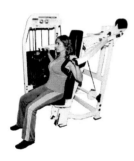

1. Adjust the weight using the pin.

2. Adjust seat so that hand bars are aligned with the top of your shoulders. Sit tall.

End

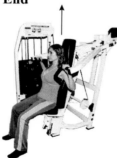

3. Slowly push up, extending your arms over your head. Avoid any snapping or locking of the elbows.

4. Slowly return to the starting position and stop just before the weights touch the stack.

Stretch

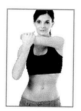

1. Cross one of your arms over your chest or shoulder.

2. Take your opposite hand and push it on the elbow. Hold for 10–15 seconds.
Repeat for the other side.

Note: *Keeping the elbow lower stretches the middle part of your shoulder, while keeping the elbow higher stretches back part of your shoulder.*

6. Bicep Curl

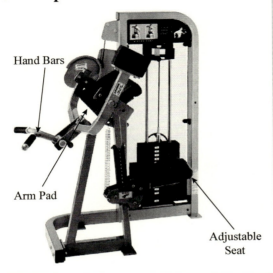

Hand Bars

Arm Pad

Adjustable
Seat

Muscles Used

Primary:

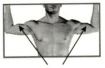

Biceps

Secondary:

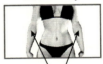

Forearms

Machine number:	
Weight:	
Seat:	
Range of Motion:	

Start

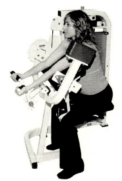

1. Adjust the weight using the pin.

2. Adjust the seat so your upper arms are resting parallel to the arm pad.

3. Stand up and reach for the hand bars, palms up.

4. Sit down with your armpits above the edge of the arm pad, keeping elbows slightly bent.

End

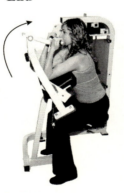

5. Curl your arms up, keeping upper arms on the arm pad. Squeeze your biceps.

6. Slowly return to the starting position and stop before locking your elbows.

Stretch

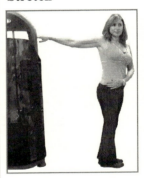

1. Lean your hand with your arm straight, palm down against the tall part of the machine.

2. Turn your body and feet away from the machine so that your hand is behind you.

3. Twist your body until you feel the stretch in your bicep. Hold for 10–15 seconds. Repeat for the other side

Keep away from moving parts.

7. Tricep Extension

Muscles Used

Primary:

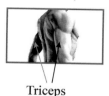

Triceps

Secondary:

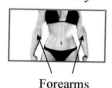

Forearms

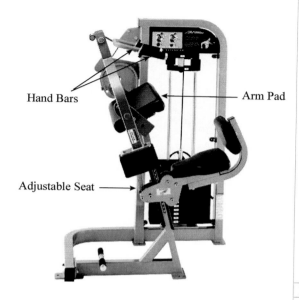

Hand Bars

Arm Pad

Adjustable Seat

Machine number:	
Weight:	
Seat:	

Start	**End**	**Stretch**
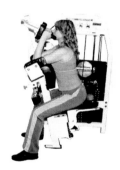	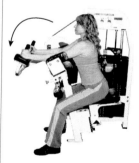	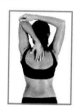

Start

1. Adjust the weight using the pin.

2. Adjust the seat so your upper arms are resting parallel to the arm pad.

3. Grab the hand bars to get starting position as shown above

End

4. Push hand bars forward-down. Keep elbows on the arm pad.

5. Slowly return to the starting position and stop just before the weights touch the stack.

Stretch

1. Bend one arm at the elbow and lift it up next to your head. Position hand so that fingers touch the shoulder blade area.

2. Place opposite arm across the top of your head, place hand on the elbow of the stretching arm, and gently push it back, supporting the arm during this stretch. Hold for 10–15 seconds.

Repeat for the other side.

437

8. Seated Leg Press

Muscles Used

Primary:

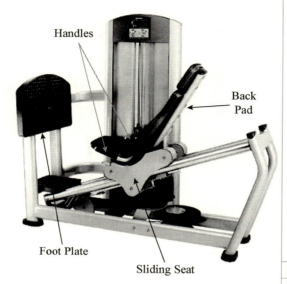

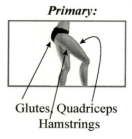

Glutes / Quadriceps
Hamstrings

Handles

Back Pad

Foot Plate

Sliding Seat

Machine number:	
Weight:	
Sliding Seat:	

Start

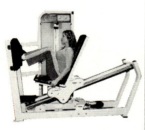

1. Adjust the weight using the pin.

2. Adjust starting position of the sliding seat so that when you sit, your knees are at 90-degree angle (or less for wider range of motion).

3. Sit, place feet on the foot plate, shoulder-width apart, and grasp the handles.

End

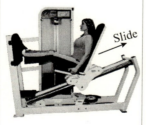

Slide

4. Push against the foot plate and slide back until your legs are almost straight—knees are not locked. Keep lower back against the back pad at all times.

5. Slowly return to the starting position and stop just before the weights touch the stack

Stretch

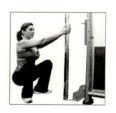

1. Grasp the tall part of the machine with both hands at your hip level.

2. Get into the full squat position, keeping your knees out, torso upright and tall. Relax your leg muscles and hold this position for 10–15 seconds.

Keep away from moving parts.

9. Leg Extension

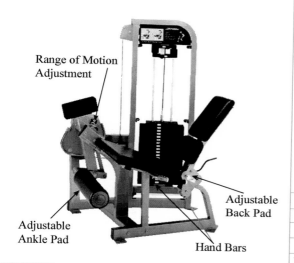

Range of Motion Adjustment

Adjustable Ankle Pad

Adjustable Back Pad

Hand Bars

Muscles Used

Primary:

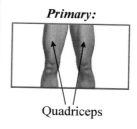

Quadriceps

Machine number:	
Weight:	
Back Pad:	
Ankle Pad:	
Range of Motion:	

Start

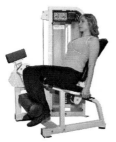

1. Adjust the weight using the pin.

2. Adjust the back pad so that when you sit, front edge of the seat feels right under your knees.

3. Adjust the ankle pad so that it is right above your ankles.

4. Adjust the preferred range of motion.

5. Sit and grab the hand bars.

End

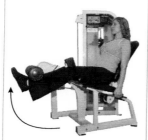

6. Straighten legs to full extension.

7. Slowly return to starting position and stop just before the weights touch the stack.

Stretch

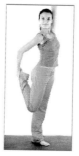

1. Stand near the machine or wall to use it for balance if needed.
2. Bend your right knee and grasp your right foot with your right hand.
3. Gently pull the foot upward toward your buttocks and hold for 10–15 seconds.
4. Repeat for your left leg.
Tip: *Keeping your knees parallel and pushing your hips slightly forward while keeping your back straight maximizes the stretch.*

10. Seated Leg Curl

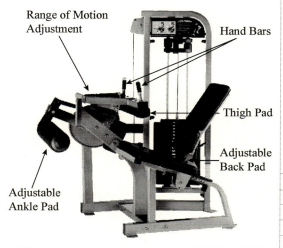

Range of Motion Adjustment

Hand Bars

Thigh Pad

Adjustable Back Pad

Adjustable Ankle Pad

Muscles Used

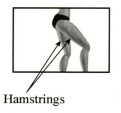

Hamstrings

Machine number:	
Weight:	
Back Pad:	
Ankle Pad:	
Range of Motion:	

Start

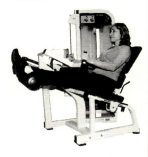

1. Adjust the weight using the pin.
2. Adjust the back pad so that when you sit, front edge of the seat feels right under your knees.
3. Adjust the ankle pad so that it is right above the back of your ankles.
4. Adjust the preferred range of motion.
5. With legs on top of the ankle pad, lower the thigh pad against your thighs and lock it. Grip the hand bars.

End

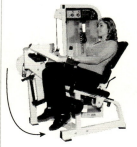

6. Slowly curl the ankle pad down, **keeping the knees tight with the thigh pad**. Keep your lower back on the back pad at all times.

7. Slowly return the ankle pad to the starting position and stop just before the weights touch the stack.

Stretch

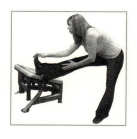

1. Stand with one foot raised onto a machine, chair, railing, or similar object. Keep your raised leg slightly bent.

2. Keep your back straight and gently move your chest toward your raised leg. Make sure your toes are pointing straight up—pull them toward your body with one hand. Hold for 10–15 seconds.
Repeat for the other leg.

Keep away from moving parts.

11. Seated Crunch

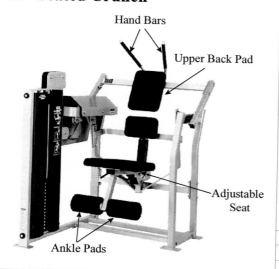

Hand Bars

Upper Back Pad

Adjustable Seat

Ankle Pads

Muscles Used

Primary:

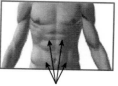

Upper and Lower Abdominals

Machine number:	
Weight:	
Seat:	

Start

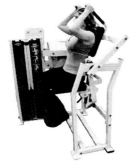

1. Adjust the weight using the pin.

2. Adjust the seat height so your upper back rests against the *upper* back pad.

3. Place your feet behind the ankle pads and grasp the hand bars.

End

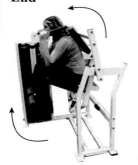

4. Curl your upper body forward. Pull with your abdominal muscles without using your legs or arms and allow the machine to guide your movements toward your knees.

5. Hold your position for one second once you reach the maximum curl.

6. Allow the weight to pull you back and stop just before the weights touch the stack.

Stretch

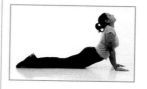

1. Lie on the mat or floor face down, hands beside your chest.

2. Slowly arch your back, assisting by a hands push. Feel the stretch in your abdomen and hold for 10–15 seconds.

Do not overextend and stop before any pain in your lower back.

441

12. Torso Rotation

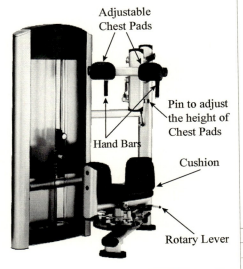

Adjustable Chest Pads

Pin to adjust the height of Chest Pads

Hand Bars

Cushion

Rotary Lever

Muscles Used

Primary:

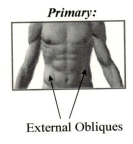

External Obliques

Machine number:	
Weight:	
Chest Pad:	

Start

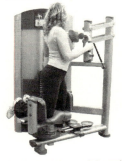

1. Adjust the weight using the pin.

2. Stand on the cushion with your knees.

3. Adjust the chest pad to align it with the top of your chest and in line with the shoulders.

4. Place your knees to the sides of the cushion, grasp the hand bars, and place your chest against the chest pad.

End

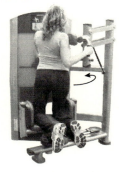

5. Rotate the cushion, keeping your lower abs tight and spine tall. Hold for one second once you reach the maximum curl.

Stretch

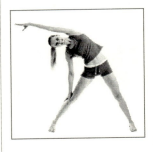

1. Place your feet wide apart. Extend your left arm above your head and stretch it to the right side as far as you can.

2. Slide your right arm down your thigh for stability. Do not lean forward or backward. Hold for 10–15 seconds.

Repeat for the other side.

Program 2 (Plate-Loaded Machines)

These machines are called plate-loaded because to select your working weight, you need to manually *load* weight *plates* on them. Those plates are the same ones that are used for barbells.

Some people, especially women, avoid using these machines finding them too complicated or designed just for bodybuilders. But, in reality, they are simpler than even selectorized machines, have fewer adjustments, and are very easy to understand. Let's take a closer look at some of them.

Chest Press Machine (Figure 41)

This machine has only two main adjustments: *weight* and *seat*.

Weight adjustment

Weight plates for all plate-loaded machines are stored on stands that are called *weight trees*. You will notice them all over the gym floor. Some machines have their own storages, but there is no particular weight plate that belongs to one or another machine.

Some plate-loaded machines are called *isolateral* machines, like this one in particular, which means that you can work one side of your body independently (iso—*isolate,* lateral—each side).

CHEST PRESS
(Plate Loaded)

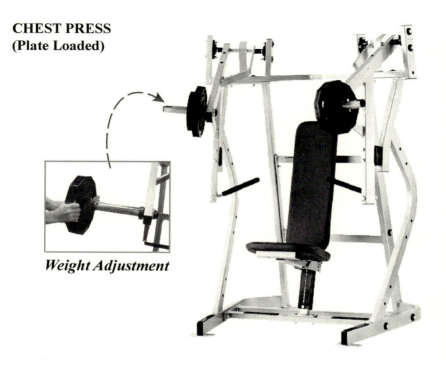

Weight Adjustment

Seat Adjustment:

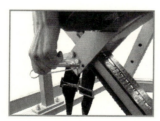

Step 1. Pull out the pin

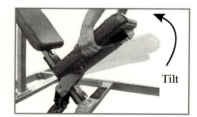

Step 2. Grab seat in the middle, tilt up
and move up or down.

Figure 41. Chest Press plate loaded machine adjustments

Seat adjustments on plate-loaded machines are very easy to use, but require some practice. Here are some main points about them:

- Some seats have *security pins*, and some don't. Those pins need to be taken out before adjusting the seat (see figure 41, bottom left). Most people don't put those pins back because they only provide extra security when using extreme weights. Normally, seats have enough security without using those pins.
- The seat needs to be slightly tilted *upward* in order to move down. For the first time, you will need to play around to understand how far up you need to tilt the seat to move it. Once you "catch" the tilting angle and your seat starts moving, keep your seat at the same angle until you get to a desired height position, and only then let go.
- If you forcefully pull the seat up by its farthest end, you will be able to move it up without tilting, but not down.
- The seat needs to be handed *in the middle* when tilting it. If you are holding it closer to its front edge, it will be easier to tilt, but impossible to move.
- Once you adjust the desired height seat, push the front end of the seat down to make sure that it sets fully on the proper spot (or alternatively insert the pin back). After you figure out your seat height, write down your settings from the label under the seat, so you don't have to experiment next time again.

High Row Machine (Figure 42)

This machine has a seat, adjusted in a similar way, and also a knee pad adjustment. Figure 42 also displays how weight plates can be stored directly on a plate-loaded machine.

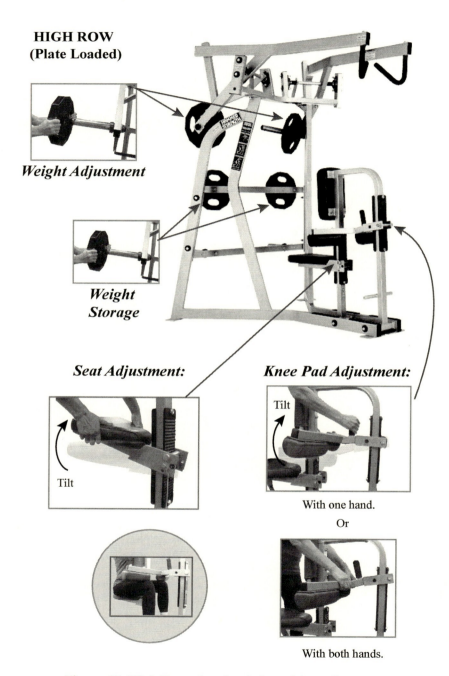

Figure 42. High Row plate loaded machine adjustments

PROGRAM 2 - Plate Loaded Machines

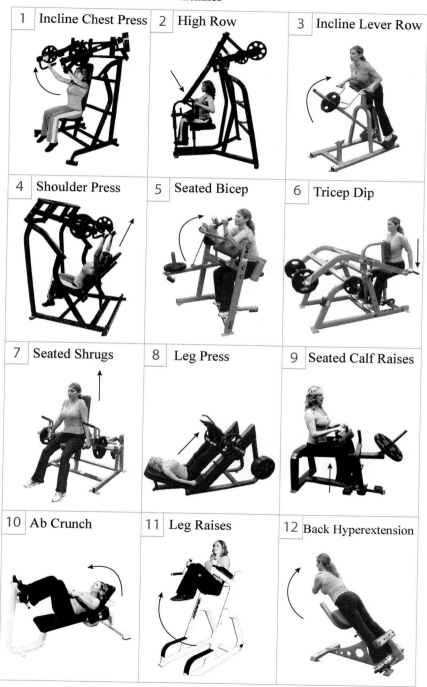

1 Incline Chest Press	2 High Row	3 Incline Lever Row
4 Shoulder Press	5 Seated Bicep	6 Tricep Dip
7 Seated Shrugs	8 Leg Press	9 Seated Calf Raises
10 Ab Crunch	11 Leg Raises	12 Back Hyperextension

1. Incline Chest Press

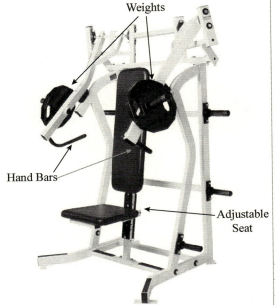

Weights

Hand Bars

Adjustable Seat

Muscles Used

Primary:

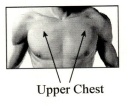

Upper Chest

Secondary:

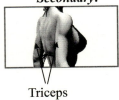

Triceps

Machine number:	
Weight:	x2
Seat:	

Start

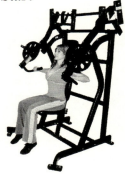

1. Load the appropriate weight using the weight plates.

2. Adjust the seat so that the hand bars are slightly below your shoulders when you sit.

End

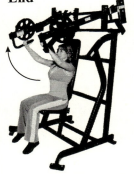

3. Place your hands on the hand bars and push them forward-up in a controlled manner. Do not lock your elbows or move your body forward.

4. Slowly return to the starting position and stop just before plate-loaded levers go at complete rest.

Stretch

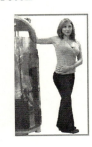

1. Bend your arm at a right angle and place elbow against machine.
2. Turn your body and feet away from machine so that your elbow is behind you.
3. Twist your body until you feel the stretch in your chest. Hold for 10–15 seconds.
Repeat for the other side.

Keep away from moving parts

2. High Row

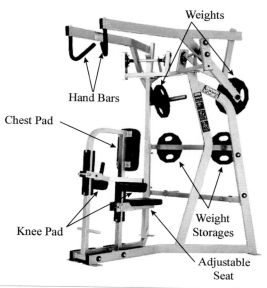

Weights

Hand Bars

Chest Pad

Knee Pad

Weight Storages

Adjustable Seat

Muscles Used

Primary:

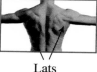

Lats

Secondary:

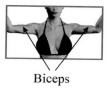

Biceps

Machine number:	
Weight:	x2
Seat:	

Start

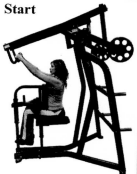

1. Load the appropriate weight using the weight plates.
2. Move the knee pad all the way up.
3. Adjust the seat so that when you sit, you can reach the hand bars only with your fingertips.
4. Stand up and grab the hand bars. Sit and kick the knee pad with one of your knees to make it fall and lock your knees.

End

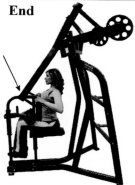

5. Pull the hand bars down toward your chest, drawing your shoulders back first. Concentrate on pulling from your elbows. Arch your lower back and puff your chest out. Keep your chest on the chest pad.
6. Slowly return to the starting position, allowing the shoulders to stretch forward without losing tension on the back.

Stretch

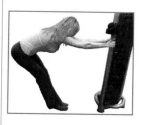

1. Stand facing any tall part of the machine approximately two feet away.

2. Grab the machine with both hands at your hips level.

3. Keeping your knees slightly bent, drop your hips backward to elongate and stretch your back muscles. Hold for 10–15 seconds.

Keep away from moving parts

449

3. Incline Lever Row

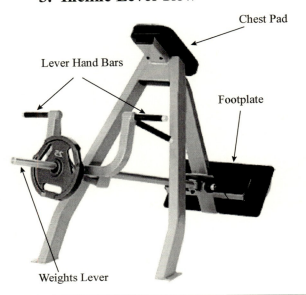

Chest Pad

Lever Hand Bars

Footplate

Weights Lever

Muscles Used

Primary:

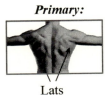

Lats

Secondary:

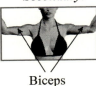

Biceps

Machine number:	
Weight:	

Start

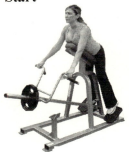

1. Load the appropriate weight onto the weight lever using the weight plate/s.

2. Lie with your chest on the chest pad and place your feet comfortably on the foot plate.

3. Grasp the lever's hand bars.

End

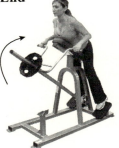

4. Pull the lever up toward your chest, drawing your shoulders back first. Concentrate on pulling from your elbows. Arch your lower back and puff your chest out.

5. Slowly return to the starting position, allowing shoulders to stretch forward without losing tension on the back.

Stretch

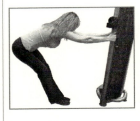

1. Stand facing any tall part of the machine approximately two feet away.
2. Grab the machine with both hands at your hips level.
3. Keeping your knees slightly bent, drop your hips backward to elongate and stretch your back muscles. Hold for 10–15 seconds.

Keep away from moving parts

4. Shoulder Press

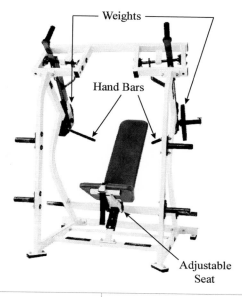

Weights

Hand Bars

Adjustable
Seat

Muscles Used

Primary:

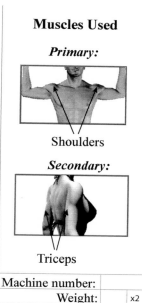

Shoulders

Secondary:

Triceps

Machine number:	
Weight:	x2
Seat:	

Start

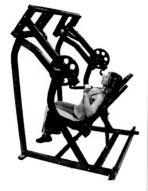

1. Load the appropriate weight using weight plates.

2. Adjust seat so that the hand bars are aligned with the top of your shoulders. (Your feet don't need to be touching the ground.)

End

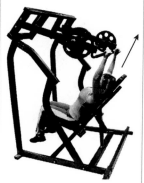

3. Place your hands on the hand bars and push up, extending your arms over your head. Avoid any snapping or locking of the elbows.

4. Slowly return to the starting position and stop just before plate-loaded levers go at complete rest.

Stretch

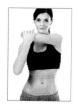

1. Cross one of your arms over your chest or shoulder.

2. Take your opposite hand and push it on the elbow. Hold for 10–15 seconds. Repeat for the other side.

Tip: *Keeping the elbow lower stretches the middle part of your shoulder, while keeping the elbow higher stretches back part of your shoulder.*

5. Seated Bicep

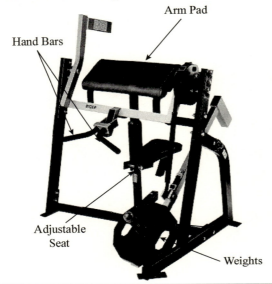

Arm Pad

Hand Bars

Adjustable Seat

Weights

Muscles Used

Primary:

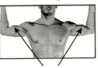

Biceps

Secondary:

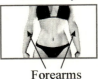

Forearms

Machine number:	
Weight:	
Seat:	

Start

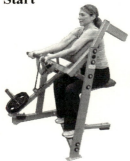

1. Load the appropriate weight using the weight plates.

2. Adjust the seat so your upper arms are resting parallel to the arm pad.

3. Stand up and reach for the hand bars, palms up.

4. Sit down with your armpits above the edge of the arm pad, keeping the elbows slightly bent.

End

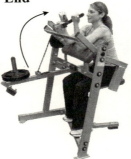

5. Curl your arms, bringing hands toward the shoulders as close as possible, keeping upper arms on the arm pad. Contract your biceps at the end of the motion.

6. Slowly return to the starting position. Do not lock your elbows.

7. When exercise is completed, rise and lower hand bars back.

Stretch

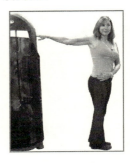

1. Lean your hand with your arm straight, palm down against the tall part of the machine.
2. Turn your body and feet away from the machine so that your hand is behind you.
3. Twist your body until you feel the stretch in your bicep. Hold for 10–15 seconds.
Repeat for the other side.

Keep away from moving parts

6. Tricep Dip

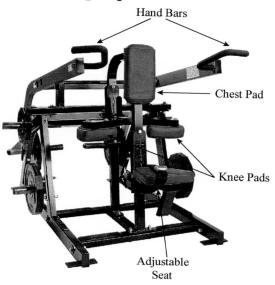

Hand Bars

Chest Pad

Knee Pads

Adjustable Seat

Muscles Used

Primary:

Triceps

Secondary:

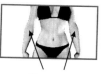

Forearms

Machine number:	
Weight:	x2
Seat:	

Start

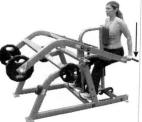

End

Stretch

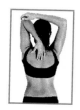

1. Load the appropriate weight using weight plates.
2. Move the knee pads all the way up.
3. Adjust the seat as low as possible to have maximum range of motion but without causing discomfort in your shoulders when you sit and place your hands on hand bars.
4. Sit, place your chest on to the chest pad, hands on hand bars, and kick the knee pad with one of your knees to make it fall and lock your knees.

5. Push the hand bars down until your arms are fully extended. Keep your elbows tucked in throughout the motion. Concentrate on your triceps.
6. Slowly return to the starting position and stop just before weight levers go at full rest.

1. Bend one arm at the elbow and lift it up next to your head. Position hand so that fingers touch the shoulder blade area.

2. Place opposite arm across the top of your head, place hand on the elbow of the stretching arm, and gently push it back, supporting the arm during this stretch. Hold for 10–15 seconds.

Repeat for the other side.

453

7. Seated Shrugs

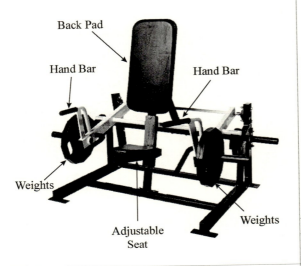

Back Pad

Hand Bar

Hand Bar

Weights

Weights

Adjustable Seat

Muscles Used

Primary:

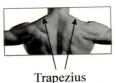

Trapezius

Secondary:

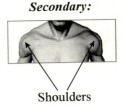

Shoulders

Machine number:	
Weight:	x2
Seat:	

Start

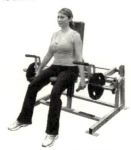

1. Load the appropriate weight using weight plates.

2. Adjust the seat so when you sit, you can reach the hand bars only with your fingertips.

3. Bend over to reach the hand bars and sit in good body alignment—chest up, back straight— abs tight. Keep arms straight, elbows fixed, and back on the back pad.

End

4. Draw your shoulders up toward the back of your head as high as possible. Contract trapezius muscles without any change in body alignment. Do not involve your arms.

5. Slowly return hand bars to the starting position.

Stretch

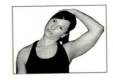

1. Sit up straight with your shoulders relaxed, looking straight ahead, and head in neutral position.

2. Bring your hand to the right side of your head and gently pull toward the left shoulder. Hold this position for 10–15 seconds.

Repeat on the other side.

454

8. Leg Press

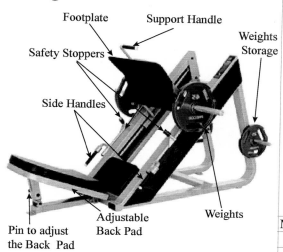

Footplate
Support Handle
Weights Storage
Safety Stoppers
Side Handles
Pin to adjust the Back Pad
Adjustable Back Pad
Weights

Muscles Used

Primary:

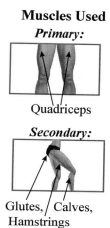

Quadriceps

Secondary:

Glutes, Calves, Hamstrings

Machine number:		
Weight:		x2
Back Pad:		

Start

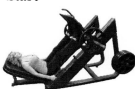

1. Load the appropriate weight using weight plates.
2. Adjust preferred back pad position.
Note: *Higher back pad position provides better support for your back, but places greater pressure on your knees and vice versa.*
3. Holding on to the support handle step into the machine, sit down and position yourself comfortably.
4. Put your feet up in the middle of the foot plate, hips-width apart, and hands on the side handles. Align your feet with knees and hips.

End

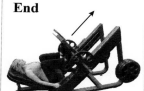

5. While keeping your back pressed against the back pad and head straight, push foot plate with your heels and turn side handles to release the safety stoppers.
6. Lower the weight until there is a 90-degree angle in your knees.
7. Slowly return to starting position until your legs are almost straight. Do not lock your knees.
8. When exercise is completed, turn side handles back to safety position and lower the foot plate onto the safety stoppers. Step out of the machine holding on to the support handle.

Stretch

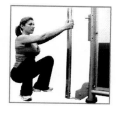

1. Grasp the tall part of the machine with both hands at your hip level.

2. Get into the full squat position, keeping your knees out, torso upright and tall. Relax your leg muscles and hold this position for 10–15 seconds.

Keep away from moving parts.

9. Seated Calf Raises

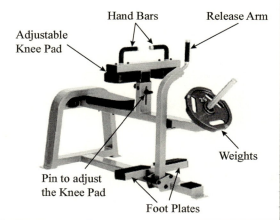

Adjustable Knee Pad

Hand Bars

Release Arm

Weights

Pin to adjust the Knee Pad

Foot Plates

Muscles Used

Primary:

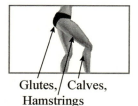

Glutes, Hamstrings

Calves,

Machine number:	
Weight:	
Knee Pad:	

Start

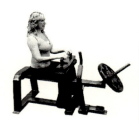

1. Load the appropriate weight using weight plates.
2. Sit on the machine and place balls of your feet on the foot plates.
3. Adjust the knee pad so that your knees are locked when heels are down. Knee pad must be placed just above your knees.
Tip: *If your knees feel loose under the knee pad, you will not have enough range of motion to perform the exercise correctly. Always adjust the knee pad so you can hardly slide your knees under the knee pad.*

End

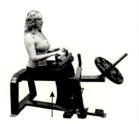

4. Raise your heels up and hold this position to release the release arm.
5. Slowly lower the heels down.
6. Raise your heels up and squeeze calf muscles at the top.
7. Lower heels back down. Keep the tension.
8. When you complete your desired number of repetitions, raise your heels up to lock the release arm.

Stretch

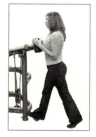

1. Raise the toes of one of your feet to the full extension up and place them against the bottom of the machine or a wall. Hold on to the machine or wall for balance.

2. Move opposite foot one step back and lift your heel off the floor.

3. Bring your body closer to the machine or the wall until you feel a stretch at the calf of the front leg. Hold for 10–15 seconds.

Repeat for the other leg.

10. Ab Crunch

Foot Bar

Hand Bars

Head Pad

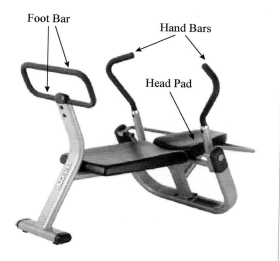

Muscles Used

Primary:

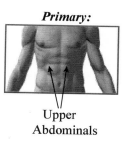

Upper
Abdominals

Machine number:

Start	End	Stretch
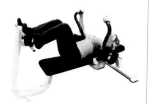	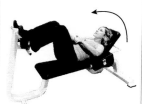	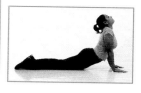

Start

1. Lie on the machine, resting your neck on the head pad.

2. Place your feet on foot bar, hands and elbows, on hand bars.

End

3. Pushing hand bars forward-down while keeping neck relaxed, lift upper torso by contracting your abdominals in a slow, controlled movement. *Keep head in contact with head pad at all times.*

4. Slowly return to the starting position and stop just before the head pad touches machine frame.

Stretch

1. Lie on the mat or floor face down, hands beside your chest.

2. Slowly arch your back, assisting by a hand push. Feel the stretch in your abdomen and hold for 10–15 seconds. Do not overextend and stop before any pain in your lower back.

11. Leg Raises

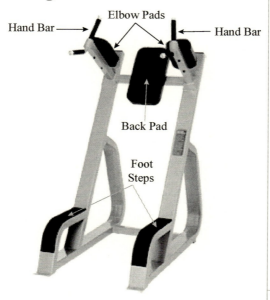

Hand Bar

Elbow Pads

Hand Bar

Back Pad

Foot Steps

Muscles Used

Primary:

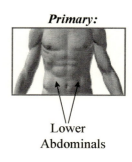

Lower
Abdominals

Machine number:

Start	End	Stretch
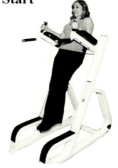	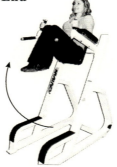	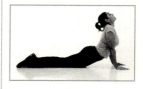

1. Stand on the foot steps, leaning on the back pad with your back.

2. Grab hand bars and place your elbows on elbow pads.

3. Tighten your torso and shoulders and let your feet hang off the foot steps.

4. Using your abdominal muscles, raise your knees up slightly higher than your belly button. Do not swing with your hips, and focus on your abdominals. Hold the peak contraction for a count of one or two.

5. Slowly lower your legs resisting on the way down.

1. Lie on the mat or floor face down, hands beside your chest.

2. Slowly arch your back, assisting by a hand push. Feel the stretch in your abdomen and hold for 10–15 seconds. Do not overextend and stop before any pain in your lower back.

12. Back Hyperextension

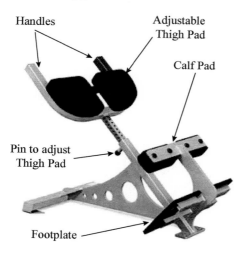

Handles

Adjustable Thigh Pad

Calf Pad

Pin to adjust Thigh Pad

Footplate

Muscles Used

Primary:

Lower Back

Assisting:

Glutes and Hamstrings

Machine number:	
Thigh Pads:	

Start	**End**	**Stretch**

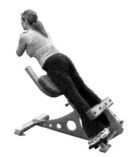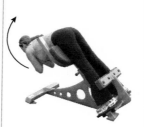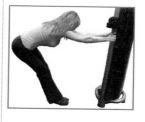

1. Adjust the thigh pad so the top of it is in line with your upper thighs, leaving enough room for you to bend at the waist without any restriction.
2. Holding on to the handles step onto the foot plate, tucking your calves securely under the calf pad.
3. Lean on the thigh pad with your thighs, straighten your body, and cross your arms on the chest.

4. Slowly bend forward, keeping your back straight. **Tip:** *Never round the back and go as far as your body allows you.*

5. Slowly raise your upper body back to the starting position.
Tip: *Avoid arching your back past a straight line.*

1. Stand facing any tall part of the machine approximately two feet away.

2. Grab the machine with both hands at your hips level.

3. Keeping your knees slightly bent, drop your hips backward to elongate and stretch your back muscles. Hold for 10–15 seconds.

Keep away from moving parts

Program 3 (Free-Motion Machines)

Free-motion machines are designed to increase performance in daily activities and also in sports. By adding resistance to these movement patterns, you can effectively train the specific muscles to enhance that activity. While fixed-isolated equipment (programs 1 and program 2) is great to enhance strength in specific muscles, this strength has not enough carryover to everyday life.

Free-motion should be looked at in respect to individual kinesiology (the study of motion), which involves pushing, pulling, squatting, rotating, stepping, lunging, bending, and balancing in a three-dimensional world. Free-motion machines allow the users to define their own movement patterns based on needs and goals.

Free-motion machines involve *multiple-joint* movements. For instance, the fixed-isolated seated bicep machine tends to immobilize the shoulder joint so that larger stress is placed on the elbow joint and musculature. Free-motion equipment allows the user to move naturally, based on their abilities and differences in limb lengths and joints.

Most movements in life are asymmetrical. Think of how we open and close doors and get in and out of cars. Integrating unilateral movement into your training is easy with free-motion equipment because the cable/pulley design allows to train at the speed of life, which is never constant.

Table 32 gives a great overview of the superior benefits of free-motion machines.

Table 32. Benefits Of FreeMotion Machines

Benefits	Traditional Equipment	Freemotion Fitness
Postural Training	No	Yes
Balance Training	No	Yes
Recruitment of Stabilizing Muscles	No	Yes
Allows for 3-dimensional Training	No	Yes
Burns Calories	Yes	More Than Traditional
Allows for Assymetrical Training	Limited	Yes
Engages the Core	No	Yes
Allows for Multi-planar/Multi-joint Training	No	Yes
Coordination Training	Yes	Yes
Machine Adjustments	2-4	0-1
Life/Sport Specific Movement Patterns	No	Yes
Population Usage	Limited	Everyone
Variety of Exercises	Limited	Many Per Machine
Time Efficient	Limited	Yes
Grip Adjustment	No	Yes
Bodybuilding	Yes	Yes
Individual Visual Feedback	Minimal	Yes
Rehabilitation Limited	Yes	Yes
Functional Development	No	Yes
Ground Foot Position Limited	Limited	Complete Line
Stand/Sit Variation	No	Yes

Source: freemotionfitness.com

Free-motion machines have very few adjustments. They allow the exerciser to choose the trajectory of his motion. From the same *start* position, the exerciser can pull or push in various *end* positions. Take a look at figure 43 to see how you can choose *end positions* from the same start—you can move the pulley at various horizontal and vertical levels.

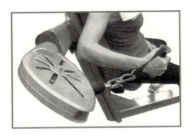 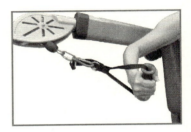

Figure 43

Weight adjustments on free-motion machines are the same as on selectorized machines—by reinserting the pin.

Most free-motion machines are with preset starting positions, which mean that their ranges of motions are not adjustable. But there are few universal multistations where you can choose from which position you would like to start. Figure 44 displays a multistation where you can train your whole body by changing positions of the adjustable levers on both sides of the machine. By readjusting the starting position of the levers, you can pull the pulley from different height directions. Levers are also adjustable horizontally, and you can rotate them.

Vertical Adjustment

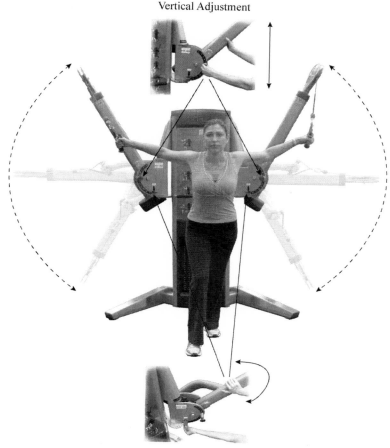

Horizontal Adjustment

Figure 44. Freemotion multi-station machine

Before you start exercising on free-motion machines, try each of them first. Set the lightest weight, take the handles in your hands, and pull. You may immediately ask yourself a question: "Which direction or height do I pull?" Further in this book you will learn some basic free-motion exercises, but in the future you can experiment with multiple directions, varying which will help you to develop muscles more evenly throughout the body.

In our daily life, we always use our muscles in a free range of motion. Free-motion machines can help you to perform certain tasks, such as lifting things from the floor, bending over, or moving things from one place to another.

PROGRAM 3 - Freemotion Machines

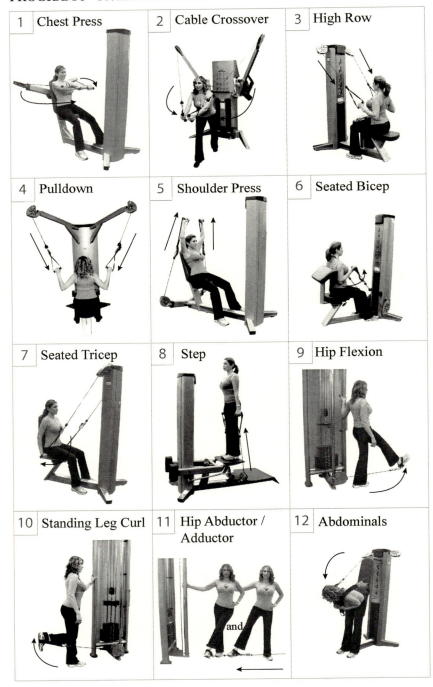

1 Chest Press	2 Cable Crossover	3 High Row
4 Pulldown	5 Shoulder Press	6 Seated Bicep
7 Seated Tricep	8 Step	9 Hip Flexion
10 Standing Leg Curl	11 Hip Abductor / Adductor	12 Abdominals

1. Chest Press

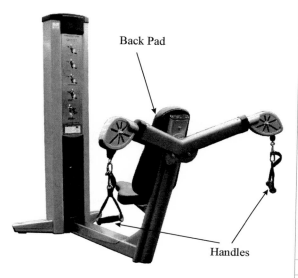

Back Pad

Handles

Muscles Used

Primary:

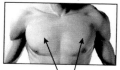

Chest

Secondary:

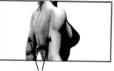

Triceps

Machine number:	
Weight:	

Start

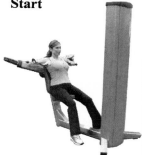

1. Adjust the weight using the pin.

2. Sit with your back tight to the back pad.

3. Grasp handles and position your elbows and hands at your chest level, palms facing down. Keep spine tall and abdominals tight.

End

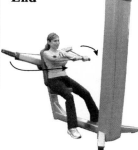

4. Push handles forward, bringing hands close to each other at the end. Do not lock elbows.

5. Contract your chest muscles once your arms are extended. Do not move your shoulders forward.

6. Slowly return to the starting position. Keep hands and elbows at chest level throughout the motion.

Stretch

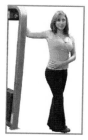

1. Bend your arm at a right angle and place elbow against machine.

2. Turn your body and feet away from machine so that your elbow is behind you.

3. Twist your body until you feel the stretch in your chest. Hold for 10–15 seconds.
Repeat for the other side.

Keep away from moving parts.

2. Cable Crossover

Handles

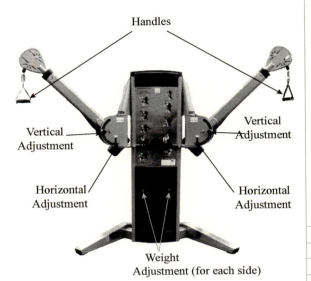

Vertical Adjustment

Vertical Adjustment

Horizontal Adjustment

Horizontal Adjustment

Weight
Adjustment (for each side)

Muscles Used

Primary:

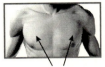

Chest

Secondary:

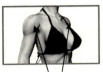

Front Shoulder

Machine number:	
Weight:	
Vertical Adj:	
Horizontal Adj:	

Start

End

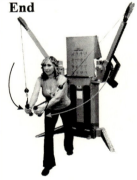

Stretch

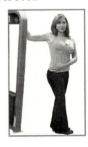

1. Adjust the weight using the pin. Adjust levers vertically and horizontally.
2. Grasp the handles and center your body between the levers of the machine.
3. Take a few small steps forward and place one foot forward-out for balance. Angle your torso forward at 15–30 degrees.
4. Slowly let the weight pull your arms out until your hands reach the chest level.

5. Keeping your elbows slightly bent and your back straight, bring handles in front of your midsection until your hands touch each other or slightly cross.

6. Pause squeezing your pectoral muscles.

7. Slowly return to the starting position.

1. Bend your arm at a right angle and place elbow against machine.

2. Turn your body and feet away from machine so that your elbow is behind you.

3. Twist your body until you feel the stretch in your chest. Hold for 10–15 seconds.
Repeat for the other side.

Keep away from moving parts.

3. High Row

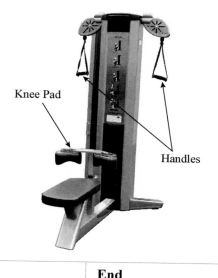

Knee Pad

Handles

Muscles Used

Primary

Lats

Secondary:

Biceps

Machine number:	
Thigh Pad:	
Weight:	

Start

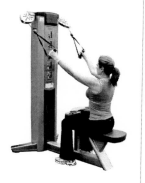

1. Adjust the weight using the pin.

2. Adjust knee pad so that when you sit, your knees are secured under it.

3. Stand up, grasp handles, and sit with your knees under the knee pad.

End

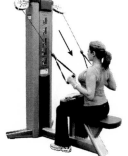

4. Pull the handles toward your chest, keeping elbows close to your sides.

5. Squeeze shoulder blades together, maintaining a neutral spine.

6. Slowly return to the starting position and stop just before the weights touch the stack.

Stretch

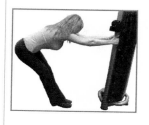

1. Stand facing any tall part of the machine approximately two feet away.

2. Grab the machine with both hands at your hips level.

3. Keeping your knees slightly bent, drop your hips backward to elongate and stretch your back muscles. Hold for 10–15 seconds.

Keep away from moving parts.

4. Pulldown

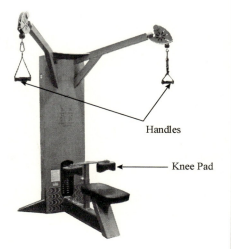

Handles

Knee Pad

Muscles Used

Primary

Lats

Secondary:

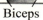

Biceps

Machine number:	
Thigh Pad:	
Weight:	

Start

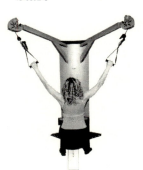

1. Adjust the weight using the pin.

2. Adjust knee pad so that when you sit, your thighs are secured under it.

3. Stand up, grasp handles, and sit with your knees under the knee pad.

End

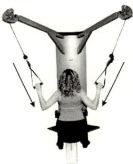

4. Pull down, leading with your elbows. Wrists should remain straight and in line with the cable as you draw elbows down toward your sides. Maintain a neutral spine.

5. Slowly return to the starting position and stop just before the weights touch the stack.

Stretch

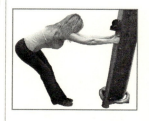

1. Stand facing any tall part of the machine approximately two feet away.

2. Grab the machine with both hands at your hips level.

3. Keeping your knees slightly bent, drop your hips backward to elongate and stretch your back muscles. Hold for 10–15 seconds.

Keep away from moving parts.

5. Shoulder Press

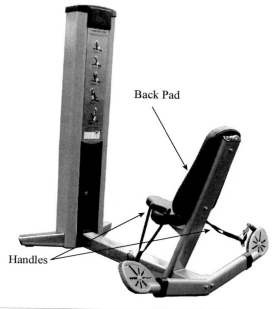

Back Pad

Handles

Muscles Used

Primary:

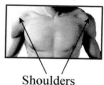

Shoulders

Secondary:

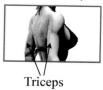

Triceps

Machine number:	
Weight:	

Start	End	Stretch
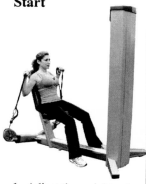	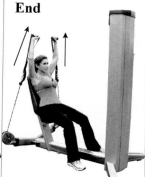	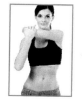

Start

1. Adjust the weight using the pin.

2. Sit with your back tight to the back pad and handles at shoulder height.

End

3. Push handles up, bringing hands close to each other directly above your head. Do not lock elbows. Keep your core tight and spine tall.

4. Slowly return to the starting position, stopping your hands at shoulder height.

Stretch

1. Cross one of your arms over your chest or shoulder.

2. Take your opposite hand and push it on the elbow. Hold for 10–15 seconds.

Repeat for the other side.

Note: *Keeping the elbow lower stretches the middle part of your shoulder, while keeping the elbow higher stretches back part of your shoulder.*

6. Seated Bicep Curl

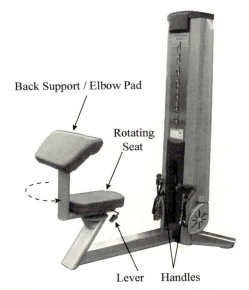

Back Support / Elbow Pad

Rotating Seat

Lever   Handles

Muscles Used

Primary:

Biceps

Secondary:

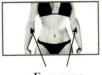

Forearms

Machine number:
Weight:

Start

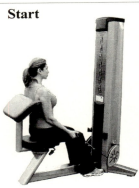

1. Adjust the weight using the pin.

2. Sit and grab the handles with palms facing up. Keep your torso straight and abdominals tight.

Note: *For alternative exercise use the lever to rotate the seat.*

End

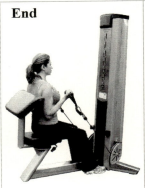

3. Keeping your elbows tight to the body, curl your arms, bringing hands toward the shoulders as close as possible. Squeeze your bicep at the top of the motion.

4. Slowly return to the starting position and stop just before weights touch the stack.

Stretch

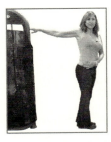

1. Lean your hand with your arm straight, palm down against the tall part of the machine.
2. Turn your body and feet away from the machine so that your hand is behind you.
3. Twist your body until you feel the stretch in your bicep. Hold for 10–15 seconds.
 Repeat for the other side.

Keep away from moving parts.

7. Seated Tricep Extension

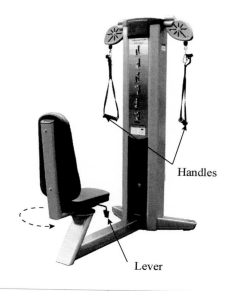

Handles

Lever

Muscles Used

Primary:

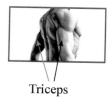

Triceps

Secondary:

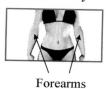

Forearms

Machine number:	
Weight:	

Start

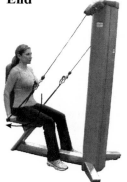

End

Stretch

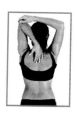

1. Adjust the weight using the pin.

2. Sit and grab the handles, palms facing down. Keep elbows tight to your body, torso straight, and abdominals tight.

Note: *For alternative exercises, use the lever to rotate the seat.*

3. Straighten your arms to full extension keeping your elbows in one place.

4. Squeeze triceps when arms are fully extended.

5. Slowly return to the starting position. Do not move your elbows.

1. Bend one arm at the elbow and lift it up next to your head. Position hand so that fingers touch the shoulder blade area.

2. Place opposite arm across the top of your head, place hand on the elbow of the stretching arm, and gently push it back, supporting the arm during this stretch. Hold for 10–15 seconds.

Repeat for the other side.

8. Step

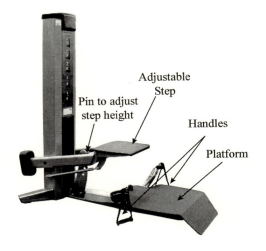

Adjustable Step

Pin to adjust step height

Handles

Platform

Muscles Used

Primary:

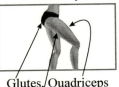

Glutes, Quadriceps
Hamstrings

Secondary:

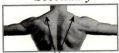

Trapezius

Machine number:	
Step:	
Weight:	

Start

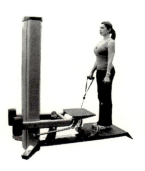

1. Adjust the weight using the pin.

2. Adjust preferable step height.

3. Stand in the middle of the platform, grasp both handles, and straighten your body.

End

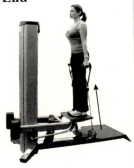

4. Step up onto the step with your left foot.
5. Without using momentum and keeping your arms and back straight, force yourself up and place right foot on the step.
6. Return left foot back onto the platform and then step down with your right foot. Keep core tight for balance.
Repeat the exercise starting from the right foot.

Stretch

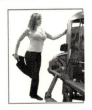

1. Stand near the machine or wall to use it for balance if needed.

2. Bend your right knee and grasp your right foot with your right hand.

3. Gently pull the foot upward toward your buttocks and hold for 10–15 seconds.
Repeat for your left leg.

Tip: *Keeping your knees parallel and pushing your hips slightly forward while keeping your back straight maximizes the stretch.*

9. Hip Flexion

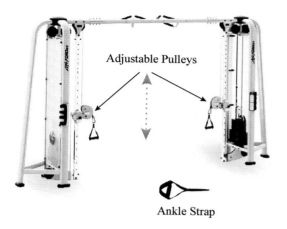

Adjustable Pulleys

Ankle Strap

Muscles Used

Primary:

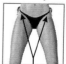

Hip Flexors

Secondary:

Glutes

Machine number:	
Weight:	

Start	End	Stretch

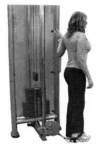

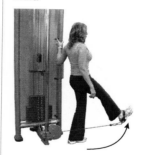

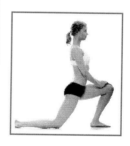

Start

1. Adjust the weight using the pin.
2. Move one of the adjustable pulleys all the way down and connect ankle strap to it.
3. Connect ankle strap to your right foot.
4. Stand with the left side of your body turned to the machine and pulley behind you. Move far enough so the used weight is not resting on the stack. Hold on to the machine for balance.

End

5. Slowly move your right leg in front of you. Keep both legs straight.
6. Slowly return to the starting position and stop just before the weights touch the stack.
7. When you complete your desired number of repetitions, connect the ankle strap to the left ankle, turn around, and repeat the exercise for your left leg.
Keep hands away from the moving parts.

Stretch

1. Step forward with your left foot while keeping your right knee on the floor. Put your hands on top of your left thigh.

2. Slide your right leg behind you and sag your body down until you feel the stretch in your hip. Hold for 10–15 seconds.

Repeat for the other side.

10. Standing Leg Curl

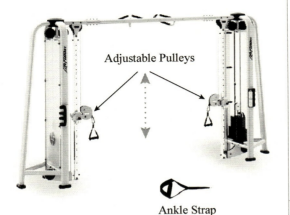

Adjustable Pulleys

Ankle Strap

Muscles Used

Primary:

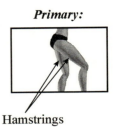

Hamstrings

Machine number: _____

Weight: _____

Start	End	Stretch

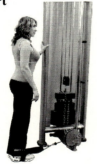 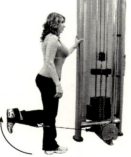 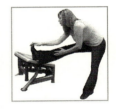

Start

1. Adjust the weight using the pin.
2. Move one of the adjustable pulleys all the way down and connect the ankle strap to it.
3. Connect the ankle strap to your right foot.
4. Stand with the left side of your body turned to the machine and pulley in front of you. Move far enough so the used weight is not resting on the stack. Hold on to the machine for balance.

End

5. Curl your right leg toward your buttocks as high as you can. Keep your right knee in one place; do not swing your body.
6. Slowly return to the starting position and stop just before the weights touch the stack.
7. When you complete your desired number of repetitions, connect the ankle strap to your left ankle, turn around and repeat the exercise for your left leg.
Keep hands away from moving parts.

Stretch

1. Stand with one foot raised onto a machine, chair, railing, or similar object. Keep your raised leg slightly bent.

2. Keep your back straight and gently move your chest toward your raised leg. Make sure your toes are pointing straight up—pull them toward your body with one hand. Hold for 10–15 seconds.

Repeat for the other leg.

Keep away from moving parts.

11. Hip Adduction / Abduction

Muscles Used

Primary:

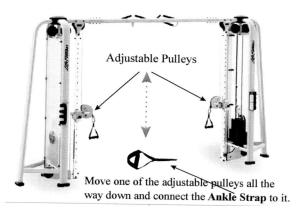

Adjustable Pulleys

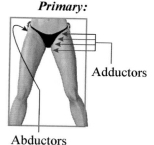

Adductors

Abductors

Move one of the adjustable pulleys all the way down and connect the **Ankle Strap** to it.

Machine number:

Weight:

Adduction

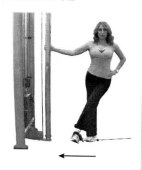

1. Adjust the weight using the pin.
2. Connect the ankle strap to your left ankle and stand on the right leg, holding on to the machine for support. Move far enough so the used weight is not resting on the stack. Resistance must be directed from the left side.
3. Keeping your both legs straight, move left leg sideways, crossing in front of the right leg.
4. Slowly return to the starting position.
Change sides and work your right leg.

Abduction

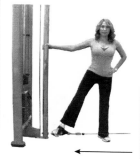

1. Adjust the weight using the pin.
2. Connect the ankle strap to your right ankle and stand on your left leg, holding on to the machine for support. The right leg will cross in front of your left leg at the start.
3. Move your right leg straight out to your right side. Do not swing.
4. Slowly return to the starting position.

Change sides and work your left leg.

Keep hands away from moving parts for both exercises.

Stretch:

Adduction

1. Stand with your legs wide apart.
2. Shift your weight to the side so one leg is bent and the other is extended straight. Hold for 10–15 seconds. Return to the starting position and repeat with the other leg.

Abduction

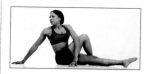

1. Sit down on the floor.
2. Cross your right leg over your left leg so the right foot is on the outside of the left knee.
3. Turn your body right and assist the stretch by pressing on your right knee with your left elbow. Hold for 10–15 seconds.
Repeat for the other leg.

12. Abdominal

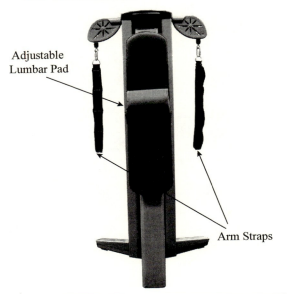

Adjustable Lumbar Pad

Arm Straps

Muscles Used

Primary:

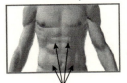

Upper and Lower Abdominals

Machine number:	
Weight:	

Start

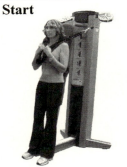

1. Adjust the weight using the pin.

2. Adjust the height of the lumbar pad where you feel more support for your lower back. Stand tight to the back pad.

3. Grasp arm straps and hold them over your shoulders at any comfort-able length where you feel resistance and used weight is off the stack.

End

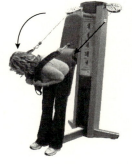

4. Crunch forward at the waist, bringing your torso toward hips.

5. Slowly return to the starting position and stop just before the weights touch the stack.

Stretch

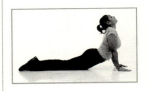

1. Lie on the mat or floor face down, hands beside your chest.

2. Slowly arch your back, assisting by a hand push. Feel the stretch in your abdomen and hold for 10–15 seconds. Do not overextend and stop before any pain in your lower back.

Program 4 (Free Weights)

Free weights are *handheld* weights that are not attached to any frame or machine. They include barbells, dumbbells, weight bars, kettle bells, etc. Free weights are often used as part of a more comprehensive exercise program, and this is the main reason why free weights program is placed as number 4 in this book. This doesn't mean that you cannot start learning free weights first. If you do not want to go to a gym, exercising with free weights in your home can be a good way to stay in shape.

Dumbbells and barbells come in different sizes and weights. Weight bars are designed to increase or decrease the weight as needed, but some weight bars are preset and are not adjustable. Barbells are also designed to allow you to add or subtract more weight, while dumbbells are usually manufactured in a fixed weight, only those that are for home use are adjustable.

Some exercises with free weights require the use of benches, supporting racks, and other accessories. To minimize expenses on your home fitness equipment and also for the simplicity of exercising, program 4 includes the use of a stability ball instead of a bench. If you usually feel intimidated by exercising in the free weight area of a gym, you can do these exercises in any place else.

Last suggestions before going to program 4:

- If you are a beginner, stay with using machines until you feel more comfortable with the movements.
- If you are always in a hurry, stick to the machines because they are generally more time efficient.
- If you work out in the gym at busy times, choose free weights so you don't have to line up for the machines.
- If you decide to work out at home, choose free weights. Home machines take up a lot of space, usually of poor quality, and cost much more than free weights.
- If you have disability or joint problems, stick with machines because they provide the most support.

- If you hate the idea of lifting weight, stick to the machines. Your positive attitude toward exercise is far more important than the exercise selection itself. Try combining machines with some of the free weights exercises.

Some of the most important advantages of using free weights are the following:

- Ability to move the body through natural motions
- Ability to train functionalities and movements of everyday life, such as bending over, squatting, moving things around, and rotating the body
- Flexibility of exercising whole body in a small space
- Better ability to build body strength

The most important disadvantages of using free weights are the following:

- Difficulty to learn without instruction
- Higher risk of injury
- Intimidation
- Confusion

RESISTANCE TRAINING PROGRAMS

PROGRAM 4 - Free Weights

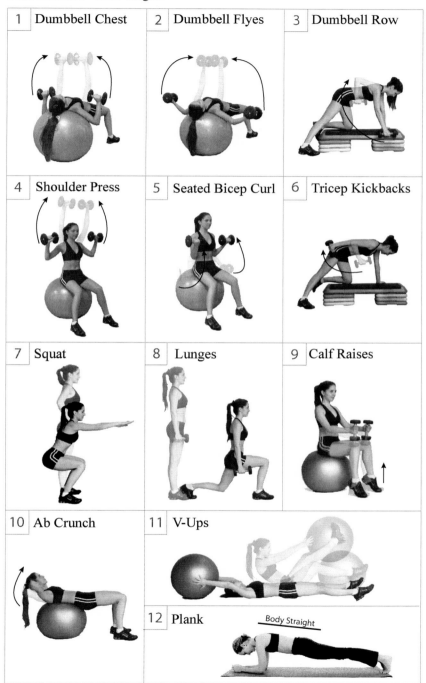

1	Dumbbell Chest	2	Dumbbell Flyes	3	Dumbbell Row
4	Shoulder Press	5	Seated Bicep Curl	6	Tricep Kickbacks
7	Squat	8	Lunges	9	Calf Raises
10	Ab Crunch	11	V-Ups	12	Plank (Body Straight)

1. Dumbbell Press

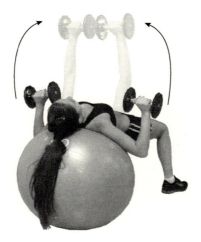

Muscles Used

Primary:

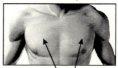

Chest

Secondary:

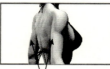

Triceps

Assisting:

Shoulders, Back, Glutes and Abs

Dumbbell Weight:

Start

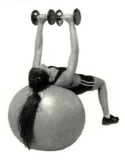

1. Lie on an exercise ball with shoulders and head supported on the ball. Form a bridge and bring dumbbells up directly above your chest.

2. Balance dumbbells and get comfortable on the ball. Keep your buttocks and abdominals tight.

End

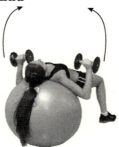

3. Lower the dumbbells down until your elbows are slightly below your shoulders. Keep forearms perpendicular to the floor.

4. Press dumbbells up, bringing them close to each other directly above your chest. Do not lock your elbows.

Stretch

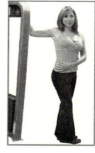

1. Bend your arm at a right angle and place elbow against machine.
2. Turn your body and feet away from machine so that your elbow is behind you.
3. Twist your body until you feel the stretch in your chest. Hold for 10–15 seconds.

Repeat for the other side.

Keep away from moving parts.

480

2. Dumbbell Flyes

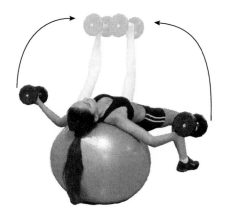

Muscles Used

Primary:

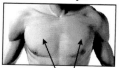

Chest

Secondary:

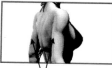

Triceps

Assisting:
Shoulders, Back, Glutes and Abs

Dumbbell Weight:

Start	End	Stretch

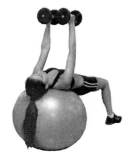

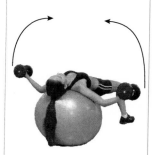

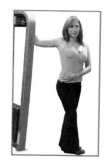

Start

1. Lie on an exercise ball with shoulders and head supported on the ball. Form a bridge and bring dumbbells up directly above your chest, palms facing each other.

2. Balance the dumbbells and get comfortable on the ball. Keep your buttocks and abdominals tight.

End

3. Bring the dumbbells out to the sides, keeping your arms almost straight (with just a slight bend at the elbows). Bending the elbows more will only make the exercise easier and less effective. Do not drop dumbbells below the shoulder level.

4. Raise dumbbells up, focusing on your chest.

Stretch

1. Bend your arm at a right angle and place elbow against machine.
2. Turn your body and feet away from machine so that your elbow is behind you.
3. Twist your body until you feel the stretch in your chest. Hold for 10–15 seconds.

Repeat for the other side.

Keep away from moving parts.

3. Dumbbell Row

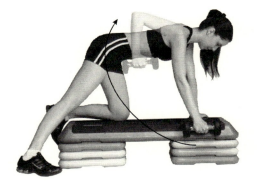

Muscles Used

Primary

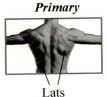

Lats

Secondary:

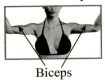

Biceps

Dumbbell Weight:

Start	**End**	**Stretch**
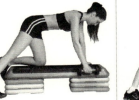	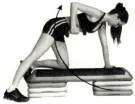	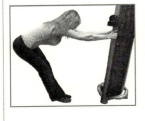

Start

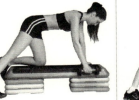

1. Position yourself on the right side of the step with your left knee and left hand resting on the step. Hold dumbbell in your right hand keeping your back straight.

2. Place your right foot to the side slightly back for balance.

End

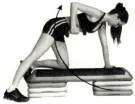

3. Pull the dumbbell up toward your abdomen, drawing your shoulder back first. Concentrate on pulling from your elbow and keeping the elbow close to the body. Pull your shoulder blade back at the end of the motion.

4. Pause, squeeze your back muscles and slowly lower the dumbbell back to the starting position, allowing the shoulder to stretch forward without losing tension on the back.

Stretch

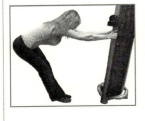

1. Stand facing any tall part of the machine approximately two feet away.

2. Grab the machine with both hands at your hips level.

3. Keeping your knees slightly bent, drop your hips backward to elongate and stretch your back muscles. Hold for 10–15 seconds.

Keep away from moving parts.

4. Dumbbell Shoulder Press

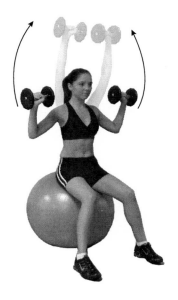

Muscles Used

Primary:

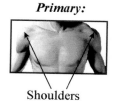

Shoulders

Secondary:

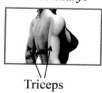

Triceps

Dumbbell Weight:

Start	**End**	**Stretch**
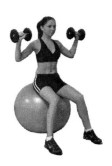	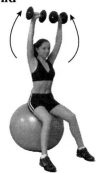	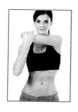

1. Cross one of your arms over your chest or shoulder.

2. Take your opposite hand and push it on the elbow. Hold for 10–15 seconds.

Repeat for the other side.

Note: *Keeping the elbow lower stretches the middle part of your shoulder, while keeping the elbow higher stretches back part of your shoulder.*

1. Sit on the ball with your feet firmly planted on the floor, wider than shoulder-width apart for balance. Keep your abdominal muscles tight and hold dumbbells to the side of your head, palms facing forward.

2. Press dumbbells up, bringing them close to each other directly above your head. Do not lock your elbows.

3. Slowly return dumbbells to the starting position.

5. Seated Bicep Curl

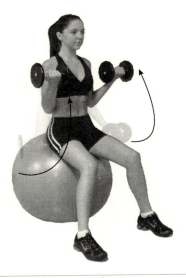

Muscles Used

Primary:

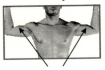

Biceps

Secondary:

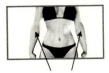

Forearms

Dumbbell Weight:

Start	End	Stretch

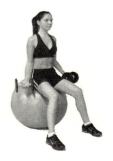

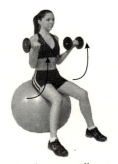

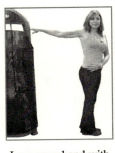

1. Sit on the ball with your feet firmly planted on the floor, wider than shoulder-width apart for balance. Keep your abdominal muscles tight and hold dumbbells down to the sides of your hips, palms facing forward, elbows slightly bent.

2. Keeping your elbows tight to the body, curl your arms, bringing hands toward the shoulders as close as possible. Squeeze your bicep at the top of the motion.

3. Slowly return dumb-bells to the starting position.

1. Lean your hand with your arm straight, palm down against the tall part of the machine.
2. Turn your body and feet away from the machine so that your hand is behind you.
3. Twist your body until you feel the stretch in your bicep. Hold for 10–15 seconds.

Repeat for the other side.

Keep away from moving parts.

484

6. Tricep Kickbacks

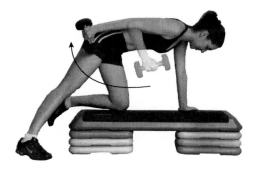

Muscles Used

Primary:

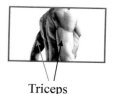

Triceps

Secondary:

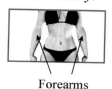

Forearms

Dumbbell Weight:

Start	**End**	**Stretch**

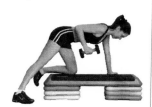

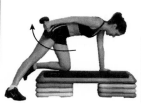

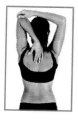

1. Position yourself on the right side of the step with your left knee and left hand resting on the step. Hold dumbbell in your right hand, keeping your upper arm parallel to the body and back straight.

2. Place your right foot to the side, slightly back for balance.

3. Slowly extend your arm until it is fully straight. Do not move your elbow.

4. Slowly return dumbbells to the starting position.

1. Bend one arm at the elbow and lift it up next to your head. Position hand so that fingers touch the shoulder blade area.
2. Place opposite arm across the top of your head, place hand on the elbow of the stretching arm, and gently push it back, supporting the arm during this stretch. Hold for 10–15 seconds.

Repeat for the other side.

7. Squat

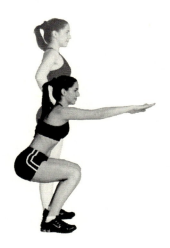

Muscles Used

Primary:

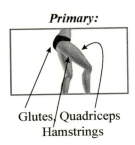

Glutes, Quadriceps
Hamstrings

Start

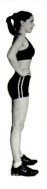

1. Stand straight, feet approximately hip-width apart and flared 15–20 degrees, hands on the hips.

End

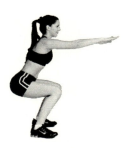

2. Squat down until your thighs are parallel to the floor. Keep your knees out, torso upright, and push your buttocks backward. Straighten your arms forward for balance. Keep knees behind the toes and shoulders in line with your ankles.

Stretch

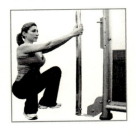

1. Grasp the tall part of the machine with both hands at your hip level.

2. Get into the full squat position, keeping your knees out, torso upright and tall. Relax your leg muscles and hold this position for 10–15 seconds.

Keep away from moving parts.

8. Lunges

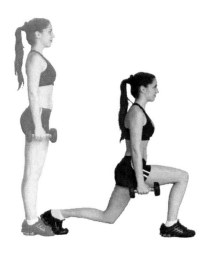

Muscles Used

Primary:

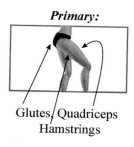

Glutes/ Quadriceps
Hamstrings

Start

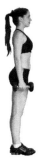

1. Stand tall with your feet shoulder-width apart, holding dumbbells to your sides.

End

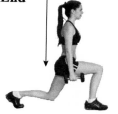

2. Step wide forward, landing with the heel first so that your knee is at 90 degrees and directly above the toes (taking a shorter step can add pressure on your knee).

3. Holding your body upright and rigid, lower yourself down until the back knee is nearly touching the ground.

4. Return to the starting position by pushing upward with the front leg.

Repeat for the other leg.

Stretch

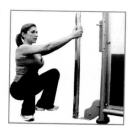

1. Grasp the tall part of the machine with both hands at your hip level.

2. Get into the full squat position, keeping your knees out, torso upright and tall. Relax your leg muscles and hold this position for 10–15 seconds.

Keep away from moving parts.

9. Calf Raises

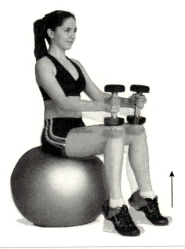

Muscles Used

Primary:

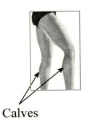

Calves

Dumbbell Weight:

Start

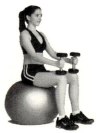

End

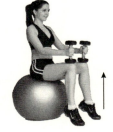

Stretch

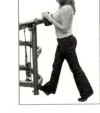

1. Sit tall on a ball with your knees at a 90-degree bend and feet shoulder-width apart.

2. Place dumbbells directly on your knees, palms facing each other.

3. Raise your heels up to the full extension and hold for one second.

4. Slowly return to the starting position.

1. Raise the toes of one of your feet to the full extension up and place them against the bottom of the machine or a wall. Hold on to the machine or wall for balance.
2. Move opposite foot one step back and lift your heel off the floor.
3. Bring your body closer to the machine or the wall until you feel a stretch at the calf of the front leg. Hold for 10–15 seconds.

Repeat for the other leg.

10. Ab Crunch

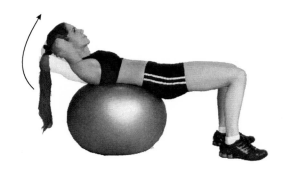

Muscles Used

Primary:

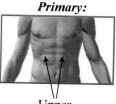

Upper
Abdominals

Assisting:
Shoulders, Back, Glutes
and Neck

Start	End	Stretch
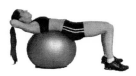	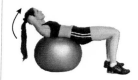	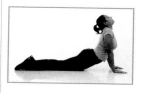

Start

1. Lie on the ball and position your lower back in the center of the ball.

2. Place your feet hip-width apart and get comfortable on the ball.

3. Make your body parallel to the floor and place your hands next to your ears.

End

4. Draw your neck up as far as you can, curling your body only at the waist. Squeeze your abdominal muscles. Focus your eyes on the ceiling and keep the ball stable.

5. Slowly return to the starting position, keeping your abdominals contracted.

.

Stretch

1. Lie on the mat or floor face down, hands beside your chest.

2. Slowly arch your back, assisting by a hand push. Feel the stretch in your abdomen and hold for 10–15 seconds. Do not overextend and stop before any pain in your lower back.

11. V-Ups

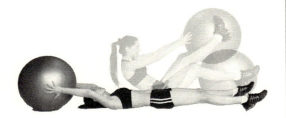

Muscles Used

Primary:

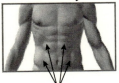

Upper and Lower
Abdominals

Start

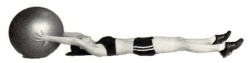

1. Lying on your back on the floor, hold the ball with your hands above your head.

Stretch

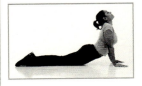

Middle

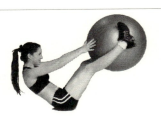

2. Swoop the ball into the air over the body, raising your upper body up, and keeping arms straight. As the arms come forward, raise the legs toward the ball. Keep them straight as well. Transfer the ball to the legs by grabbing it with your ankles, calves, and feet.

1. Lie on the mat or floor face down, hands beside your chest.

2. Slowly arch your back, assisting by a hand push. Feel the stretch in your abdomen and hold for 10–15 seconds. Do not overextend and stop before any pain in your lower back.

End

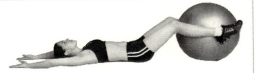

3. Lower the ball slowly to the ground. Be sure to keep the abdominals tight.

12. Plank

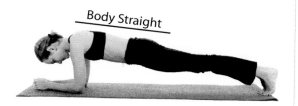

Body Straight

Muscles Used

Core:

Upper, Lower, External
and Internal Abdominals;
Back, Pelvic, Glutes,
Trapezius, Diaphragm
and some others.

Start

1. Lie face down on the floor or exercise mat.

2. Place your elbows right underneath your shoulders, arching your back, forearms parallel to each other.

End

3. Raise yourself up and form a straight bridge using your toes and forearms.

4. Maintain a straight line from your shoulders to your hips and knees. Keep your head aligned with your body.

Do not let your body sag down or raise your hips up. Remember to breathe.

In each program, exercises are performed involving different parts of muscles, using different angles, positions, or hand grips. The purpose of this is to develop the symmetry and balance between muscles.

Once you learn all four programs, you can start alternating them. For example, program 1—Monday, program 2—Wednesday, and program 3—on Friday.

To create even more variety, you can mix and match exercises between programs. For example, you can do chest exercises from program 1, back exercises from program 2, arms exercises from program 3, and leg exercises from program 4. This will bring muscle confusion for your workouts, forcing your body to spend more calories. The possibilities of variations between these four programs are endless.

As you get more experienced, you will learn more exercises watching other people exercising or reading more books. For more information, visit our website: www.gymbagbooks.com

Many gyms offer an equipment orientation, a 20-60 minute lesson on how to use gym equipment. Ask.

Part 3

Soul

CHAPTER 41

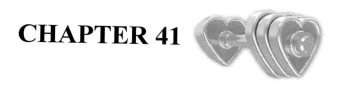

MOTIVATION

When I was working as a personal trainer, I had one very unique client—a thirty-year-old female from Australia who was paying for my personal training sessions and spent most of them on conversations between us sitting on the gym floor. Every time I tried to make her exercise, she would say:

"Let's just talk. I had a rough day, and I need some emotional relief."

"But I am a personal trainer. I am supposed to be training your muscles, not your brain," I joked. "Remember, every session costs you sixty-five dollars. C'mon! Let's get your monies worth!"

"But I don't feel that I am wasting my money," she usually answered. "My sessions are worth every penny to me. Let's not waste time and have a chat!"

All other trainers were laughing at us how we were exercising our tongues sitting on the gym floor, but what could I do?—this was what she needed.

It lasted like this for about six months. Eventually I managed to turn her sessions into physical ones, but what I have learned from this experience is that many times in life it doesn't matter what you do along the way to keep you going. As long as you don't stop and don't give up. Once you've developed the habit, then it's easy. Through our conversations on the gym floor, my client hasn't learned much of the exercise for a while, but what she developed was the most important for her—a habit of regularly going to the gym.

She left back to Australia next year. Few months later I called her to find out how she was doing. She told me that she immediately joined a local gym there, already lost twenty pounds and got happily married.

Different things *motivate* different people on doing different things.

What is motivation?

Motive means *an emotion*, desire, psychological need, or similar impulse that acts as *stimulation to action*, and we all need that something that will drive us into action.

Motivation can be *internal* and *external*.

Internal motivation is something that pushes us from our inside, and it is determined by our own goals.

Some of the examples of internal motivations are the following:

- Education
- Skills
- Passion
- Attitude
- Confidence

External motivation is the outer sources that *make us do things*. Some of the examples of external motivations:

- Money
- Health
- Clothes

- Appearance
- Language

While competing, the crowd may cheer on the performer, which may motivate him or her to do well. Competition, in general, is external because it encourages the performer to win and beat others, not to enjoy the internal rewards of the activity.

Once I was training my wife and her girlfriend. At the very beginning of our lesson, I told them both to go on the treadmill to warm up and was about to leave to make some phone calls. But they asked me to stay with them.

"We hate treadmills, so if you want us to do it, you'd better be beside us, otherwise we will quit."

I agreed, and after they walked for about five minutes, I told them to start running.

"I feel like a buffalo when I run," said my wife's girlfriend. We all laughed.

About three minutes later, they both slowed down and started to walk again.

"What's wrong? Your warm-up is not finished. Go on! Keep going!" I said.

"Yeah, but for some reason we don't have the motivation to do it. Let's do something else instead," said my wife.

"C'mon, guys! Motivation is something that can be found from the inside of you. It is really easy—just think of something good—something very pleasant and what would make you do anything."

"Ice cream!" they yelled together.

Everyone is different. What motivates some people doesn't motivate others. According to various theories, motivation may be rooted in the basic need to either

- *minimize physical pain and maximize pleasure*;
- include *specific needs* such as eating and resting;
- to have a *desired object*, hobby, goal, state of being;
- be attributed to less-apparent reasons such as *altruism, selfishness, morality*; *or*
- *avoid death.*

Conceptually, motivation should not be confused with either volition or optimism.

Self-Control

Self-control is understood as an *emotional intelligence*.

Emotional intelligence may have nothing to do with intelligence itself. A person may be highly intelligent but not able to pursue a particular goal because of his inability to exert his self-control. This doesn't always mean that this person is lacking willpower or self-discipline. He or she can be simply unmotivated.

To activate behavior toward our goals, we need a *drive* or *desire*. These desires often originate inside of us and may not always require external influence. For example, simple desires such as hunger makes people search for food, necessity to sleep for a shelter. But desire to be praised or approved by other people makes people to learn, study, or simply act in a manner to please other people.

Animals get motivated by a treat to perform specific tasks. People are the same. The treat that people receive doesn't have to always be something tangible. Very often it is something that people feel inside—a personal satisfaction.

A *reward* after completing the task motivates people do things. If reward comes sooner, people tend to be motivated more, but if achieving the goal takes time, the desire to pursue those goals may get lost.

The motivational techniques to pursue goals vary from person to person, but everyone can create his/her own reward system to achieve goals. There are a number of drive theories to do that:

Drive reduction theory is based on the concept that we all have certain biological drives, such as hunger, for example. As times passes, the strength of hunger increases, and as we eat, it reduces.

Cognitive dissonance theory suggested by Leon Festinger occurs when an individual experiences some degree of discomfort resulting from a conflict between two decisions to make. For example, when you may want to buy something, you may be feeling otherwise to make another decision.

Another example of cognitive dissonance is when a *belief and a behavior are in conflict*. A person may wish to be healthy, believes smoking is bad for one's health, and yet continues to smoke.

Abraham Maslow's theory is one of the most widely discussed theories of motivation. The theory can be summarized as follows:

- Human beings have wants and desires that influence their behavior. *Only unsatisfied needs influence behavior, satisfied needs do not*.
- Since needs are many, *they are arranged in order of importance*, from the basic to the complex.
- The person advances to the next level of needs *only after the lower level need is at least minimally satisfied*.
- *The further the progress up the hierarchy, the more individuality, humanness, and psychological health a person will show.*

The needs, listed from basic (lowest-earliest) to most complex (highest-latest) are as follows:

1. Physiology (hunger, thirst, sleep, etc.)

2. Safety/security/shelter/health
3. Belongingness/love/friendship
4. Self-esteem/recognition/achievement
5. Self-actualization

People cannot survive without first two levels of needs, and this is only natural. But the problem is that trying hard for those two levels, people do repetitive things, and those things develop many habits. When it comes to the move to the next level of needs, old habits might contradict with new habits to develop. Eventually people may end up on the crossroads to choose—either break old habits or not take another level. They make those choice based on how much value they give to one or another. If going into a new level of needs has more value for them, they break old habits; if not, everything stays unchanged.

To work even further, on levels 4 and 5, requires even more effort and also adjustments of all habits from levels 1, 2, and 3. Many people get stuck here, especially when they get married, fall in love, or get into serious relationships. Belongingness, love, and friendship are very important to people, and sometimes due to lack of support, the person who wanted to achieve something in life for himself gets completely "drowned" by the first three levels and can't move any further.

Every time I talk to a new person who comes to join the gym, the very first question I usually ask is this: "Is your family supporting you in making this decision?" If the answer is no or if I see some hesitation, chances that I will see that person in the gym again are getting very slim.

The further we move up on the hierarchy of those five levels, the more human we become, the more individuality we acquire, and the more psychologically balanced and happy our life gets.

People are not motivated unless they get rewarded. Either way— physical or psychological, but the reward must be there. Many of my workouts I'd rather skip, but my immediate rewards are the amazing feeling after each workout, eating without feeling guilty, and also my health and my body that I hope to keep in good condition until I die.

The pleasure after completing the task is not always immediate. Sometimes it needs to be worked on for a while, but when you achieve something substantial in your life, you acquire a feeling of self-worth that fulfills your soul with pleasure that never goes away.

Since we are all so different, it is very hard to suggest the types of motivations, and everyone needs to create his own reward system to move further up in the hierarchy of life. Some people have more willpower and patience—they can wait longer, but some have less, and those need every day's rewards.

Think of what would motivate you to stay on track and how often do you need your motivation. If you did well in something, always reward yourself. And don't be afraid if your rewards contradict with what you are trying to accomplish. As long as there is progress, that's all that counts.

Surround yourself with people like you or read about those people, watch TV shows. One of the reasons why some people are more successful is their feeling of *belongingness* to a group.

When we are aware of everything what drives us in life, we can learn how to operate those drives to move us further and further. It doesn't have to be perfect, smooth, and easy, and most likely, it won't be. But if we motivate our unsatisfied needs with proper rewards, we can reach the unlimited.

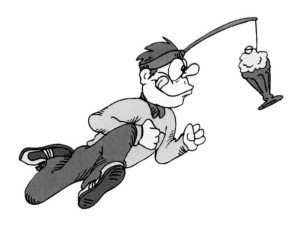

CHAPTER 42

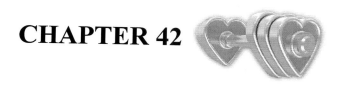

SOUL, TIME, AND MONEY

"Life is a precious gift—which we tend to take for granted. Rather than stop to appreciate what a miracle existence is, we dwell on our problems, resentments, fears or responsibilities. We think about the future, we think about the past and we forget what incredible present we have. But the present is the only time we have—and we should make an effort to see it as such." Jonathan Cainer

Being able to accomplish things in life is great, and that's what separates us, humans, from any other living kind. But there is something else inside of us that makes us also unique—our souls. We are not brought in to this world just to become working robots and get things done one after another. We are also able to feel and experience emotions when going through life.

There are millions of extremely successful people who still don't know how to enjoy their lives. They know how to use their minds and might even have great bodies but still go through life being unsatisfied.

Besides our main life goals, we need things that give us pleasure of experiencing them at the present without expecting anything in return or thinking of the future. It's like being in love. When you truly love somebody, your love is always there regardless if you are rewarded for it or not, and you are not thinking of the future because you like your present.

Some might say this: "Oh, I love my work." But do you love your work that much so you can work without getting paid for it? If your answer is negative, then your work is not a pure pleasure, and you just like being praised or rewarded.

There must be something in everyone's life that he/she would do without tracking time or waiting for a reward, and that something has to feel like a reward itself.

When I was learning music, my teacher was always telling me: "If you want to get good at music, you have to learn how to play with your heart, not with your fingers! Music is not a skill, it is a feeling! Anyone can learn how to move his fingers, but only few know how to sync them with their soul!"

Sometimes we get so tied up with our daily duties, goals, and responsibilities that we completely forget about ourselves. Slowly but surely we are getting drowned into an idea that life is about paying bills, doing daily chores, working out, or striving for success and money. Trying to catch up with more and more of the materialistic demands and constantly raising the bar, we often end up being exhausted, frustrated, and unhappy.

Why do we sometimes become so soulless? Because we plan our life that way. We often think of only big plans and forget about simple pleasures—going to a concert, football, hockey game, meeting with friends, family, or just taking enough vacations. These things give balance in life and make us happy.

Even in my worst financial times, I tried to take two to three vacations per year. They were not always luxury vacations, and sometimes we had to stay in cheap motels instead of the fancy resorts, but those vacations fulfilled my life with big meaning. I've learned how to think outside the box, and this brought balance and more success into my life.

I have never believed that vacations are luxuries. They are our necessities—just like shelter, clothes, and food, they make us feel like humans and not like animals that care only for survival. Vacations for the soul are like the sleep for the body; you need it so you don't "collapse," getting sick or emotionally drained. It works like a computer that gets frozen when you open too many files on it or perform too many tasks. Any computer pro will tell you that the best way to fix frozen computer is to restart it. When we take vacations, we restart and refresh ourselves too. Then everything shapes up better in our life because we get reenergized to continue and do more.

Everyone needs to have something for the soul—something that takes your mind away and makes you forget about all your problems. And that something has to be done every day, just like everything else, because our soul needs to work together with our goals. No matter how many great things you achieve in life, you still won't feel satisfied with your life if you have nothing for your soul to do. Soul supports what you achieve with much greater value. It's like singing or dancing. Anyone can learn notes or dance moves, but only those who succeed are those who put their souls into their performance. Sometimes when people get successful at something, they start putting enormous amount of time toward their successes hoping that one day—in the future (supposedly when they achieve everything), they will have time for themselves, and they will do things that they have always wanted to do. But as time passes, very often, things that those people wanted to do, they cannot do anymore because of either their age, some kind of disability, or just body changes. Then the achieved successes lose their values, and life feels wasted regardless of how much of the success you have achieved.

Balance Between Time and Money

I have a friend whose brother is a very successful lawyer. Once we were together driving in my car through the downtown of Toronto. At one intersection, while we were waiting for the light to turn green, my friend's brother sadly looked out of the window at one of the local coffee shops where people were sitting outside and said, "One day I will be able to do that—just go for a coffee and sit there—just like them."

"What do you mean?" I asked him. "You are making 300 bucks an hour, why can't you go for a coffee?"

"It's not the money part," he answered. "It's the time."

I think I understood how he was thinking: "Every hour of my work is worth 300 dollars. So if I go for an hour and sit there, this is going to cost me 300 dollars plus the cost of coffee . . ."

We never met with him until ten years later when he had to have a heart surgery. At the hospital, he smiled at me and said, "You know what? I still didn't go for that coffee . . ."

Sure, money is important to us, but sometimes, we get so tied up thinking about it that we forget why we are trying so hard. I like seeing the balance between time and money as both of my legs that have to be of equal length. If I start working too hard toward my money and don't have time for anything else, one of my "legs" gets shorter, and I start feeling lopsided.

To help each other deal with overworking, my sons and I came up with a trick. When we see how one of us "forgets to stop" working, we say to each other: "What if you had five minutes left to live? Would you still be doing what you are doing now?" It works for all of us, and we often go in our family room to take a break and do something fun.

No matter how paradoxical it may sound, but we need willpower to start enjoying things in life. Very often, our habits to work or study hard prevent us from enjoying simple things in life. For some people to disconnect from daily duties can be just as difficult as for others to start doing them.

Life works in balance. Mind, body, and soul are interconnected with each other and complement each other.

Statistically, about 80 percent of the population on our planet is experiencing some kind of depression. This usually happens due to misbalance between mind, body, and soul—those 80 percent are either not successful enough, unhealthy, or just unhappy not knowing how to enjoy simple pleasures. But happiness is a state of mind, and not something that can be measured. Happiness is what you feel, and not what you have. You can start feeling happy anytime while striving for all your successes and even when going through difficulties.

Don't ever feel guilty for having a good time or doing things that you love to do, even when you have other important things. Learn how to disconnect yourself from problems for moments of your pleasures because those pleasures are part of your life too. Enjoy your life because you have only one to live.

This is **yin** and **yang**. In Chinese philosophy, the concept of **yin and yang** is used to describe how polar or seemingly contrary forces are interconnected and interdependent in the natural world and how they give rise to each other in turn. The concept lies at the origins of many branches of classical Chinese science and philosophy, as well as being a primary guideline of traditional Chinese medicine and a central principle of different forms of Chinese martial arts and exercise. According to Chinese philosophy, **yin** and **yang** are the forces that animate the universe and your body. If these two interdependent forces are out of balance, you get sick. To prevent illness, you need to balance all aspects of your *mental*, *physical*, *spiritual*, and *communal* life.

INDEX

INDEX

C

calcium, 158-64, 166, 168-69
Campbell, T. Colin, 160
campylobacter, 358
cancer, 169-70, 191-97, 199-200,
    205, 274, 362-63
Cancer Care Ontario, 199-200
canola oil, 345-47
carbohydrates, 270, 272-73, 275-
    77, 288, 292-93, 366-67, 369-
    71, 378, 380, 385
  complex, 277, 290-91, 293
  glycemic index of, 294
  glycemic load of, 295
  simple, 290-91
carcinogens, 192-97
Carlin, Sara, 216, 219-20
CDC (Centers for Disease Control
    and Prevention), 196, 318
chickens, 357-59
chlorophyll, 289
cholesterol, 319, 323-28, 356, 371
chylomicrons, 171
cis configurations, 329, 331, 333
concentration, 106-7, 403
coordination, 259, 344, 398-99

D

deep-frying, 335-36
dependency, 33
DES (diethylstilbestrol), 359
DHEA (dehydroepiandrosterone),
    206
diets, 37-38, 40, 313-15, 317, 322-
    23
  balanced, aspects to consider in
    balance of carbohydrates,

proteins, and fats, 366-67, 369
    making of better choices, 375
    nutritional balance, 365
    proper food combination, 377,
      380
  dangers of, 277-78
  examples of
    Bernstein, 273, 275
    Dean Ornish, 274
    high-complex-carbohydrate,
      low-fat, 274-75
    high-protein, high-fat, 273
    Paavo Airola, 274
    Pritikin, 273-75
  misconceptions about, 278-79
discipline, 33-34
drive, 498-99

E

ego, 121-25
emotions, 35, 121, 124, 129-32,
    139-40
Enig, Mary, 346
erucic acid, 345
estrogen, 161-62, 189, 319
exercises, 13, 80, 82, 224-29, 234-
    39
  correlation between age and, 187,
    189
  correlation between cancer and,
    199
  correlation between sex drive
    and, 203, 205, 207
  correlation between smoking and,
    201
  examples of, 109-10, 112, 115,
    117
  finding time for, 61, 64, 66

510